T0358951

Severe Sepsis Care in the Emergency Department

Editors

JACK PERKINS
MICHAEL E. WINTERS

EMERGENCY MEDICINE CLINICS OF NORTH AMERICA

www.emed.theclinics.com

Consulting Editor
AMAL MATTU

February 2017 • Volume 35 • Number 1

ELSEVIER

1600 John F. Kennedy Boulevard • Suite 1800 • Philadelphia, Pennsylvania, 19103-2899
http://www.theclinics.com

EMERGENCY MEDICINE CLINICS OF NORTH AMERICA Volume 35, Number 1
February 2017 ISSN 0733-8627, ISBN-13: 978-0-323-49646-9

Editor: Katie Pfaff
Developmental Editor: Casey Potter

Emergency Medicine Clinics of North America (ISSN 0733-8627) is published quarterly by Elsevier Inc., 360 Park Avenue South, New York, NY, 10010-1710. Months of issue are February, May, August, and November. Business and Editorial Offices: 1600 John F. Kennedy Boulevard, Suite 1800, Philadelphia, PA 19103-2899. Customer Service Office: 6277 Sea Harbor Drive, Orlando, FL 32887-4800. Periodicals postage paid at New York, NY, and additional mailing offices. Subscription prices are $100.00 per year (US students), $323.00 per year (US individuals), $608.00 per year (US institutions), $220.00 per year (international students), $455.00 per year (international individuals), $747.00 per year (international institutions), $220.00 per year (Canadian students), $389.00 per year (Canadian individuals), and $747.00 per year (Canadian institutions). International air speed delivery is included in all *Clinics'* subscription prices. All prices are subject to change without notice. **POSTMASTER:** Send address changes to *Emergency Medicine Clinics of North America*, Elsevier Periodicals Customer Service, 11830 Westline Industrial Drive, St. Louis, MO 63146. Customer Service (orders, claims, online, change of address): Elsevier Periodicals **Customer Service, 11830 Westline Industrial Drive, St. Louis, MO 63146. Tel: 1-800-654-2452 (U.S. and Canada); 314-453-7041 (outside U.S. and Canada). Fax: 314-453-5170. E-mail: journalscustomerservice-usa@elsevier.com (for print support); journalsonlinesupport-usa@elsevier.com (for online support).**

Reprints. For copies of 100 or more of articles in this publication, please contact the Commercial Reprints Department, Elsevier Inc., 360 Park Avenue South, New York, NY 10010-1710. Tel.: 212-633-3874; Fax: 212-633-3820; E-mail: reprints@elsevier.com.

Emergency Medicine Clinics of North America is covered in *MEDLINE/PubMed (Index Medicus), Current Contents/Clinical Medicine, EMBASE/Excerpta Medica, BIOSIS, SciSearch, CINAHL, ISI/BIOMED,* and *Research Alert.*

Contributors

CONSULTING EDITOR

AMAL MATTU, MD, FAAEM, FACEP
Professor and Vice Chair, Department of Emergency Medicine, University of Maryland School of Medicine, Baltimore, Maryland

EDITORS

JACK PERKINS, MD, FACEP, FAAEM, FACP
Associate Professor of Emergency Medicine; Assistant Program Director of Emergency Medicine Residency, Virginia Tech Carilion School of Medicine, Roanoke, Virginia

MICHAEL E. WINTERS, MD, FACEP, FAAEM
Associate Professor of Emergency Medicine and Medicine; Co-Director, Critical Care Program, Internal Medicine, Emergency Medicine, University of Maryland School of Medicine, Baltimore, Maryland

AUTHORS

MICHAEL G. ALLISON, MD
Attending Physician, Critical Care Medicine, St. Agnes Hospital, Baltimore, Maryland

JOHN E. ARBO, MD
Divisions of Emergency Medicine; Division of Pulmonary and Critical Care Medicine, New York Presbyterian Hospital/Weill Cornell Medical Center, New York, New York

DAVID A. BERLIN, MD
Division of Pulmonary and Critical Care Medicine, New York Presbyterian Hospital/Weill Cornell Medical Center, New York, New York

MATTHEW P. BORLOZ, MD, FACEP
Assistant Professor, Department of Emergency Medicine, Virginia Tech Carilion School of Medicine, Roanoke, Virginia

DANIEL BOUTSIKARIS, MD
Attending Physician, Department of Emergency Medicine, Saint Peters University Hospital; Assistant Professor, Departments of Emergency Medicine and Medicine, Division of Pulmonary and Critical Care, Rutgers Robert Wood Johnson Medical School, New Brunswick, New Jersey

KARIN CHASE, MD
Assistant Professor, Pulmonary and Critical Care Medicine Division, Department of Medicine; Department of Emergency Medicine, University of Rochester Medical Center, Rochester, New York

AUDREY P. CHEN, PNP
Department of Emergency Medicine, Carilion Clinic, Roanoke, Virginia

JEREMY S. FAUST, MD, MS
Clinical Instructor, Department of Emergency Medicine, Brigham and Women's Hospital, Harvard Medical School, Boston, Massachusetts

JOHN C. GREENWOOD, MD
Departments of Emergency Medicine, Anesthesiology & Critical Care, Perelman School of Medicine, University of Pennsylvania, Philadelphia, Pennsylvania

KHALIEF E. HAMDEN, MD, MS, FAAEM
Assistant Professor, Department of Emergency Medicine, Virginia Tech Carilion School of Medicine, Roanoke, Virginia

BRYAN D. HAYES, PharmD
Clinical Associate Professor, Department of Emergency Medicine, University of Maryland Medical Center, University of Maryland School of Medicine, Baltimore, Maryland

EMILY L. HEIL, PharmD
Infectious Diseases Clinical Pharmacy Specialist, University of Maryland Medical Center, Baltimore, Maryland

JERRILYN JONES, MD, MPH
Assistant Professor, Department of Emergency Medicine, University of Maryland School of Medicine, Baltimore, Maryland

ALEX KOYFMAN, MD, FAAEM
Clinical Assistant Professor, Attending Physician, Department of Emergency Medicine, Parkland Memorial Hospital, UT Southwestern Medical Center, Dallas, Texas

BENJAMIN J. LAWNER, DO, MS, EMT-P
Assistant Professor, Department of Emergency Medicine, University of Maryland School of Medicine; Deputy EMS Director, Baltimore City Fire Department, Baltimore, Maryland

ROB LOFLIN, MD
Critical Care Medicine Fellow, University of Rochester Medical Center, Rochester, New York

BRIT LONG, MD
Attending Physician, Department of Emergency Medicine, San Antonio Uniformed Services Health Education Consortium (SAUSHEC) Emergency Medicine, San Antonio Military Medical Center, Fort Sam Houston, Texas

BRIAN MEIER, MD
Global Health Research Fellow, Division of Emergency Medicine, Department of Surgery, Duke University Medical Center; Duke Global Health Institute, Durham, North Carolina

ZEKE P. OLIVER, MD
Resident Physician, Department of Emergency Medicine, Carilion Clinic Virginia Tech School of Medicine, Roanoke, Virginia

CLINTON J. ORLOSKI, MD
Department of Emergency Medicine, Hospital of the University of Pennsylvania, Philadelphia, Pennsylvania

JACK PERKINS, MD, FACEP, FAAEM, FACP
Associate Professor of Emergency Medicine; Assistant Program Director of Emergency
Medicine Residency, Virginia Tech Carilion School of Medicine, Roanoke, Virginia

LARS-KRISTOFER N. PETERSON, MD
Assistant Professor, Department of Medicine; Department of Emergency Medicine,
Cooper Medical School of Rowan University, Camden, New Jersey

MELANIE K. PRUSAKOWSKI, MD
Associate Professor, Departments of Emergency Medicine and Pediatrics, Assistant
Dean for Admissions, Virginia Tech Carilion School of Medicine, Roanoke, Virginia

MICHAEL S. PULIA, MD, MS, FAAEM, FACEP
Assistant Professor; Director, Emergency Medicine Antimicrobial Stewardship Program,
BerbeeWalsh Department of Emergency Medicine, University of Wisconsin School of
Medicine and Public Health, Madison, Wisconsin

JARED RADBEL, MD
Pulmonary and Critical Care Fellow, Division of Pulmonary and Critical Care, Department
of Medicine, Rutgers Robert Wood Johnson Medical School, New Brunswick,
New Jersey

ROBERT REDWOOD, MD, MPH
Chairperson, Antibiotic Stewardship Committee; Emergency Physician, Divine Savior
Healthcare, Portage, Wisconsin

MICHAEL C. SCOTT, MD
Attending Physician, Adult Intensive Care Unit, Saint Agnes Hospital, Baltimore, Maryland

BRIAN SHARP, MD, FACEP
Assistant Professor; Associate Vice Chair of Quality; Medical Director, The American
Center, BerbeeWalsh Department of Emergency Medicine, University of Wisconsin
School of Medicine and Public Health, Madison, Wisconsin

CATHERINE STATON, MD, MScGH
Assistant Professor of Surgery and Global Health, Division of Emergency Medicine,
Department of Surgery, Duke University Medical Center; Duke Global Health Institute,
Durham, North Carolina

LEEANNE STRATTON, MD
Division of Emergency Medicine, New York Presbyterian Hospital/Weill Cornell Medical
Center, New York, New York

SCOTT D. WEINGART, MD
Clinical Associate Professor; Chief, Division of Emergency Critical Care, Department of
Emergency Medicine, Stony Brook Hospital, Stony Brook, New York

MICHAEL E. WINTERS, MD, FACEP, FAAEM
Associate Professor of Emergency Medicine and Medicine; Co-Director, Critical Care
Program, Internal Medicine, Emergency Medicine, University of Maryland School of
Medicine, Baltimore, Maryland

Contents

> Sepsis is a heterogeneous clinical syndrome that encompasses infections of many different types and severity. Not surprisingly, it has confounded most attempts to apply a single definition, which has also limited the ability to develop a set of reliable diagnostic criteria. It is perhaps best defined as the different clinical syndromes produced by an immune response to infection that causes harm to the body beyond that of the local effects of the infection.

> Recent literature continues to refine which components of the early goal-directed therapy (EGDT) algorithm are necessary. Given it utilizes central venous pressure, continuous central venous oxygen saturation, routine blood transfusions, and inotropic medications, this algorithm can be timely, invasive, costly, and potentially harmful. New trials highlight early recognition, early fluid resuscitation, appropriate antibiotic treatment, source control, and the application of a multidisciplinary evidence-based approach as essential components of current sepsis management. This article discusses the landmark sepsis trials that have been published over the past several decades and offers recommendations on what should currently be considered 'usual care'.

> Prescribing antibiotics is an essential component of initial therapy in sepsis. Early antibiotics are an important component of therapy, but speed of administration should not overshadow the patient-specific characteristics that determine the optimal breadth of antimicrobial therapy. Cultures should be drawn before antibiotic therapy if it does not significantly delay administration. Combination antibiotic therapy against gram-negative infections is not routinely required, and combination therapy involving vancomycin and piperacillin/tazobactam is associated with an increase in acute kidney injury. Emergency practitioners should be aware of special considerations in the administration and dosing of antibiotics in order to deliver optimal care to septic patients.

> Identifying sources of infection and establishing source control is an essential component of the workup and treatment of sepsis. Investigation with history, physical examination, laboratory tests, and imaging can in identifying sources of infection. All organ systems have the potential to develop sources of infection. However, there are inherent difficulties presented by some that require additional diligence, namely, urinalysis, chest radiographs, and intraabdominal infections. Interventions include administration of antibiotics and may require surgical or other specialist intervention. This is highlighted by the Surviving Sepsis Campaign with specific recommendations for time to antibiotics and expeditious time to surgical source control.

> Since its original description in 1832, fluid resuscitation has become the cornerstone of early and aggressive treatment of severe sepsis and septic shock. However, questions remain about optimal fluid composition, dose, and rate of administration for critically ill patients. This article reviews pertinent physiology of the circulatory system, pathogenesis of septic shock, and phases of sepsis resuscitation, and then focuses on the type, rate, and amount of fluid administration for severe sepsis and septic shock, so providers can choose the right fluid, for the right patient, at the right time.

> Vasopressor and inotropes are beneficial in shock states. Norepinephrine is considered the first-line vasopressor for patients with sepsis-associated hypotension. Dobutamine is considered the first-line inotrope in sepsis, and should be considered for patients with evidence of myocardial dysfunction or ongoing signs of hypoperfusion. Vasopressor and inotrope therapy has complex effects that are often difficult to predict; emergency providers should consider the physiology and clinical trial data. It is essential to continually reevaluate the patient to determine if the selected treatment is having the intended result.

> Resuscitation goals for the patient with sepsis and septic shock are to return the patient to a physiologic state that promotes adequate end-organ perfusion along with matching metabolic supply and demand. Ideal resuscitation end points should assess the adequacy of tissue oxygen delivery and oxygen consumption, and be quantifiable and reproducible. Despite years of research, a single resuscitation end point to assess adequacy of resuscitation has yet to be found. Thus, the clinician must rely on multiple end points to assess the patient's overall response to therapy. This review will discuss the role and limitations of central venous pressure (CVP), mean arterial pressure (MAP), and cardiac output/index as macrocirculatory resuscitation targets along with lactate, central venous oxygen

saturation (ScvO$_2$), central venous-arterial CO$_2$ gradient, urine output, and capillary refill time as microcirculatory resuscitation endpoints in patients with sepsis.

Sepsis is a common condition managed in the emergency department. Current diagnosis relies on physiologic criteria and suspicion of a source of infection using history, physical examination, laboratory studies, and imaging studies. The infection triggers a host response with the aim to destroy the pathogen, and this response can be measured. A reliable biomarker for sepsis should assist with earlier diagnosis, improve risk stratification, or improve clinical decision making. Current biomarkers for sepsis include lactate, troponin, and procalcitonin. This article discusses the use of lactate, procalcitonin, troponin, and novel biomarkers for use in sepsis.

Pediatric sepsis is distinct from adult sepsis in its definitions, clinical presentations, and management. Recognition of pediatric sepsis is complicated by the various pediatric-specific comorbidities that contribute to its mortality and the age- and development-specific vital sign and clinical parameters that obscure its recognition. This article outlines the clinical presentation and management of sepsis in neonates, infants, and children, and highlights some key populations who require specialized care.

Sepsis is recognized by the presence of physiologic and laboratory changes that reflect the inflammatory response to infection on cellular and systemic levels. Comorbid conditions, such as cirrhosis, end-stage renal disease, and obesity, alter patients' susceptibility to infection and their response to it once present. Baseline changes in vital signs and chronic medications often mask clues to the severity of illness. The physiologic, hematologic, and biochemical adjustments that accompany pregnancy and the puerperium introduce similar challenges. Emergency providers must remain vigilant for subtle alterations in the expected baseline for these conditions to arrive at appropriate management decisions.

Our evolving understanding of the physiologic processes that lead to sepsis has led to updated consensus guidelines outlining priorities in the recognition and treatment of septic patients. However, an enormous question remains when considering how to best implement these guidelines in settings with limited resources, which include rural US emergency departments and low- and middle-income countries. The core principles of sepsis management should be a priority in community emergency

regardless of the size of the emergency department where the patient is being treated. SEP-1 does not necessarily follow the best current evidence available. Nevertheless, a thorough understanding of SEP-1 is crucial because all hospitals and emergency providers will be accountable for meeting the requirements of this measure. SEP-1 is the first national quality measure on early management of sepsis care. This article provides a review of SEP-1 and all its potential implications on sepsis care in the United States.

EMERGENCY MEDICINE
CLINICS OF NORTH AMERICA

RELATED INTEREST

Clinics in Geriatric Medicine, May 2016 (Vol. 32, Issue 2)
Managing Chronic Conditions in Older Adults with Cardiovascular Disease
Michael W. Rich, Cynthia Boyd, and James T. Pacala, *Editors*

THE CLINICS ARE NOW AVAILABLE ONLINE!
Access your subscription at:
www.theclinics.com

PROGRAM OBJECTIVE

The goal of *Emergency Medicine Clinics of North America* is to keep practicing emergency medicine physicians and emergency medicine residents up to date with current clinical practice in emergency medicine by providing timely articles reviewing the state of the art in patient care.

LEARNING OBJECTIVES

Upon completion of this activity, participants will be able to:
1. Review the definition and diagnosis of sepsis.
2. Recognize therapies and management strategies for sepsis in the emergency department.
3. Discuss sepsis in special populations such as pediatrics, among others.

ACCREDITATION

The Elsevier Office of Continuing Medical Education (EOCME) is accredited by the Accreditation Council for Continuing Medical Education (ACCME) to provide continuing medical education for physicians.

The EOCME designates this enduring material for a maximum of 15 *AMA PRA Category 1 Credit*(s)™. Physicians should claim only the credit commensurate with the extent of their participation in the activity.

All other health care professionals requesting continuing education credit for this enduring material will be issued a certificate of participation.

DISCLOSURE OF CONFLICTS OF INTEREST

The EOCME assesses conflict of interest with its instructors, faculty, planners, and other individuals who are in a position to control the content of CME activities. All relevant conflicts of interest that are identified are thoroughly vetted by EOCME for fair balance, scientific objectivity, and patient care recommendations. EOCME is committed to providing its learners with CME activities that promote improvements or quality in healthcare and not a specific proprietary business or a commercial interest.

The planning committee, staff, authors and editors listed below have identified no financial relationships or relationships to products or devices they or their spouse/life partner have with commercial interest related to the content of this CME activity:

Michael G. Allison, MD; John E. Arbo, MD; David A. Berlin, MD; Matthew P. Borloz, MD, FACEP; Daniel Boutsikaris, MD; Karin Chase, MD; Audrey P. Chen, PNP; Jeremy S. Faust, MD, MS; Anjali Fortna; John C. Greenwood, MD; Khalief E. Hamden, MD, MS, FAAEM; Bryan D. Hayes, PharmD; Emily L. Heil, PharmD; Jerrilyn Jones, MD, MPH; Alex Koyfman, MD, FAAEM; Indu Kumari; Benjamin J. Lawner, DO, MS, EMT-P; Rob Loflin, MD; Brit Long, MD; Amal Mattu, MD, FAAEM, FACEP; Brian Meier, MD; Zeke P. Oliver, MD; Clinton J. Orloski, MD; Jack Perkins, MD, FACEP, FAAEM, FACP; Lars-Kristofer N. Peterson, MD; Katie Pfaff; Melanie K. Prusakowski, MD; Jared Radbel, MD; Robert Redwood, MD, MPH; Michael C. Scott, MD; Brian Sharp, MD, FACEP; Catherine Staton, MD, MScGH; Leeanne Stratton, MD; Megan Suermann; Scott D. Weingart, MD; Michael E. Winters, MD, FACEP, FAAEM.

The planning committee, staff, authors and editors listed below have identified financial relationships or relationships to products or devices they or their spouse/life partner have with commercial interest related to the content of this CME activity:

Michael S. Pulia, MD, MS, FAAEM, FACEP is a consultant/advisor for Thermo Fisher Scientific Inc. and Cempra.

UNAPPROVED/OFF-LABEL USE DISCLOSURE

The EOCME requires CME faculty to disclose to the participants:
1. When products or procedures being discussed are off-label, unlabelled, experimental, and/or investigational (not US Food and Drug Administration [FDA] approved); and
2. Any limitations on the information presented, such as data that are preliminary or that represent ongoing research, interim analyses, and/or unsupported opinions. Faculty may discuss information about pharmaceutical agents that is outside of FDA-approved labelling. This information is intended solely for CME and is not intended to promote off-label use of these medications. If you have any questions, contact the medical affairs department of the manufacturer for the most recent prescribing information.

TO ENROLL

To enroll in the *Emergency Medicine Clinics* Continuing Medical Education program, call customer service at 1-800-654-2452 or sign up online at http://www.theclinics.com/home/cme. The CME program is available to subscribers for an additional annual fee of $235 USD.

METHOD OF PARTICIPATION

In order to claim credit, participants must complete the following:

1. Complete enrolment as indicated above.
2. Read the activity.
3. Complete the CME Test and Evaluation. Participants must achieve a score of 70% on the test. All CME Tests and Evaluations must be completed online.

CME INQUIRIES/SPECIAL NEEDS

For all CME inquiries or special needs, please contact elsevierCME@elsevier.com.

Foreword

Severe Sepsis Care in the Emergency Department

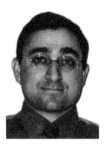

Amal Mattu, MD
Consulting Editor

A senior medical student was recently telling me about a lecture he did just 2 years ago for his medical school classmates. He talked about early goal-directed therapy, $ScVO_2$, the use of Edwards catheters, transfusion and steroid protocols, and the use of normal saline and dopamine for shock. This was an impressive work by a student, and by all rights, it was as cutting edge as it gets...for 2 years ago. He was disappointed to find out, however, that sepsis care is now completely different. The changing landscape of sepsis care during just the past few years has been quite extraordinary, with new updates and recommendations arriving almost monthly. Anyone that has not been diligent about keeping up with the literature will find himself quickly out of touch with best practice recommendations. Given that sepsis is one of the leading causes of death worldwide, a cutting-edge knowledge of sepsis is crucial to insure optimal care of patients.

In this issue of *Emergency Medicine Clinics of North America*, Guest Editors Drs Jack Perkins and Michael Winters have assembled an outstanding group of authors to address the current diagnostic and management issues pertaining to sepsis. They begin the issue by discussing the definitions (sepsis, severe sepsis, septic shock) and provide a nice overview of the "new" usual care. Articles follow that focus on source identification and source control, optimal antibiotic use, and resuscitation with fluids and vasopressors. Novel biomarkers of sepsis are also addressed. Special articles are provided that focus on pediatric patients and other special populations as well as prehospital care. Finally, articles are provided that address pitfalls in sepsis care and quality measures.

This issue of *Emergency Medicine Clinics of North America* is an invaluable addition to the library of emergency physicians and other health care providers that diagnose and manage patients with sepsis. This issue should be considered must-reading for all emergency health care providers in order to maintain a sound knowledge regarding one of the leading killers in modern medicine. Knowledge and practice of the concepts

Emerg Med Clin N Am 35 (2017) xv–xvi
http://dx.doi.org/10.1016/j.emc.2016.11.002
0733-8627/17/© 2016 Published by Elsevier Inc.

that are discussed in the following pages are certain to save lives. The guest editors and authors are to be commended for providing this outstanding resource for our specialty.

Amal Mattu, MD, FAAEM, FACEP
Department of Emergency Medicine
University of Maryland School of Medicine
Baltimore, MD 21201, USA

E-mail address:
amalmattu@comcast.net

Preface

An Introduction to the Most Complex Disease in Emergency Medicine

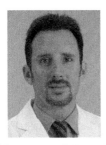 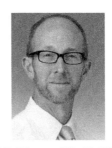

Jack Perkins, MD, FACEP, FAAEM, FACP   Michael E. Winters, MD, FACEP, FAAEM

Editors

Sepsis is one of the most complex and challenging diseases in medicine. Timely diagnosis and initiation of therapy are required in order to prevent unnecessary increases in patient morbidity and mortality. Unfortunately, the clinical presentation of sepsis is often nonspecific and may lead to delays in diagnosis and treatment. Since the majority of patients with sepsis initially present to the emergency department, it is imperative for the emergency provider (EP) to be knowledgeable regarding current concepts and controversies in sepsis management. Recent literature has improved our understanding of numerous critical aspects in sepsis management. In addition, the Centers for Medicare and Medicaid Services recently implemented a sepsis core measure (SEP-1) in the United States. SEP-1 contains several measures that are a matter of intense debate across the United States. Given these recent developments, we have dedicated this issue of *Emergency Medicine Clinics of North America* to a current evidence-based review of more than a dozen sepsis-related topics.

The initial articles of this special issue are dedicated to a discussion of the new definitions of sepsis and septic shock, the new "usual care," current recommendations on appropriate antimicrobial therapy, fluid administration, source control, vasoactive medications for septic shock, and endpoints of sepsis resuscitation. Additional articles are dedicated to the prehospital resuscitation of septic patients, pearls in pediatric sepsis resuscitation, sepsis in austere settings, biomarkers, and sepsis care in special patient populations. The final three articles in this issue discuss common pearls and pitfalls in emergency department sepsis care, antimicrobial stewardship, and SEP-1. EPs should have a detailed understanding of SEP-1, as every hospital in the United States will be accountable to meet these metrics. Unfortunately, it appears that significant monetary penalties may be assessed against those hospitals that fail to achieve adequate compliance.

Emerg Med Clin N Am 35 (2017) xvii–xviii
http://dx.doi.org/10.1016/j.emc.2016.11.001
0733-8627/17/© 2016 Published by Elsevier Inc.

emed.theclinics.com

The authors of these articles represent more than a dozen institutions across the United States. They were selected based on their expertise and recognition as outstanding educators in emergency medicine and critical care. They have provided cutting-edge, up-to-date reviews of the critical concepts in sepsis recognition and treatment. Undoubtedly, sepsis will continue to be one of the most common critical illnesses encountered by the EP. We feel that this issue of *Emergency Medicine Clinics of North America* will be an essential resource for community and academic EPs alike. Ultimately, our goal is to provide each EP with the most up-to-date information so that emergency department patients with sepsis continue to receive outstanding care.

Jack Perkins, MD, FACEP, FAAEM, FACP
Virginia Tech Carilion School of Medicine
Department of Emergency Medicine
1 Riverside Circle, 4th Floor
Roanoke, VA 24014, USA

Michael E. Winters, MD, FACEP, FAAEM
University of Maryland School of Medicine
110 South Paca Street, 6th Floor, Suite 200
Baltimore, MD 21201, USA

E-mail addresses:
Jcperkins@carilionclinic.org (J. Perkins)
mwinters@em.umaryland.edu (M.E. Winters)

Defining and Diagnosing Sepsis

Michael C. Scott, MD

KEYWORDS

- Sepsis • Severe sepsis • Septic shock • SOFA • qSOFA

KEY POINTS

- Sepsis is a heterogeneous clinical syndrome that has defied attempts to create an exact definition or develop specific clinical diagnostic criteria.
- Sepsis is characterized by the immune response to an infection that creates harmful effects beyond the local site of the infection.
- The difficulty in defining sepsis has created significant challenges in the determination of reliable epidemiologic data for the disease.
- Despite an increased incidence, the mortality for sepsis has decreased over the past several decades.
- According to the most recent publication on the definitions for sepsis and septic shock, sepsis is life-threatening organ dysfunction caused by a dysregulated host response to infection.

INTRODUCTION

The syndrome of sepsis includes an incredibly wide variety of infections and clinical presentations, from the 85-year-old patient with a urinary tract infection with mild confusion to the 18-year-old patient with multiorgan failure from meningitis. Any attempt to define sepsis must incorporate these disparate and heterogeneous manifestations under 1 syndromic banner. The incredible difficulty of this task is reflected in the interplay between conceptual, diagnostic, and research definitions of sepsis.

It is generally accepted that worldwide sepsis represents a large burden of illness, morbidity, and mortality. In 2011, it was estimated that sepsis represented the most expensive single condition treated in US hospitals and accounted for more than $20 billion dollars in health care costs (5.2% of aggregate US hospital costs).[1] A 2009 study estimated that more than 3 million cases of sepsis occur annually in the United States and result in more than 200,000 deaths.[2] It is clear that the incidence of sepsis has increased. It is believed that increases in the aging population along with an

The author has nothing to disclose.
Adult Intensive Care Unit, Saint Agnes Hospital, 900 S. Caton Ave, Baltimore, MD 21229, USA
E-mail address: mikescott@umem.org

Emerg Med Clin N Am 35 (2017) 1–9
http://dx.doi.org/10.1016/j.emc.2016.08.002
0733-8627/17/© 2016 Elsevier Inc. All rights reserved.

emed.theclinics.com

increase in patients that have select comorbidities, such as immunosuppressive conditions, may account for the increased incidence of disease. In addition to the increased elderly population and patients with complex comorbidities, it is also postulated that increased awareness of the condition has contributed to the increase in the incidence of sepsis.[3] Despite an increased incidence of sepsis, mortality has decreased. In fact, mortality rates in the 3 most recent studies comparing the use of an early goal-directed therapy protocol with current usual care ranged from 19% to 29%. This is markedly reduced from the mortality rate of greater than 46% in the original 2001 early goal-directed therapy study.[4–7]

This article discusses the evolution of sepsis definitions that have been published over the past several decades, with attention to the most recent publication by Singer and colleagues.

SEPSIS 1: AN INITIAL DEFINITION

Sepsis is generally accepted to be an advanced, life-threatening infection that produces organ dysfunction and increases morbidity and mortality. The first formal definition of sepsis came in 1992, when a consensus conference defined sepsis as "the systemic response to infection."[8] The conference committee believed that much of the harm and damage to the body in sepsis is not the result of the microorganism causing infection, but rather the damage to various organs that are distant from the actual site of infection. Importantly, this is not necessarily owing to a systemic infection itself (ie, bacteremia), but rather to the patient's immune system response to the infection. An example of this process is the development of the acute respiratory distress syndrome in a patient with a foot abscess. One would not be expected to detect bacteria in sputum cultures that match those in wound cultures from the abscess itself.

Based on the understanding of sepsis at that time, the 1992 conference committee felt that this systemic response to infection was the result of overwhelming inflammation. They named this response the systemic inflammatory response syndrome (SIRS). SIRS is the presence of at least 2 of the 4 criteria listed in **Box 1**.[8] Importantly, the committee emphasized that the SIRS criteria needed to be both (1) a change from the patient's baseline and (2) part of the systemic response to the presence of an infectious process.[8] This highlighted that the presence of SIRS was not unique to sepsis, but

---

Box 1
Systemic inflammatory response syndrome

Defined as the presence of at least 2 of the following 4 criteria:

Body temperature greater than 38°C or less than 36°C

Heart rate greater than 90 bpm

Tachypnea: RR >20 breaths per minute; or

Hyperventilation: $Paco_2$ less than 32 mm Hg

WBC greater than 12,000/mm^3 or less than 4000/mm^3 or greater than 10% immature neutrophils

Abbreviations: bpm, beats per minute; $Paco_2$, partial pressure CO_2 in arterial blood gas sample; RR, respiratory rate; WBC, white blood cell count.
    Data from Bone RC, Balk RA, Cerra FB, et al. Definitions for sepsis and organ failure and guidelines for the use of innovative therapies in sepsis. The ACCP/SCCM Consensus Conference Committee. American College of Chest Physicians/Society of Critical Care Medicine. Chest 1992;101(6):1644–55.

rather could be present in many other inflammatory conditions, such as pancreatitis, ischemia, trauma and tissue injury, hemorrhagic shock, and immune-mediated organ injury[8] (**Fig. 1**).

Importantly, the conference committee also recognized that the syndrome of sepsis encompassed a wide range of clinical severities. The committee stated that, as SIRS develops and progresses untreated, it produces organ dysfunction.[8] As such, they identified 2 discrete clinical conditions that were important indicators of the progression of sepsis toward death. The first of these clinical conditions was severe sepsis, defined as a subset of patients with sepsis who also had organ dysfunction, hypoperfusion abnormalities, or sepsis-induced hypotension[8] (**Box 2**). Finally, the 1992 committee defined septic shock as those patients with severe sepsis who also had sepsis-induced hypotension and evidence of hypoperfusion or organ dysfunction that persisted despite adequate fluid resuscitation.[8]

In addition, these initial terms and definitions were meant to clarify confusion that existed around the use of the words "sepsis" or "septic." In fact, these terms were often used by providers interchangeably with the term "toxic" to describe a patient who seemed to be ill. Furthermore, the term "sepsis" was often used interchangeably with the term "septicemia." Importantly, the committee recommended that the term "septicemia" no longer be used in everyday clinical discussion. This change was used to emphasize that sepsis is defined not by a systemic infection, but rather by a systemic immune response to infection, whether or not that infection was local or had spread systemically. Put another way, patients may have bacteremia, viremia, or fungemia without necessarily having sepsis.

A final goal of the 1992 conference committee was to standardize the framework for everyday clinical application and for research studies. The landmark sepsis study by

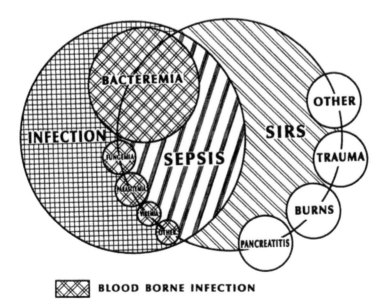

BLOOD BORNE INFECTION

Fig. 1. The interrelationship between systemic inflammatory response syndrome (SIRS), sepsis, and infection. (*From* Bone RC, Balk RA, Cerra FB, et al. Definitions for sepsis and organ failure and guidelines for the use of innovative therapies in sepsis. The ACCP/SCCM Consensus Conference Committee. American College of Chest Physicians/Society of Critical Care Medicine. Chest 1992;101(6):1645; with permission.)

Box 2
Severe sepsis

Defined as the presence of sepsis plus at least one of the following:

Organ dysfunction (not specifically defined)

Hypoperfusion abnormality, including but not limited to one of:
   Lactic acidosis
   Oliguria
   Acute alteration in mental status

Sepsis-induced hypotension:
   Systolic blood pressure <90 mm Hg or a reduction of greater than 40 mm Hg from baseline in the absence of a cause of hypotension besides sepsis

Data from Bone RC, Balk RA, Cerra FB, et al. Definitions for sepsis and organ failure and guidelines for the use of innovative therapies in sepsis. The ACCP/SCCM Consensus Conference Committee. American College of Chest Physicians/Society of Critical Care Medicine. Chest 1992;101(6):1644–55.

Rivers and colleagues[4] used the definitions put forth in this first sepsis definitions conference to evaluate an intense treatment protocol for patients with sepsis. The remarkable results of this study effectively solidified these inclusion criteria as the de facto definitions of severe sepsis and septic shock for the majority of the subsequent research.[5–7,9,10] Importantly, they also established that severe sepsis and septic shock represent a distinct clinical entity from sepsis that has not progressed to organ dysfunction, hypoperfusion, or shock.

SEPSIS 2: AN UPDATED DEFINITION

Shortly after the early goal-directed therapy publication by Rivers and colleagues, a second sepsis definitions conference was held to update the initial work published in 1992. Interestingly, there was no mention of the Rivers trial, or the research definitions of severe sepsis and septic shock used by Rivers and colleagues, in the updated version. Instead, the committee upheld the initial definition of sepsis as a "clinical syndrome defined by the presence of both infection and a systemic inflammatory response syndrome."[11] However, the committee did feel that the SIRS criteria lacked sufficient specificity to identify patients with sepsis. As a result, the committee broadened the list of clinical and laboratory findings to facilitate the usefulness of criteria for the bedside clinician.[11] The expanded list of sepsis criteria are listed in **Box 3**. It is important to note that these criteria were chosen based on expert opinion. In fact, the authors state that, in the "day-to-day reality, a bedside clinician does not use rigid criteria to diagnose sepsis, but instead, the clinician identifies a myriad of symptoms, and regardless of an evident infection declares the patient to look septic."[11] In addition, the committee members specifically emphasized that these additional criteria are not specific to infection and must be interpreted in light of the provider's opinion on whether an infection is present and whether that infection is the cause of these abnormalities.

This expanded list of clinical and laboratory findings was the precursor for the clinical definition of severe sepsis used by the Surviving Sepsis Campaign (SSC) to identify patients who should receive their sepsis resuscitation bundle.[12,13] This tool uses history suggestive of infection, the presence of SIRS criteria (with altered mental status or hyperglycemia being additional criteria), and organ dysfunction (defined by the presence of any of hypotension, hypoxia, elevated creatinine/oliguria,

---

Box 3
Expanded list of sepsis criteria from the 2001 consensus conference

Sepsis is defined as infection plus some of the following:

Hyperthermia or hypothermia

Tachycardia or tachypnea

Altered mental status

Edema or positive fluid balance

Elevated glucose (without a history of diabetes)

Leukocytosis or leukopenia or bandemia

Elevated C-reactive protein level or procalcitonin level

Hypotension

Low mixed venous oxygen saturation or cardiac index

Hypoxia

Oliguria or elevated creatinine level

Coagulation abnormalities

Ileus

Thrombocytopenia

Elevated bilirubin level

Elevated lactate level

Decreased capillary refill time

Data from Levy MM, Fink MP, Marshall JC, et al. 2001 SCCM/ESICM/ACCP/ATS/SIS international sepsis definitions conference. Intensive Care Med 2003;29(4):530–8.

---

thrombocytopenia, coagulopathy, elevated bilirubin, or elevated lactate) to identify a severe sepsis population. Although some authors have criticized the SSCs broader definition of severe sepsis as being significantly divergent from the definitions used in large sepsis trials,[4–7] it should be noted that the SSC bundles do use a more narrow research definition (ie, lactate of ≥4 mmol/L or mean arterial pressure of <65 mm Hg after fluid administration) to define the subset of severe sepsis patients that need to proceed to the more advanced form of the SSC resuscitation bundle.[13,14] Importantly, there are also trials that suggest the possibility that implementation of the SSC screening tool and resuscitation bundles correlates with decreased mortality in this patient population.[13,14]

CENTERS FOR MEDICARE AND MEDICAID SERVICES

In October 2015, the US Centers for Medicare and Medicaid Services implemented a quality measure called the Sepsis Bundle Project. The Sepsis Bundle Project details a specific metric for patients with severe sepsis and septic shock, with diagnostic criteria for severe sepsis that have a significant overlap with those used in the SSC bundles.[13] Although the US Centers for Medicare and Medicaid Services definition of sepsis may not be evidence based, it is important for providers to be familiar with these specific criteria, because provider reimbursement may be tied to the achievement of these metrics.

It is not surprising that coding for sepsis diagnoses has been fraught with questions, inconsistencies, and controversies. Until 2003, there was no *International Statistical Classification of Diseases and Related Health Problems* (ICD) code specific to sepsis, SIRS, severe sepsis, or septic shock. Although coding for an infection plus an organ dysfunction could substitute for severe sepsis, or coding for an infection plus shock could approximate septic shock, the closest thing to code for sepsis that was not complicated by organ dysfunction or shock was to code for septicemia (ICD-9 code 0.38.**). Although the coding literature specifically delineates that equating septicemia (a systemic infection) with sepsis is erroneous, it continues to recommend using the 0.38 code for a systemic infection as the principal diagnostic code in sepsis, severe sepsis, or septic shock, despite the existence now of the secondary diagnoses specific to these conditions.[15] Even after creating diagnostic codes specific to these systemic responses, the coding agencies still recommend coupling them with a code for a systemic infection in essentially all cases.

As imagined, it seems that sepsis coding is far from uniformly accepted by bedside clinicians. Aside from the potential problems created with regard to tracking quality and reimbursement, this messy coding practice also makes it nearly impossible to accurately determine any population-wide epidemiology of sepsis. It has been noted many times and in multiple geographic areas that using coding data to determine sepsis incidence or mortality rates creates a situation where the rates can vary by a factor as high as 3.5, depending on which coding extraction method is used.[2,16–18]

SEPSIS 3: A NEW DEFINITION

Recently, the Society of Critical Care Medicine and the European Society of Intensive Care Medicine sponsored a 19-member Task Force to update the definitions of sepsis and septic shock. The results and recommendations of this task force where published in a February 2016 issue of the *Journal of the American Medical Association*.[19] The recommendations of this task force marked a significant change from the conferences held in 1992 and 2001. Owing to an increased understanding of the harmful systemic response to infection, members of the multidisciplinary task force proposed that sepsis now be defined as "life threatening organ dysfunction caused by a dysregulated host response to infection."[19] This underscores the current belief that the presence of a systemic inflammatory response does not necessarily reflect an inappropriate, dysregulated host response, and that this dysregulation is better identified by organ dysfunction. In proposing this definition, the authors emphasized that sepsis, in the absence of organ dysfunction, hypotension, and hypoperfusion, is a clinically distinct entity from severe sepsis or septic shock and may not necessarily warrant the same aggressive therapeutic approach. With the new proposed definitions and criteria, the authors eliminated the term "severe sepsis," because this term in previous definitions is made up by patients now defined simply by the term "sepsis." This means that the group of "uncomplicated sepsis" patients identified by previous definitions would not qualify under any cohort on the spectrum that is the syndrome of sepsis. Instead, these patients would simply qualify as having an infection.

To standardize the assessment of organ dysfunction, the Task Force members propose that provider use the Sequential Organ Failure Assessment (SOFA) score. The components of the SOFA score are listed in **Box 4**. Patients who have an increase of 2 or more points above their baseline SOFA score would be classified as having organ dysfunction.[19] The recommendation to adopt the SOFA score was the result of a comparison of the performance of the SIRS criteria, the SOFA, and the Logistic Organ Dysfunction System.[20] The comparison found SOFA and Logistic Organ Dysfunction

---

Box 4
Sequential Organ Failure Assessment (SOFA) score

Respiration: low $Pao_2:Fio_2$ ratio

Coagulation: thrombocytopenia

Liver: elevated bilirubin

Cardiovascular: hypotension

Central nervous system: altered mental status

Renal: elevated creatinine or low urine output

Data from Singer M, Deutschman CS, Seymour CW, et al. The third international consensus definitions for sepsis and septic shock (sepsis-3). JAMA 2016;315(8):801–10.

System to have the best receiver operating curve with regard to in-hospital mortality prediction in patients in the intensive care unit (ICU). The Task Force felt that the SOFA score was less complicated and more widely used than the Logistic Organ Dysfunction System, and therefore it was chosen as the best definition of organ dysfunction to define the new term of sepsis. Because the SOFA score is not widely used, if at all, outside of the ICU, the task force retrospectively derived a new score, the quick SOFA (qSOFA) score. The qSOFA score is composed of 3 variables: the respiratory rate (1 point if >22/min), systolic blood pressure (1 point if <100 mm Hg), and mentation (1 point if the Glasgow Coma Scale is <15). When applied, the receiver operating curve of qSOFA in patients outside the ICU approached that of SOFA for ICU patients. Thus, the task force recommended implementation of the qSOFA score as a method to quickly identify adult patients with suspected infection who are likely to have poor outcomes.[19] Importantly, the qSOFA score has not been validated prospectively, a primary concern of critics of these newly proposed definitions. Similar to the term severe sepsis, the task force recommended that the SIRS criteria no longer be used to screen patients for suspected sepsis.

Finally, the task force proposed that septic shock be defined as "a subset of sepsis in which underlying circulatory and cellular metabolism abnormalities are profound enough to substantially increase mortality."[19] After examining the mortality associated with 6 different proposed clinical criteria to define a clinical population of septic shock,[21] the committee decided on the following clinical criteria to define septic shock: persistent hypotension requiring vasopressors to maintain a mean arterial pressure of greater than or equal to 65 mm Hg and a serum lactate of greater than 2 mmol/L despite adequate volume resuscitation.[19]

Although a significant number of national and international organizations endorsed these definitions as part of the peer review and publishing process, some groups did not endorse the new definitions. Perhaps most notably, the American College of Chest Physicians (ACCP), a title sponsor of the first 2 iterations of the definitions at the conferences held in 1991 and 2001, published a statement in opposition to the newly proposed definitions.[22] They cite a number of concerns with the new definitions that are especially noteworthy. First, the ACCP is concerned with changing definitions that have previously been shown to predict mortality and that have been used in studies to apply interventions that have reduced global sepsis mortality.[22] Second, the ACCP is concerned with the recommendation to stop using the SIRS criteria, and the resultant shift that does not recognize the start of the continuum of the sepsis syndrome until the patient has progressed to organ dysfunction. Specifically, they hypothesize that this shift could lead to failure to recognize the signs of potentially lethal infection until the combination is significantly more likely to be deadly.[22]

Finally, the ACCP specifically calls for a reconvening of the definitions conference, specifically with greater representation from emergency medicine and hospitalist physicians, to address a principle concern that the new definition deemphasizes intervention at earlier stages of sepsis when the syndrome is actually at its most treatable.[22]

SUMMARY

The syndrome of sepsis covers a myriad of infections and the wide range of clinical severity those infections produce. The breadth and heterogeneity of the clinical entities contained in this syndrome, and the evolution of the understanding of the syndrome, have led to multiple different, and to some extent competing, definitions over the past decades. This has come to a head recently with the submission of a new, revised definition for the syndrome, which has been met with significant resistance by some parts of the medical community.

REFERENCES

1. Torio C, Andrews R. National inpatient hospital costs: the most expensive conditions by payer, 2011. Washington, DC: Agency for Health Care Policy and Research (US); 2013.
2. Gaieski DF, Edwards JM, Kallan MJ, et al. Benchmarking the incidence and mortality of severe sepsis in the United States. Crit Care Med 2013;41(5): 1167–74.
3. Walkey AJ, Lagu T, Lindenauer PK. Trends in sepsis and infection sources in the United States. A population-based study. Ann Am Thorac Soc 2015;12(2): 216–20.
4. Rivers E, Nguyen B, Havstad S, et al. Early goal-directed therapy in the treatment of severe sepsis and septic shock. N Engl J Med 2001;345(19):1368–77.
5. Investigators TA. Randomized trial of protocol-based care for early septic shock. N Engl J Med 2014;370(18):1683–93.
6. Investigators A, Group A, Peake S, et al. Goal-directed resuscitation for patients with early septic shock. N Engl J Med 2014;371(16):1496–506.
7. Mouncey PR, Osborn TM, Power GS, et al. Trial of early, goal-directed resuscitation for septic shock. N Engl J Med 2015;372(14):1301–11.
8. Bone RC, Balk RA, Cerra FB, et al. Definitions for sepsis and organ failure and guidelines for the use of innovative therapies in sepsis. The ACCP/SCCM Consensus Conference Committee. American College of Chest Physicians/Society of Critical Care Medicine. Chest 1992;101(6):1644–55.
9. Nguyen HB, Rivers EP, Knoblich BP. Early lactate clearance is associated with improved outcome in severe sepsis and septic shock. Crit Care Med 2004; 32(8):1637–42.
10. Jones AE, Shapiro NI, Trzeciak S, et al. Lactate clearance vs central venous oxygen saturation as goals of early sepsis therapy: a randomized clinical trial. JAMA 2010;303(8):739–46.
11. Levy MM, Fink MP, Marshall JC, et al. 2001 SCCM/ESICM/ACCP/ATS/SIS international Sepsis Definitions Conference. Intensive Care Med 2003;29(4):530–8.
12. Dellinger RP, Levy M, Carlet J, et al. Surviving Sepsis Campaign: international guidelines for management of severe sepsis and septic shock: 2008. Intensive Care Med 2008;34(1):17–60.

13. Levy MM, Dellinger RP, Townsend SR, et al. The Surviving Sepsis Campaign: results of an international guideline-based performance improvement program targeting severe sepsis. Intensive Care Med 2010;36(2):222–31.

14. Levy M, Rhodes A, Phillips G, et al. Surviving Sepsis Campaign: association between performance metrics and outcomes in a 7.5-year study. Intensive Care Med 2014;40(11):1623–33.

15. Wiedemann L. Coding sepsis and SIRS. J AHIMA 2007;78(4):76–8.

16. Wilhelms SB, Huss FR, Granath G, et al. Assessment of incidence of severe sepsis in Sweden using different ways of abstracting international classification of diseases codes: difficulties with methods and interpretation of results. Crit Care Med 2010;38(6):1442–9.

17. Liu V, Escobar GJ, Greene JD, et al. Hospital deaths in patients with sepsis from 2 independent cohorts. JAMA 2014;312(1):90–2.

18. Fleischmann C, Scherag A, Adhikari NK, et al. Assessment of global incidence and mortality of hospital-treated sepsis. current estimates and limitations. Am J Respir Crit Care Med 2016;193(3):259–72.

19. Singer M, Deutschman CS, Seymour CW, et al. The third international consensus definitions for sepsis and septic shock (sepsis-3). JAMA 2016;315(8):801–10.

20. Seymour CW, Liu VX, Iwashyna TJ, et al. Assessment of clinical criteria for sepsis: for the third international consensus definitions for sepsis and septic shock (sepsis-3). JAMA 2016;315(8):762–74.

21. Shankar-Hari M, Phillips GS, Levy ML, et al. Developing a new definition and assessing new clinical criteria for septic shock: for the third international consensus definitions for sepsis and septic shock (sepsis-3). JAMA 2016;315(8):775–87.

22. Simpson SQ. New sepsis criteria: a change we should not make. Chest 2016; 149(5):117–8.

The New Usual Care

Jared Radbel, MD[a], Daniel Boutsikaris, MD[b,c],*

KEYWORDS

- Sepsis • Early goal-directed therapy (EGDT) • Usual care • ProCESS trial
- ARISE trial • ProMISe trial

KEY POINTS

- Current sepsis trials have not shown a benefit from protocolized early goal-directed care, as opposed to usual care.
- Early recognition of sepsis, fluid resuscitation, appropriate antibiotic treatment, source control, and the application of multidiscipline evidence-based medicine are essential components of sepsis care.
- Central venous pressure and continuous central venous saturation measurements, placement of central venous catheters, and routine blood transfusions are not necessary for all patients with sepsis.

INTRODUCTION

Sepsis is a common and deadly disease, in which many survivors are burdened with life altering effects.[1] In order to deliver current evidence-based treatment and avoid unnecessary, costly, and harmful therapy, it is imperative that emergency and acute care providers be knowledgeable about current treatments that affect outcomes in septic patients. In 2001, a landmark trial by Rivers and colleagues[2] was published, which showed that an early and aggressive treatment approach to patients with sepsis was associated with a significant mortality benefit. In the period following this study, along with the efforts of the Surviving Sepsis Campaign (SSC), there was the emergence of protocolized, evidence-based care for patients with sepsis and septic shock.[3] Although the SSC provided an evidence-based approach, the largest

Disclosures: The authors have nothing to disclose.
[a] Division of Pulmonary and Critical Care, Department of Medicine, Rutgers Robert Wood Johnson Medical School, 1 Robert Wood Johnson Place/MEB 568, New Brunswick, NJ 08901, USA; [b] Department of Emergency Medicine, Saint Peters University Hospital, 254 Easton Ave, New Brunswick, NJ 08901, USA; [c] Division of Pulmonary and Critical Care, Department of Medicine, Rutgers Robert Wood Johnson Medical School, One Robert Johnson Place, New Brunswick, NJ 08903, USA
* Corresponding author. Division of Pulmonary and Critical Care, Department of Emergency Medicine, Rutgers Robert Wood Johnson Medical School, Rutgers RWJMS, MEB 104, One Robert Johnson Place, New Brunswick, NJ 08903.
E-mail address: boutsida@rwjms.rutgers.edu

Emerg Med Clin N Am 35 (2017) 11–23
http://dx.doi.org/10.1016/j.emc.2016.08.007
0733-8627/17/© 2016 Elsevier Inc. All rights reserved.

impact from this work is likely the increased awareness for early identification of septic patients.

So-called usual' sepsis care has evolved over the past 3 decades as knowledge of the disease and its treatment has been refined. The term usual care (UC), represents a consensus of what is needed to effectively combat this syndrome. Early goal-directed therapy (EGDT), as described in the Rivers and colleagues[2] study and the Surviving Sepsis Guidelines from the SSC, can be especially taxing in resource-limited settings. Further, additional literature over the past several years has questioned whether all components are necessary or even harmful,[4–7] prompting the ProCESS (A Protocolized Care for Early Septic Shock),[8] ARISE (The Australasian Resuscitation in Sepsis Evaluation)[9] and ProMISe (A Protocolised Management in Sepsis)[10] trials. These studies evaluated the various elements of EGDT, and it is anticipated that these data will further refine the components that should be routinely applied in the care of septic patients. This article discusses the landmark sepsis trials that have been published over the past several decades and offers recommendations on what should currently be considered UC.

MORTALITY IN THE ERA BEFORE EARLY GOAL-DIRECTED THERAPY

In the roughly 35 years leading up to the introduction of the SSC, the overall mortality for patients with sepsis was 49.7%.[11] Most publications over that time reported mortalities between 40% and 80%.[11] Although there had been some improvements in mortality, the trend was small.[11] Although it is easy to assume that this was the result of outdated treatments, the therapies delivered then were similar to modern interventions. Despite this, recent studies have suggested dramatic improvements in survival, with current mortalities ranging from 20% to 35%.[8–10,12,13] Note that just as sepsis care has changed, its definition has changed as well.[14] As a result, this can present some challenges to interpreting current and historical data. Regardless of which definition is used, mortality has clearly improved.

EARLY GOAL-DIRECTED THERAPY

In 2001, Rivers and colleagues[2] published a landmark article that challenged contemporary sepsis care. The investigators theorized that if patients could be treated in a timely and targeted manner to correct the imbalance between oxygen delivery and demand, the progression to multiorgan failure and death could be halted. They did this by targeting specific central hemodynamic end points during the initial 6 hours of treatment of severe sepsis (defined by the presence of 2 systemic inflammatory response syndrome criteria and end-organ damage) and septic shock (defined by a lack of blood pressure response to adequate fluid resuscitation).

The study randomized 263 patients to 2 study arms. Those in the standard therapy (ST) arm were treated at physician discretion according to a protocol for hemodynamic support. This treatment included placement of central venous and arterial catheters. Patients randomized to the EGDT arm were resuscitated according to a protocol that designated preset hemodynamic end points. This protocol included placement of a central venous catheter capable of continuous central venous oxygen saturation ($Scvo_2$) monitoring.

Importantly, treatments in the 2 arms varied. The EGDT group used prespecified hemodynamic targets to assess success of resuscitation and as triggers for additional interventions. The first hemodynamic variable targeted was a central venous pressure (CVP) of 8 to 12 mm Hg. In order to achieve this, patients were given 500 mL of a crystalloid every 30 minutes until this target was reached. If the mean arterial pressure (MAP) remained less than 65 mm Hg despite a CVP of 8 to 12 mm Hg, vasopressor therapy was initiated to achieve this goal. If, despite achieving a goal CVP and

MAP, the $Scvo_2$ was less than 70%, the patient was transfused red blood cells to a hematocrit of 30%. If, despite transfusion, the $Scvo_2$ remained less than the target, inotropic therapy was initiated with dobutamine. In addition, if the $Scvo_2$ goal was still not achieved in a nonventilated patient, the patient was intubated and sedative agents were administered.

The results of this study suggested that a timely, targeted approach conferred a significant mortality benefit, because the EGDT group had statistically significant improvements in in-hospital, 28-day, and 60-day mortalities. Some of the significant differences between the treatment arms included fluid administration, continuous $Scvo_2$ monitoring, vasopressor use, inotropic support, and blood transfusions (**Table 1**). The total amount of fluids at 72 hours administered to both groups was not statistically significant. However, the amount that the EGDT group received in the first 6 hours was significant, compared with patients in the ST arm. Also, during the initial 6 hours, the EGDT group received continuous $Scvo_2$ monitoring, and significantly more inotropic medications and red blood cell transfusions.

The investigators of this study postulated that the improved mortality seen in the EGDT group was caused by improved matching of oxygen delivery to oxygen demand during the earliest stages of sepsis and septic shock. This improved matching was accomplished with improved preload via volume resuscitation and increased oxygen carrying capacity from blood transfusions and inotropy. Patients in the ST group, after the 6-hour intervention period, received more fluids, required more vasopressors, and were mechanically ventilated at higher rates. This finding suggested that providers may have missed an opportunity for hemodynamic optimization during the essential early phase of resuscitation. There were no measurements of time-to-antibiotic administration in each group. However, more patients received antibiotic therapy in the first 6 hours in the ST group than in the EGDT group.

A SHIFT IN SEPSIS CARE

After publication of the Rivers and colleagues[2] trial, EGDT was viewed as cornerstone to successful sepsis management.[15] In 2002, EGDT was suggested as a guideline for care by an expert sepsis panel.[16] In 2004, the SSC, a committee composed of critical care and infectious disease experts representing 11 international organizations, recommended the following EGDT hemodynamic targets with grade B evidence: CVP of 8 to 12 mm Hg, MAP greater than or equal to 65 mm Hg, central venous or mixed venous oxygen saturation of greater than 70% via the use of fluids, red blood cells, and dobutamine to achieve these goals.[3]

The SSC guidelines established goals of care across various therapeutic modalities for sepsis. These guidelines were expansive and included recommendations on initial resuscitation; diagnostic goals; timing and regimens of antibiotic administration; vasopressor and inotropic use; corticosteroids; sedation strategies; ventilation strategies; blood product administration; and preventive measures against ventilator-acquired pneumonia, stress ulcers, and deep vein thrombosis (DVT).

Clearly, more integrated care for sepsis developed from the EGDT trial. However, despite the mortality benefit noted in this study population, there were concerns that certain elements of the EGDT protocol may be unnecessary, or potentially harmful. For instance, restrictive transfusion protocols have shown improved mortality, whereas other literature has simply shown noninferiority.[4,17] This finding suggests that transfusing to a goal hematocrit of 30% to improve the $Scvo_2$ and oxygen delivery did not confer the observed benefit seen in the River and colleagues[2] EGDT algorithm. In addition, CVP and other static cardiac filling pressures can be poor predictors of

Table 1 Results of early goal-directed therapy				
Variable	EGDT vs ST at 6 h	P Value	EGDT vs ST at 7–72 h	P Value
CVP (mm Hg)	13.8 ± 4.4 vs 11.8 ± 6.8	.007	11.6 ± 6.1 vs 11.9 ± 5.6	.68
Total fluids (mL)	4981 ± 2984 vs 3499 ± 2438	<.001	8625 ± 5162 vs 10,602 ± 6216	.01
MAP (mm Hg)	95 ± 19 vs 81 ± 18	<.001	87 ± 15 vs 80 ± 15	<.001
Vasopressor (%)	27.4 vs 30.3	.62	29.1 vs 42.9	.03
Scvo$_2$ (%)	77.3 ± 10 vs 66.0 ± 5.5	<.001	70.4 ± 10.7 vs 65.3 ± 11.4	<.001
Red cell transfusion (%)	64.1 vs 18.5	<.001	11.1 vs 32.8	<.001
Inotropic therapy (%)	13.7 vs 0.8	<.001	14.5 vs 8.4	.14
Lactate (mmol/L)	4.3 ± 4.2 vs 4.9 ± 4.7	.01	3.0 ± 4.4 vs 3.9 ± 4.4	.02
Arterial pH	7.35 ± 0.11 vs 7.31 ± 0.15	<.001	7.40 ± 0.12 vs 7.36 ± 0.12	<.001
APACHE II	16.0 ± 6.9 vs 17.6 ± 6.2	<.001	13.0 ± 6.3 vs 15.9 ± 6.4	<.001
SAPS II	42.2 ± 13.2 vs 45.5 ± 12.3	<.001	36.9 ± 11.3 vs 42.6 ± 11.5	<.001
MODS	5.9 ± 3.7 vs 6.8 ± 3.7	<.001	5.1 ± 3.9 vs 6.4 ± 4.0	<.001
Mechanical ventilation (%)	53.0 vs 53.8	.90	2.6 vs 16.8	<.001
			EGDT vs ST	P Value
Mortality (%)				
In-hospital			30.5 vs 46.5	.009
28-d			33.3 vs 49.2	.01
60-d			44.3 vs 56.9	.03
Cause of In-hospital Death				
Cardiovascular collapse (%)			10.3 vs 21	.02
Multiorgan failure (%)			16.2 vs 21.8	.27

Plus-minus values are ± standard deviation.

Abbreviations: APACHE II, Acute Physiology and Chronic Health Evaluation score II; MODS, Multiple Organ Dysfunction Score; SAPS II, Simplified Acute Physiology Score II.

Data from Rivers E, Nguyen B, Havstad S, et al. Early goal-directed therapy in the treatment of severe sepsis and septic shock. N Engl J Med 2001;345(19):1368–77.

fluid responsiveness.[5,18,19] Further, there are some retrospective data that suggested increased mortality in patients who are over-resuscitated because of implementation of EGDT.[6] In addition, placement of central venous catheters is not completely benign and carries inherent risks of mechanical complications and infection. When catheter-related infections do occur, they increase morbidity and mortality, length of stay, and health care cost.[7]

There were also criticisms of the external validity of the EGDT study, because this was a single-center trial. Although mortality of the control group for this single-center study was 48.3%, control arms of multicenter, randomized controlled trials conducted in a similar time period were only 30% to 35%, highlighting a possible overestimation of treatment benefit with EGDT.[20] These patients may also have been sicker or arrived to the emergency room in later stages of disease, creating results that may, at best, only translate to a small and specific subset of septic patients.[21]

In addition, there are many barriers to implementation of EGDT. A survey of medical directors and nurse managers from high-volume, urban hospitals in the United States found common barriers to be nursing staff requirements, monitoring CVP in the emergency department, and identification of septic patients.[22] Regarding the use of continuous Scvo$_2$, not all settings are equipped to use these catheters, and further study found lactate trends to be a noninferior surrogate.[23] Other barriers to EGDT that have been reported include reluctance of physicians, availability of and training for new technology, and the extensive time and resources needed to implement the protocol.[24]

THE ProCESS, ARISE, AND ProMISe TRIALS

Given the criticisms, 3 multicenter, randomized, independent but collaborative trials were conducted in the United States (ProCESS), Australia (ARISE), and United Kingdom (ProMISe) to evaluate the benefits of EGDT.[8–10] Each trial used the definitions of severe sepsis and septic shock used in the original EGDT trial. However, the definition of refractory hypotension was changed from unresponsive to 20 to 30 mL/kg over 30 minutes (as in the original EGDT trial) to unresponsive to a 1-L fluid bolus over 30 to 60 minutes.[25] In contrast with the original EGDT trial, it was specified that antibiotics should be administered before randomization in the ARISE and ProMISe trials. Each center selected in these trials lacked routine protocolized emergency department sepsis care.[25] Investigators in each trial chose leading academic and regional centers that were thought to follow best evidence for sepsis care in order to maximize the likelihood of best current practice in the UC arms.[25] The EGDT arms of each study required a central venous catheter with Scvo$_2$ monitoring, administration of fluids, use of vasopressors, and red blood cells targeting CVP, MAP, and Scvo$_2$ goals in the same fashion as the original EGDT study. The ProCESS trial included a third arm, protocolized standard care (PSC), which used a 6-hour protocol but did not require central venous catheters, inotropes, or blood products. Volume status decisions were based on clinical signs of perfusion, in contrast with triggered fluid administration of the EGDT arm, and used a systolic blood pressure goal of 100 mm Hg rather than the MAP.

In total 1351, 1600, and 1260 patients underwent randomization in the ProCESS, ARISE, and ProMISe trials, respectively. The primary outcome of the ProCESS trial was 60-day mortality. The primary outcomes for the ARISE and ProMISe trials were 90-day mortality. The secondary outcomes of all 3 trials included the use of mechanical ventilation, dialysis, prolonged vasopressor or cardiac support, and the duration of intensive care unit (ICU) and hospital stay.

The key results of the 3 trials are included in **Tables 2** and **3**. There were no significant differences in mortality between arms in any of the 3 trials. There were no differences in the need for mechanical ventilation and dialysis between groups, except for the PSC group in the ProCESS trial, in which more patients received dialysis (see **Table 3**). With the exception of a shorter ICU stay in the UC arm of the ProMISe trial, there were otherwise no differences in ICU or hospital length of stay. There was more use of vasopressors and advanced cardiovascular support, fluids, central venous catheters, dobutamine, and red blood cell transfusions in the EGDT arms of all 3 trials.

WHAT MAKES A DIFFERENCE?

The results of these 3 large trials provide a wealth of evidence to further refine current sepsis management. Importantly, strict adherence to the original goals of the initial

Table 2
Mortality data from the ProCESS, ARISE, and ProMISe trials

Outcome	EGDT	UC	PSC	P Value
ProCESS				
60-d mortality (%)	21	18.9	18.2	.83
90-d mortality (%)	31.9	33.7	30.8	.66
ARISE				
90-d mortality (%)	18.6	18.8	—	.90
28-d mortality (%)	14.8	15.9	—	.53
Death in ICU (%)	10.9	12.9	—	.28
Death in hospital (%)	14.5	15.7	—	.53
ProMISe				
90-d mortality (%)	29.5	29.2	—	a
28-d mortality (%)	24.8	24.5	—	a
Death in hospital (%)	25.6	24.6	—	a

Abbreviations: ARISE, The Australasian Resuscitation in Sepsis Evaluation; ProCESS, A Protocolized Care for Early Septic Shock; ProMISe, A Protocolised Management in Sepsis.
[a] No significant difference in relative risk or odds ratio.

EGDT trial and the methods implemented to reach central hemodynamic end points does not seem to result in a significant difference in patient outcomes. However, the mortality data from these 3 studies indicate a clear overall improvement in mortality compared with previous data and the original EGDT trial, which suggests that there are other causes influencing the observed improvement in sepsis care.

Table 3
Secondary outcomes from the selected trials

Outcome	EGDT	UC	PSC	P Value
ProCESS				
Mechanical ventilation (%)	38.0	32.4	36.5	.19
Vasopressor support (%)	61.3	56.1	63.7	.06
Dialysis (%)	3.1	2.8	6.0	.04
ICU days	5.1	4.7	5.1	.63
Hospital days	11.1	11.3	12.3	.25
ARISE				
Mechanical ventilation (%)	30.0	31.5	—	.52
Vasopressor support (%)	76.3	65.8	—	<.001
Dialysis (%)	13.4	13.5	—	.94
ICU days	2.8	2.8	—	.81
Hospital days	8.2	8.5	—	.89
ProMISe				
Mechanical/positive pressure ventilation (%)	28.9	28.5	—	.90
Cardiovascular support (%)	37	30.9	—	.026
Dialysis (%)	14.2	13.2	—	.62
ICU days	2.6	2.2	—	.005
Hospital days	9	9	—	.46

Bundled Therapy

Perhaps the greatest impact of the SSC guidelines was the recommendation to screen patients early and apply comprehensive, evidence-based bundles of therapy. These bundles selected specific interventions that make it easier to bring these guidelines into practice, while reducing mortality and creating objective measures of quality of care.[26] Using bundles decreased absolute mortality from 37% to 30.8% in a multicenter study that included 15,022 patients from the United States, Europe, and South Africa.[27] Individual items included in this bundle were the administration of antibiotics within 6 hours, obtaining blood cultures before antibiotic initiation, blood glucose control, and achieving plateau pressure control if patients were mechanically ventilated. Lactate levels, corticosteroids, or achieving CVP or $Scvo_2$ goals were not associated with a mortality improvement.[27]

A mainstay of bundled therapy for sepsis is the administration of intravenous fluids for signs of organ hypoperfusion. Although the markers for volume repletion are controversial, the Rivers and colleagues[2] trial suggested that giving fluids early helped improve outcomes. Multiple smaller studies that examined bundled therapy also revealed an almost 50% mortality reduction.[28–32] Rivers and colleagues[2] noted a nearly 1500-mL difference in the amount of fluids administered in favor of the EGDT arm during the intervention period. In the more recent trials, the EGDT arms received only 200 to 500 mL more fluid during the intervention period compared with the UC arms. This observation across all 3 recent studies suggests that overall sepsis care has transitioned toward more aggressive and timely treatment, regardless of implemented protocols. This is supported by the fact that, although the centers in the newer EGDT trials did not have a protocol in place, they were chosen based on their higher likelihood to follow best practice and the bundles put forth by the SSC.[25]

Early Antibiotics and Source Control

Antibiotic administration generally occurs simultaneously with fluid resuscitation. Studies published after the original EGDT trial revealed a mortality benefit of antibiotic administration within 1 hour of recognized hypotension in septic patients, with an increase in mortality of 7.6% for each hour of antibiotic delay.[33,34] This evidence resulted in a level 1C recommendation for antibiotic therapy in the latest version of the SSC guidelines (**Table 4**).[35] Early administration of antibiotics was not controlled for, or measured, in the original EGDT trial but was achieved before randomization in the ARISE and ProMISe trials, which suggests that, as with aggressive volume repletion, early antibiotic administration has likely contributed to the improvement in mortality.

Note that a recent meta-analysis suggested no difference in mortality when antibiotics are administered from less than 1 hour to more than 5 hours following recognition of sepsis or septic shock.[36] However, early antibiotic administration must continue to be a goal, because this is one of the few interventions that treats the underlying cause. Further, there is clearly a point at which delayed antibiotic administration results in increased mortality. As such, the goal of antibiotic administration in less than 1 hour from recognition continues to be imperative. Despite the data presented in this article, the investigators caution the interpretation of its data stating, "We believe an incorrect interpretation of this report would be that early administration of antibiotics is not of substantial importance."[36]

Along with early antibiotics, source control within 12 hours is recommended in the current SSC guidelines, based on studies that examined improved outcomes with

Table 4
Current Surviving Sepsis Campaign guideline recommendations

Intervention	Recommendation	GRADE[a]
Initial resuscitation	• CVP: 8–12 mm Hg • MAP: $\geq$65 mm Hg • Urine output: $\geq$0.5 ml/kg/h • Scvo$_2$ or mixed venous oxygen saturation: $\geq$70%	1C
Screening for sepsis and performance improvement	Routine screening of potentially infected seriously ill patients for severe sepsis to allow earlier implementation of therapy	1C
Diagnosis	At least 2 blood cultures should be obtained	1C
Antibiotic therapy	• IV antibiotics within first hour of septic shock or severe sepsis • Antibiotics should be readdressed daily for de-escalation	1B 1C 1B
Source control	Every patient should be evaluated for a source that can be intervened on and, if present, intervened on within 12 h	1C
Fluids	Challenge with sepsis-induced hypoperfusion	1C
Vasopressors	Norepinephrine should be the first-choice agent	1B
Glucose	Protocolized glucose management with goal glucose level 180 mg/dL	1A

Abbreviation: IV, intravenous.
[a] GRADE system classifies recommendations as strong or weak (1 or 2 respectively) and incorporates a letter scale (A–D, highest to lowest, respectively) for quality of evidence.
Data from Dellinger RP, Levy MM, Rhodes A, et al. Surviving Sepsis Campaign: international guidelines for management of severe sepsis and septic shock, 2012. Intensive Care Med 2013;39(2):165–228.

surgical interventions on soft tissue infections and intra-abdominal abscesses and guidelines pushing for removal of potentially infected catheters.[37–40] When indwelling catheters have been in place for more than 48 hours and are thought to be a possible source, additional blood cultures should include a sample drawn through each lumen of each vascular access.[35]

Prophylactic Care

In protecting patients from known complications of care while they are treated for sepsis it is also important to optimize the best chances of survival. Recommendations with consistent strong evidence are those addressing preventive measures. These recommendations are based on several large trials examining DVT, gastrointestinal stress ulcer, and ventilator-associated pneumonia prophylaxis.[41–48] Moreover, when a bundle of ventilator care that includes stress ulcer disease prophylaxis, DVT prophylaxis, elevation of the head of bed, and sedation vacation was applied to 35 ICUs, there was an average 44.5% reduction in ventilator-acquired pneumonias.[49]

Mechanical Ventilation and Sedation

The SSC guidelines provide strong recommendations with regard to mechanical ventilation. These recommendations include lung protective ventilation even when acute respiratory distress syndrome (ARDS) is not present, the use of daily spontaneous breathing trials, and current sedation strategies to limit ventilator time. These recommendations are based on studies showing the efficacy of spontaneous breathing trials and decreased duration of mechanical ventilation using this strategy.[50–52] The endorsement of low-tidal-volume ventilation was derived from the landmark work of the ARDS Network.[53]

Sedation regimens are an integral part of mechanical ventilation and can strongly influence spontaneous breathing trials, and patient morbidity. Several studies showed prolonged mechanical ventilation with antiquated sedation techniques and improvements when targeted sedation protocols and daily interruptions were implemented.[54–56] Thus, such strategies may also have influenced the observed improvement in mortality in these trials.

Glucose Control

Since the original EGDT trial there have been changes in the management of hyperglycemia. Initial evidence suggested that intensive intravenous insulin with goal glucose level of 80 to 110 mg/dL is beneficial.[57] However, since the initial SSC guidelines there has been a myriad of evidence suggesting that these intensive regimens cause harm and increase mortality.[58–61] Based on outcomes in the NICE-SUGAR (The Normoglycemia in Intensive Care Evaluation–Survival Using Glucose Algorithm Regulation) trial, the SSC now gives a 1C recommendation to target glucose concentrations less than 180 mg/dL.[59] It is important to control blood glucose level but avoid hypoglycemia.

Vasopressor Selection

The increased use of vasopressors in the recent 3 trials examining EGDT did not influence mortality. However, several studies before and after the first EGDT trial show that norepinephrine is superior to dopamine and confers a lower risk of arrhythmogenic events. Further, norepinephrine may improve mortality compared with dopamine, especially in patients with a cardiogenic component of shock.[35,62] The current recommendations now select norepinephrine as the sole first-line agent.[35]

THE NEW USUAL CARE

The use of continuous Scvo$_2$ has now failed to show mortality benefit in 3 multicenter, randomized controlled trials when implemented in the routine care of patients with sepsis.[8–10] Similarly the transfusion of red blood cells to target a hematocrit of 30%, either alone or with inotropic support with the goal of increasing oxygen delivery, is also unlikely to provide any additional benefit.[8–10] Therefore, as with the use of continuous Scvo$_2$, this practice is anticipated to become less favored.

The new UC is characterized by early recognition and early intervention. Although previous goals of fluid resuscitation used CVP and other static markers of volume responsiveness, these are being replaced with better dynamic markers of volume responsiveness that include pulse-pressure variation, stroke volume variation, passive leg raise, and respirophasic changes in the inferior vena cava measured by ultrasonography.[63] Regardless of which of these methods is chosen, early aggressive crystalloid administration remains a cornerstone of sepsis resuscitation. This fact was highlighted in the ProCESS, ARISE, and ProMISe trials, because all treatment arms received similar resuscitation volumes before randomization, and it is true for early antibiotics as well. This advice was not emphasized in the Rivers and colleagues[2] trial, but was a prerequisite before randomization in the ARISE and ProMISe trials. Both of these interventions are likely a product of earlier recognition and screening for this potentially deadly disease process. When early identification, fluid resuscitation, and appropriate antibiotic administration are combined with source control, lung protective ventilation, evidence-based sedation strategies, and implementation of prophylactic interventions, patients are given the best chance of survival.

SUMMARY

UC before the major EGDT trials[2,8-10] was characterized by a delayed response in the treatment of sepsis and septic shock. EGDT has evolved over the past 2 decades. Therapeutic modalities such as CVP and continuous $Scvo_2$ measurements, placement of central venous catheters, routine blood transfusions, and inotropic support are no longer viewed as prerequisites in the treatment of sepsis. Notwithstanding, the current sepsis trials have established a culture of early recognition of sepsis, early fluid resuscitation, appropriate antibiotic treatment, source control, and the application of multi-discipline evidence-based medicine to the most current sepsis care. This culture has created a new UC.

REFERENCES

1. Centers for Disease Control and Prevention (CDC). 2016. Available at: Www.hcup-Us.ahrq.gov/nisoverview.jsp. Accessed February 22, 2016.
2. Rivers E, Nguyen B, Havstad S, et al. Early goal-directed therapy in the treatment of severe sepsis and septic shock. N Engl J Med 2001;345(19):1368–77.
3. Dellinger RP, Carlet JM, Masur H, et al. Surviving Sepsis Campaign guidelines for management of severe sepsis and septic shock. Crit Care Med 2004;32(3):858–73.
4. Hébert PC, Wells G, Blajchman MA, et al. A multicenter, randomized, controlled clinical trial of transfusion requirements in critical care. Transfusion Requirements in Critical Care Investigators, Canadian Critical Care Trials Group. N Engl J Med 1999;340(6):409–17.
5. Osman D, Ridel C, Ray P, et al. Cardiac filling pressures are not appropriate to predict hemodynamic response to volume challenge. Crit Care Med 2007;35(1):64–8.
6. Kelm DJ, Perrin JT, Cartin-Ceba R, et al. Fluid overload in patients with severe sepsis and septic shock treated with early goal-directed therapy is associated with increased acute need for fluid-related medical interventions and hospital death. Shock 2015;43(1):68–73.
7. DePalo VA, McNicoll L, Cornell M, et al. The Rhode Island ICU collaborative: a model for reducing central line-associated bloodstream infection and ventilator-associated pneumonia statewide. Qual Saf Health Care 2010;19(6):555–61.
8. ProCESS Investigators, Yealy DM, Kellum JA, et al. A randomized trial of protocol-based care for early septic shock. N Engl J Med 2014;370(18):1683–93.
9. ARISE Investigators, ANZICS Clinical Trials Group, Peake SL, et al. Goal-directed resuscitation for patients with early septic shock. N Engl J Med 2014;371(16):1496–506.
10. Mouncey PR, Osborn TM, Power GS, et al. Trial of early, goal-directed resuscitation for septic shock. N Engl J Med 2015;372(14):1301–11.
11. Friedman G, Silva E, Vincent JL. Has the mortality of septic shock changed with time. Crit Care Med 1998;26(12):2078–86.
12. Dellinger RP. Cardiovascular management of septic shock. Crit Care Med 2003;31(3):946–55.
13. Kaukonen K-M, Bailey M, Suzuki S, et al. Mortality related to severe sepsis and septic shock among critically ill patients in Australia and New Zealand, 2000-2012. JAMA 2014;311(13):1308–16.
14. Singer M, Deutschman CS, Seymour CW, et al. The Third International Consensus Definitions for Sepsis and Septic Shock (Sepsis-3). JAMA 2016;315(8):801–10.

15. Patel GP, Gurka DP, Balk RA. New treatment strategies for severe sepsis and septic shock. Curr Opin Crit Care 2003;9(5):390–6.
16. Vincent J-L, Abraham E, Annane D, et al. Reducing mortality in sepsis: new directions. Crit Care 2002;6(Suppl 3):S1–18.
17. Holst LB, Haase N, Wetterslev J, et al. Lower versus higher hemoglobin threshold for transfusion in septic shock. N Engl J Med 2014;371(15):1381–91.
18. Kumar A, Anel R, Bunnell E, et al. Pulmonary artery occlusion pressure and central venous pressure fail to predict ventricular filling volume, cardiac performance, or the response to volume infusion in normal subjects. Crit Care Med 2004;32(3):691–9.
19. Michard F, Teboul J-L. Predicting fluid responsiveness in ICU patients: a critical analysis of the evidence. Chest 2002;121(6):2000–8.
20. Peake S, Webb S, Delaney A. Early goal-directed therapy of septic shock: we honestly remain skeptical. Crit Care Med 2007;35(3):994–5 [author reply: 995].
21. Perel A. Bench-to-bedside review: the initial hemodynamic resuscitation of the septic patient according to Surviving Sepsis Campaign guidelines–does one size fit all? Crit Care 2008;12(5):223.
22. Carlbom DJ, Rubenfeld GD. Barriers to implementing protocol-based sepsis resuscitation in the emergency department–results of a national survey. Crit Care Med 2007;35(11):2525–32.
23. Jones AE, Shapiro NI, Trzeciak S, et al. Lactate clearance vs central venous oxygen saturation as goals of early sepsis therapy: a randomized clinical trial. JAMA 2010;303(8):739–46.
24. Jones AE, Shapiro NI, Roshon M. Implementing early goal-directed therapy in the emergency setting: the challenges and experiences of translating research innovations into clinical reality in academic and community settings. Acad Emerg Med 2007;14(11):1072–8.
25. ProCESS/ARISE/ProMISe Methodology Writing Committee, Huang DT, Angus DC, et al. Harmonizing international trials of early goal-directed resuscitation for severe sepsis and septic shock: methodology of ProCESS, ARISE, and ProMISe. Intensive Care Med 2013;39(10):1760–75.
26. Levy MM, Pronovost PJ, Dellinger RP, et al. Sepsis change bundles: converting guidelines into meaningful change in behavior and clinical outcome. Crit Care Med 2004;32(11 Suppl):S595–7.
27. Levy MM, Dellinger RP, Townsend SR, et al. The Surviving Sepsis Campaign: results of an international guideline-based performance improvement program targeting severe sepsis. Crit Care Med 2010;38(2):367–74.
28. Gao F, Melody T, Daniels DF, et al. The impact of compliance with 6-hour and 24-hour sepsis bundles on hospital mortality in patients with severe sepsis: a prospective observational study. Crit Care 2005;9(6):R764–70.
29. Kortgen A, Niederprüm P, Bauer M. Implementation of an evidence-based "standard operating procedure" and outcome in septic shock. Crit Care Med 2006; 34(4):943–9.
30. Nguyen HB, Corbett SW, Steele R, et al. Implementation of a bundle of quality indicators for the early management of severe sepsis and septic shock is associated with decreased mortality. Crit Care Med 2007;35(4):1105–12.
31. El Solh AA, Akinnusi ME, Alsawalha LN, et al. Outcome of septic shock in older adults after implementation of the sepsis "bundle.,". J Am Geriatr Soc 2008; 56(2):272–8.
32. Barochia AV, Cui X, Vitberg D, et al. Bundled care for septic shock: an analysis of clinical trials. Crit Care Med 2010;38(2):668–78.

33. Kumar A, Roberts D, Wood KE, et al. Duration of hypotension before initiation of effective antimicrobial therapy is the critical determinant of survival in human septic shock. Crit Care Med 2006;34(6):1589–96.

34. Ferrer R, Artigas A, Suarez D, et al. Effectiveness of treatments for severe sepsis: a prospective, multicenter, observational study. Am J Respir Crit Care Med 2009; 180(9):861–6.

35. Dellinger RP, Levy MM, Rhodes A, et al. Surviving sepsis campaign: international guidelines for management of severe sepsis and septic shock, 2012. Intensive Care Med 2013;39(2):165–228.

36. Sterling SA, Miller WR, Pryor J, et al. The impact of timing of antibiotics on outcomes in severe sepsis and septic shock: a systematic review and meta-analysis. Crit Care Med 2015;43(9):1907–15.

37. Moss RL, Musemeche CA, Kosloske AM. Necrotizing fasciitis in children: prompt recognition and aggressive therapy improve survival. J Pediatr Surg 1996;31(8): 1142–6.

38. Boyer A, Vargas F, Coste F, et al. Influence of surgical treatment timing on mortality from necrotizing soft tissue infections requiring intensive care management. Intensive Care Med 2009;35(5):847–53.

39. Bufalari A, Giustozzi G, Moggi L. Postoperative intraabdominal abscesses: percutaneous versus surgical treatment. Acta Chir Belg 1996;96(5):197–200.

40. O'Grady NP, Alexander M, Burns LA, et al. Summary of recommendations: guidelines for the prevention of intravascular catheter-related infections. Clin Infect Dis 2011;52(9):1087–99.

41. Drakulovic MB, Torres A, Bauer TT, et al. Supine body position as a risk factor for nosocomial pneumonia in mechanically ventilated patients: a randomised trial. Lancet 1999;354(9193):1851–8.

42. Cade JF. High risk of the critically ill for venous thromboembolism. Crit Care Med 1982;10(7):448–50.

43. Belch JJ, Lowe GD, Ward AG, et al. Prevention of deep vein thrombosis in medical patients by low-dose heparin. Scott Med J 1981;26(2):115–7.

44. Samama MM, Cohen AT, Darmon JY, et al. A comparison of enoxaparin with placebo for the prevention of venous thromboembolism in acutely ill medical patients. Prophylaxis in Medical Patients with Enoxaparin Study Group. N Engl J Med 1999;341(11):793–800.

45. Borrero E, Bank S, Margolis I, et al. Comparison of antacid and sucralfate in the prevention of gastrointestinal bleeding in patients who are critically ill. Am J Med 1985;79(2C):62–4.

46. Bresalier RS, Grendell JH, Cello JP, et al. Sucralfate suspension versus titrated antacid for the prevention of acute stress-related gastrointestinal hemorrhage in critically ill patients. Am J Med 1987;83(3B):110–6.

47. Cook D, Guyatt G, Marshall J, et al. A comparison of sucralfate and ranitidine for the prevention of upper gastrointestinal bleeding in patients requiring mechanical ventilation. Canadian Critical Care Trials Group. N Engl J Med 1998;338(12): 791–7.

48. Stothert JC, Simonowitz DA, Dellinger EP, et al. Randomized prospective evaluation of cimetidine and antacid control of gastric pH in the critically ill. Ann Surg 1980;192(2):169–74.

49. Resar R, Pronovost P, Haraden C, et al. Using a bundle approach to improve ventilator care processes and reduce ventilator-associated pneumonia. Jt Comm J Qual Patient Saf 2005;31(5):243–8.

50. Ely EW, Baker AM, Dunagan DP, et al. Effect on the duration of mechanical ventilation of identifying patients capable of breathing spontaneously. N Engl J Med 1996;335(25):1864–9.
51. Esteban A, Alía I, Gordo F, et al. Extubation outcome after spontaneous breathing trials with T-tube or pressure support ventilation. The Spanish Lung Failure Collaborative Group. Am J Respir Crit Care Med 1997;156(2 Pt 1):459–65.
52. Esteban A, Alía I, Tobin MJ, et al. Effect of spontaneous breathing trial duration on outcome of attempts to discontinue mechanical ventilation. Spanish Lung Failure Collaborative Group. Am J Respir Crit Care Med 1999;159(2):512–8.
53. Ventilation with lower tidal volumes as compared with traditional tidal volumes for acute lung injury and the acute respiratory distress syndrome. The Acute Respiratory Distress Syndrome Network. N Engl J Med 2000;342(18):1301–8.
54. Kollef MH, Levy NT, Ahrens TS, et al. The use of continuous I.V. sedation is associated with prolongation of mechanical ventilation. Chest 1998;114(2):541–8.
55. Kress JP, Pohlman AS, O'Connor MF, et al. Daily interruption of sedative infusions in critically ill patients undergoing mechanical ventilation. N Engl J Med 2000; 342(20):1471–7.
56. Brook AD, Ahrens TS, Schaiff R, et al. Effect of a nursing-implemented sedation protocol on the duration of mechanical ventilation. Crit Care Med 1999;27(12): 2609–15.
57. van den Berghe G, Wouters P, Weekers F, et al. Intensive insulin therapy in critically ill patients. N Engl J Med 2001;345(19):1359–67.
58. COIITSS Study Investigators, Annane D, Cariou A, et al. Corticosteroid treatment and intensive insulin therapy for septic shock in adults: a randomized controlled trial. JAMA 2010;303(4):341–8.
59. NICE-SUGAR Study Investigators, Finfer S, Chittock DR, et al. Intensive versus conventional glucose control in critically ill patients. N Engl J Med 2009; 360(13):1283–97.
60. Preiser J-C, Devos P, Ruiz-Santana S, et al. A prospective randomised multicentre controlled trial on tight glucose control by intensive insulin therapy in adult intensive care units: the Glucontrol study. Intensive Care Med 2009;35(10): 1738–48.
61. Wiener RS, Wiener DC, Larson RJ. Benefits and risks of tight glucose control in critically ill adults: a meta-analysis. JAMA 2008;300(8):933–44.
62. De Backer D, Biston P, Devriendt J, et al. Comparison of dopamine and norepinephrine in the treatment of shock. N Engl J Med 2010;362(9):779–89.
63. Marik PE, Monnet X, Teboul J-L. Hemodynamic parameters to guide fluid therapy. Ann Intensive Care 2011;1(1):1.

Appropriate Antibiotic Therapy

Michael G. Allison, MD[a], Emily L. Heil, PharmD[b], Bryan D. Hayes, PharmD[c],*

KEYWORDS

- Sepsis • Antibiotics • Antifungals • Obesity • Resistance • Acute kidney injury
- Dosing

KEY POINTS

- Although early retrospective studies found decreased survival associated with each 1-hour delay in antibiotics, prospective studies have not validated these findings; the optimal time benefit of antibiotic delivery within the first 6 hours is not known.
- Inappropriate initial antibiotic therapy is associated with an increase in mortality; it is appropriate to start broad-spectrum antibiotic therapy that provides coverage of the most likely pathogens.
- The use of 2 antibiotics to double-cover gram-negative infections is not routinely required, especially if empiric therapy involves an antipseudomonal penicillin, cephalosporin, or carbapenems.
- Patients who receive both vancomycin and piperacillin/tazobactam may be at greater risk for acute kidney injury.
- The loading dose of antibiotics is the same in patients with and without renal dysfunction. Subsequent doses need to be adjusted in patients with renal dysfunction.

INTRODUCTION

The timely use of appropriate antimicrobials is a cornerstone therapy for patients with sepsis syndromes. Recent publications have sparked debate regarding how the selection and timing of antimicrobial therapy affect the outcomes of patients with severe sepsis and septic shock. The selection of empiric antibiotics for septic patients in the emergency department (ED) likely plays a significant role in patient mortality. Practitioners need to consider many patient-specific factors when tailoring an

Disclosure: The authors have nothing to disclose.
The article was copyedited by Linda J. Kesselring, MS, ELS, the technical editor/writer in the Department of Emergency Medicine at the University of Maryland, School of Medicine.
[a] Critical Care Medicine, St. Agnes Hospital, 900 South Caton Avenue, Baltimore, MD 21229, USA; [b] Department of Pharmacy, University of Maryland Medical Center, 29 South Greene Street, Room 400, Baltimore, MD 21201, USA; [c] Department of Emergency Medicine, University of Maryland Medical Center, University of Maryland School of Medicine, 22 South Greene Street, Baltimore, MD 21201, USA
* Corresponding author.
E-mail address: bryanhayes13@gmail.com

Emerg Med Clin N Am 35 (2017) 25–42
http://dx.doi.org/10.1016/j.emc.2016.08.003
0733-8627/17/© 2016 Elsevier Inc. All rights reserved.

antibiotic regimen to a patient's' clinical presentation. Attention should be directed toward administering the selected antimicrobials in a timely manner. However, recommendations about the timing of administration are lacking: the Surviving Sepsis Campaign (SSC) guidelines have been criticized for their lack of timing advice founded on feasibility trials.[1] Many EDs now stock empiric antimicrobial regimens within the confines of the department rather than in a central pharmacy to enhance the speed and appropriateness of initial therapy. These empiric antimicrobials are often chosen according to local susceptibility patterns and antibiograms. Regimens for appropriate coverage vary according to the suspected disease process, so speed and breadth need to be weighed against the need for a thorough diagnostic work-up to localize the source of infection. The addition of antiviral and antifungal coverage to antibacterial therapy must be considered in certain at-risk patients. Patient-specific characteristics such as renal function, weight, and allergies necessitate antibiotic substitution or dosing adjustments for many critically ill patients.

TIMING OF ANTIMICROBIAL THERAPY

Sepsis has been defined as "life-threatening organ dysfunction due to a dysregulated host response to infection," so it makes intuitive sense that the earlier antimicrobial therapy is instituted, the better outcomes patients will have.[2] Kumar and colleagues[3] found that each hour's delay in antimicrobial administration was associated with a mean decrease in survival of 7.6%. Their multicenter, retrospective study included 2154 patients with hypotension as the start-time marker for septic shock. A second retrospective evaluation, this time of the SSC database, also showed increased in-hospital mortality with each hour's delay in antibiotic administration.[4] Similarly, a retrospective observational study in pediatric intensive care unit (ICU) patients showed an increased mortality risk with each hour's delay from sepsis recognition to antibiotic administration.[5] Note that time-to-intervention studies provide information primarily on correlation, not causation. Given the inherent limitations of retrospective studies and the complex variables that can confound time-to-intervention studies, caution is warranted when interpreting the results.[6]

Prospective studies have failed to validate an increased risk of mortality with delayed antibiotics, as long as they are administered within 6 hours after the diagnosis of sepsis.[7–9] A systematic review and meta-analysis found no significant mortality benefit of administering antibiotics within 3 hours after ED triage or within 1 hour after shock recognition in patients with severe sepsis and septic shock.[10] These data do not suggest that early antibiotic administration is not important, but that the exact time of maximum benefit is yet unknown. Because sepsis is a complex spectrum of illness, many factors affect the risk of death and the length of stay in an ICU. The arbitrarily assigned markers of time to antibiotic administration that are currently used as quality metrics might not be supported by the evidence that emerges from future studies.

APPROPRIATE ANTIBIOTIC SELECTION

After appropriate cultures are obtained, prompt initiation of broad-spectrum empiric antibiotic therapy is essential. Individualizing therapy in the ED is difficult, especially when empiric antimicrobials must be chosen without culture data. Reports suggest that 10% to 40% of initial empiric antimicrobial therapy is inadequate.[11–14] Antibiotic selection should be driven by multiple factors, including the suspected site of infection, local susceptibility patterns, and patient-specific factors. The suspected site of infection suggests common potential pathogens and thus indicates the antibiotics that can achieve an adequate concentration at the site. Local susceptibility patterns, guided by institutional antibiograms, aid in the identification of antibiotics with the highest likelihood of coverage for suspected pathogens. Patient-specific factors include organ function, infection history, antibiotic exposure history, surveillance cultures, and allergies.[15] There is little margin for error in patients with severe sepsis, so it is appropriate to start broad-spectrum antibiotic therapy that provides coverage of the most likely gram-positive and gram-negative pathogens.[1] Recommendations for empiric antibiotic regimens for septic patients are presented in **Table 1**.

Inappropriate initial antibiotic therapy is associated with an increase in the mortality. A single-center study of patients with bacteremia found a 34% difference (28% vs 62%) in the mortality among patients given inappropriate antibiotics on the first day of therapy and those given the right antibiotics.[13] In one of the first observational studies on the adequacy of antibiotics specific to patients in the ICU, the mortality was significantly higher in those who received inadequate antimicrobial therapy initially.[11] Further studies have confirmed these findings in patients with gram-negative sepsis, severe sepsis, and septic shock.[12,16]

Although it is important to consider the antimicrobial stewardship principle of using the most narrow-spectrum agent possible for an infection, this practice does not apply in the management of sepsis until culture data are available. However, it is still important to use very broad-spectrum agents such as the carbapenems judiciously, reserving them for patients who have a high likelihood of multidrug-resistant (MDR) infections and in communities in which local susceptibility patterns warrant them.

A classification of infections as health care–associated infections had been used to describe patients at higher risk for MDR organisms. The most recent guidelines have removed this category due to its lack of ability to accurately describe patients who required broad spectrum antibiotic coverage.[17–19] A lack of consensus regarding the power of these risks exists, and recent studies have delineated even more risk factors, including an immunocompromised state, hospitalization during the previous year, previous antibiotic therapy, age greater than 60 years, and Karnofsky index score less than 70.[20–22] Because these risk factors might be overly broad in identifying patients with resistant organisms, Shorr and colleagues[23] designed a clinical score that can be used to assess ED patients' risk of harboring a resistant pathogen (**Table 2**). In a cohort of 977 patients, resistant organisms, defined as methicillin-resistant *Staphylococcus aureus*, *Pseudomonas aeruginosa*, and extended-spectrum β-lactamases, were isolated 46.7% of the time. The risk score was higher in those with a resistant organism (median 4) than in those without a resistant organism (median 1) ($P<.001$). A score greater than 0 had a high positive predictive value of 84.5% for resistant organisms.[24] In addition, not all risk factors for MDR organisms are equivalent in their prediction of pneumonia caused by resistant pathogens in the community. Hospitalization in the preceding 90 days and residence in a long-term care facility were independent predictors of infection with a resistant pathogen in an observational prospective cohort of patients from the community who were hospitalized with pneumonia.[24,25] Most of the studies using the health care–associated infection classification are limited to respiratory and bloodstream infections. Of note, the health-care associated pneumonia designation was removed from the updated hospital-acquired pneumonia and ventilator-associated pneumonia guidelines as there is increasing evidence that many patients defined as having HCAP are not at high risk for MDRA pathogens and do not account for underlying patient characteristics that are also important determinates for risk of MDR pathogens.[19]

Another important factor in the selection of empiric antibiotic therapy is the patient's reported allergies. Between 15% and 20% of patients report an allergy to β-lactam antibiotics. Patients' self-report of antibiotic allergy has been associated with antimicrobial resistance, increased length of stay, ICU admission, increased costs, and even

Table 1
Common empiric antibiotic regimens

Suspected Source	Regimen	Comments

Sepsis of unknown origin	• Gram-negative/pseudomonal coverage
	  ○ Piperacillin/tazobactam, 4.5 g IV q 6 h, or cefepime, 2 g IV q 8 h, or a carbapenem (eg, meropenem, imipenem/cilastatin)
	    ■ Reported β-lactam allergy, but low suspicion for severe or anaphylactic reaction: cefepime, 2 g IV q 8 h, or meropenem, 1 g IV q 8 h. Monitor for reaction
	    ■ Known severe β-lactam allergy: ciprofloxacin, 400 mg IV q 8 h, or aztreonam, 2 g IV q 8 h, if resistance to fluoroquinolones is suspected (eg, prior exposure)
	    ■ Unknown reaction: if critically ill (intubated, pressors), the benefits of appropriately broad/effective antibiotics often outweigh the risk of anaphylaxis
	  ○ Add amikacin, 25 mg/kg ideal body weight IV × 1, if patient has risk factors for resistant GNR infection. Consult pharmacy for patients with CrCl<30 mL/min or on renal replacement therapy
	• Gram-positive/MRSA coverage
	  ○ Vancomycin, 25–30 mg/kg IV ABW load, followed by 15 mg/kg IV q 12 h, or
	  ○ Linezolid if history of VRE, 600 mg IV q 12 h
		A broad-spectrum β-lactam antibiotic should be administered before the anti-MRSA coverage because of its faster infusion times and broader coverage of potential pathogens

Sepsis – Suspected pulmonary source	• CAP
	○ Ceftriaxone, 1–2 g IV q 24 h, and azithromycin, 500 mg daily, or
	○ Ceftriaxone, 1–2 g IV q 24 h, and doxycycline, 100 mg PO BID, or
	○ Levofloxacin, 750 mg, or moxifloxacin, 400 mg, IV/PO daily
	○ Necrotizing or cavitary pneumonia: add MRSA coverage
	  ■ Add linezolid, 600 mg IV/PO q 12 h, to above regimen
	  ■ Note: doxycycline is inadequate for MRSA pneumonia coverage
	• HCAP
	○ For patients with recent (within last 90 days) intravenous antibiotic exposure
	○ Resistant gram-negative organism coverage
	○ Resistant gram-negative coverage
	  ■ Piperacillin/tazobactam, 4.5 g IV q 6 h, or
	  ■ Cefepime, 2 g IV q 8 h, or
	  ■ Carbapenem (eg, meropenem, 1 g IV q 8 h)
	  ■ Penicillin allergy: fluoroquinolone (eg, cipro-floxacin, 400 mg IV q 8 h)
	  ■ Plus optional gentamicin, 7 mg/kg daily, or amikacin, 20 mg/kg daily (for patients with septic shock while cultures are pending)
	
	• HCAP was a former designation for patients with exposure to health-care settings. The distinction from CAP served to identify patients with a theoretically higher risk for infection with MDR organisms. However, the distinction has been removed from current guidelines because the risk factors for HCAP (below) might not be predictive of infection with resistant pathogens. New guidelines indicate recent intravenous antibiotic use to be the risk factor for resistant pathogens with the most supporting literature
	• Risk factors for resistant gram-negative organisms:
	○ Hospitalization for ≥2 d within the past 90 d
	○ Residence in a long-term care facility
	○ Infusions (eg, home IV antibiotics, chemotherapy)
	○ Hemodialysis patient
	○ Wound care
	○ Family member with MDR organism
	○ Immunocompromised

Sepsis: suspected meningitis	• Vancomycin, 25 mg/kg loading dose, followed by 15 mg/kg q 8–12 h; ceftriaxone, 2 g IV q 12 h, and acyclovir, 10 mg/kg ideal body weight IV q 8 h • After neurosurgery or penetrating trauma, use cefepime, 2 g IV q 8 h, instead of ceftriaxone to cover *Pseudomonas* • Age>50 y, alcohol abuse, or immunocompromised: add ampicillin, 2 g IV q 4 h, to cover *Listeria monocytogenes*

(continued on next page)

Table 1
(continued)

Suspected Source	Regimen	Comments
Sepsis: suspected urinary source	• Community patients/no MDR risk factors 　○ Ceftriaxone, 1 g IV q 24 h 　○ PCN allergic: ciprofloxacin, 500 mg PO BID, or levofloxacin, 750 mg PO daily (renal dose adjustment required) • Foley catheter/risk factors for MDR gram negatives 　○ Cefepime, 1 g IV q 8 h, or piperacillin-tazobactam, 3.375 mg IV q 6 h, or levofloxacin, 500 IV q 24 h + gentamicin, 5 mg/kg IBW IV once	Fluoroquinolones (eg, ciprofloxacin and levofloxacin) should be avoided if local antibiogram shows significant resistance to *Escherichia coli* (threshold >10% per IDSA guidelines)
Sepsis: related to central line	Treat as above for sepsis of unknown origin, tailor antibiotics based on blood culture Gram stain	
Sepsis: intra-abdominal source	Treat as above for sepsis of unknown origin; ensure anaerobe coverage is included in the regimen (eg, piperacillin/tazobactam, a carbapenem, or add metronidazole)	

Doses listed in this table are for patients with normal renal function.

Abbreviations: ABW, adjusted body weight; BID, twice a day; CAP, community-acquired pneumonia; CrCl, creatinine clearance; GNR, gram-negative rods; HCAP, health care–associated pneumonia; IBW, ideal body weight; IDSA, Infectious Diseases Society of America; IV, intravenous; MDR, multidrug resistant; MRSA, methicillin-resistant *Staphylococcus aureus*; PCN, penicillin; PO, by mouth; q, every; VRE, vancomycin-resistant enterococci.

Table 2
Risk of resistant pathogens for pneumonia

Risk Factor	Point Value
Recent hospitalization (within 90 d)	4
Presenting from long-term care facility	3
Chronic hemodialysis	2
Admission to ICU within 24 h of ED evaluation	1

death.[24–28] To optimize therapy, a thorough allergy history should be documented, because some so-called reactions to antibiotics are frequently diagnosed inaccurately as allergies. The risk of cross reactivity with cephalosporins, particularly third- and fourth generation, and carbapenems is very low, so the risk/benefit of giving a septic patient potentially suboptimal therapy such as a fluoroquinolone versus a β-lactam with a low risk of cross reactivity should be considered carefully.[29,30]

Empiric antifungal coverage is not indicated for most patients, because fungal infections are typically diagnosed late in the course of hospitalization. The mortality associated with candidal infections can reach as high as 60%.[31,32] Risk factors for invasive candidiasis are categorized as host-related factors (eg, immunosuppressive disease or therapy, neutropenia, age, solid organ transplant) and health care–associated factors (eg, catheter use, total parenteral nutrition, recent surgical interventions, use of broad-spectrum antimicrobial drugs).[33] The Candida Score developed by León and colleagues[34] uses 4 variables for diagnosing probable candidal infection in non-neutropenic hosts: multifocal candida colonization (1), surgery (1), receipt of total parenteral nutrition (1), and clinical signs of severe sepsis (2). A score greater than 2.5 is associated with a greater than 7-fold increase in the likelihood of a documented candida infection. Notably, there was no association between the presence of a central venous catheter and candidal bloodstream infection. The combination of infrequent need for antifungal therapy and delayed culture results leads to delayed treatment and a high mortality among patients with candidal infection. Using the Candida Score in at-risk patients might assist in deciding whether fluconazole or an echinocandin should be ordered preemptively for a critically ill patient.

Irrespective of the conflicting data on time to antibiotic administration, the choice of antibiotics is vital. The use of appropriate antibiotics is associated with a lower mortality and a shorter ICU length of stay.[14,16,35,36] Broad-spectrum antibiotics should be initiated as early as possible. Delays are common, with risk factors including not being seen by an emergency physician, not considering the diagnosis of sepsis initially, and delay of therapy while waiting for diagnostic tests to be performed.[37] Several groups have implemented strategies to remove specific barriers to the timely administration of appropriate antibiotics. Kalich and colleagues[38] implemented an antibiotic-specific sepsis bundle and reported a significant improvement in the initiation of appropriate initial antibiotic therapy for severe sepsis in the ED. Adding appropriate antibiotics to unit-based cabinets also reduced order-to-administration time for first doses.[38,39]

THE ROLE OF CULTURES

Obtaining appropriate blood or tissue cultures before initiating antibiotic therapy is important in identifying the causative organisms. The SSC recommends obtaining cultures before the start of antimicrobial therapy if it can be done without delaying therapy more than 45 minutes (grade 1C).[1] In practice, 2 culture sets, each containing an aerobic and anaerobic culture bottle, should be drawn from 2 sites. Although the sepsis guidelines recommend that the volume of blood drawn into culture bottles should be greater than or equal to 10 mL, other infectious disease guidelines suggest that 20 to 40 mL of blood should be drawn, because the volume collected is directly proportional to the yield of pathogens.[1,40] Skin antisepsis can be achieved with tincture of iodine or chlorhexidine gluconate, and the aerobic bottle should be filled first.[40]

Fungal infection can cause delays in growth and difficulty in identification of organisms with routine blood cultures. In addition to cultures, the SSC gives a moderate recommendation for obtaining a 1,3B-D-glucan or antimannan antibody assay when fungal infection is suspected, noting that false-positive results are caused by colonization and advising that the utility of this test in critical care settings needs further investigation.[41] Blood culture yield in sepsis syndromes is variable based on the underlying source of infection. **Table 3** shows rates of positive blood cultures according to suspected site of infection.[42–47]

MISCELLANEOUS
Gram-negative Double Coverage

The use of double coverage as empiric treatment of gram-negative organisms in sepsis remains controversial.[48] Combination therapy can increase the probability of appropriate empiric coverage, improve antibiotic activity through synergy, and potentially prevent or delay the development of resistance.[49] As discussed earlier in this article, the timely initiation of antibiotic therapy with activity against the causative pathogen is essential to decrease mortality and improve outcomes in patients with gram-negative sepsis; therefore, double coverage that increases the likelihood of choosing an effective agent with empiric therapy is the most important consideration for ED patients. A large propensity-matched cohort study of 28 ICUs evaluated the benefit of empiric combination therapy using a broad-spectrum β-lactam plus either an aminoglycoside, fluoroquinolone, or macrolide/clindamycin compared with β-lactam monotherapy in cases of culture-positive septic shock. Although the combination group had a lower 28-day mortality than the β-lactam monotherapy group (36% vs 29%; $P = .0002$), if the β-lactam used was an antipseudomonal penicillin, cephalosporin, or carbapenem, no benefit was seen with the addition of a second agent.[50]

In a study of 593 patients with bacteremia caused by *P aeruginosa*, including MDR and extensively drug-resistant strains, Peña and colleagues[51] found no difference in the 30-day mortality in the group treated with combination therapy (most often a β-lactam plus an aminoglycoside) and those who received single-drug therapy. There was also no association of combination therapy with survival among patients who received 2 antibiotics that both covered the infecting organism, an observation that questions the clinical utility of synergy. However, the study included multiple antibiotic

Table 3	
Blood culture yield according to infectious source	
Site of Infection	**Blood Cultures Positive (%)**
CAP	6–14[42,43]
Pyelonephritis/complicated UTI	20–30[44]
Meningitis	80–90[45]
Cellulitis	5–8[46]
Neutropenia	10[47]

Abbreviation: UTI, urinary tract infection.

combinations and was not designed to establish whether synergy is drug dependent. Prevention of resistance is an important goal of combination therapy, but this strategy is probably best reserved for MDR organisms, which require a longer duration of treatment. In vitro data showed that monotherapy is associated with a more rapid increase in minimum inhibitory concentration (MIC) and therefore development of resistance isolates compared with combination therapy, although in vivo data are lacking.[52] If the infecting organism has an increased MIC to the drug being used, and if it is unknown whether pharmacokinetic and pharmacodynamic targets can be attained, the addition of a second agent could help overcome the deficit.[53] Ultimately, the decision to use empiric combination therapy for sepsis should be made with consideration of local epidemiology and individual patient characteristics. In areas in which resistance to broad-spectrum β-lactam therapy is anticipated, the addition of an aminoglycoside until culture data and susceptibilities are available is reasonable but must be considered in conjunction with risks (eg, the presence or risk of renal dysfunction) and benefits (eg, for patients with previous antibiotic and hospital exposure or colonized with MDR organisms).

Acute Kidney Injury Risk with the Combination of Vancomycin and Piperacillin/Tazobactam

Two abstracts presented at the 2012 meeting of the Society of Critical Care Medicine suggested that patients who receive vancomycin plus piperacillin-tazobactam or piperacillin-tazobactam alone have a higher risk of developing acute kidney injury (AKI) than do patients who receive vancomycin alone. Hellwig and colleagues[54] performed a retrospective evaluation of all adult patients who were admitted to Sanford USD Medical Center over a 6-month period and who then received vancomycin plus or minus piperacillin-tazobactam for more than 48 hours. AKI was defined as an increase of serum creatinine level greater than 0.5 mg/dL or a 50% increase from baseline. Among the 735 patients whose records were analyzed, the incidence of AKI was 4.9% for those who received vancomycin alone, 11.1% for those who received piperacillin-tazobactam alone, and 18.6% for those who received a combination of vancomycin plus piperacillin-tazobactam (vancomycin vs piperacillin-tazobactam, $P = .014$; vancomycin vs combination, $P = .005$). Similar results were found when only the ICU patients were considered: 6.0%, 12.2%, and 21.2%, respectively (vancomycin vs piperacillin-tazobactam, $P = .279$; vancomycin vs combination, $P = .005$). Min and colleagues[55] evaluated 140 surgical ICU patients over the course of a year who received vancomycin plus or minus piperacillin-tazobactam for at least 48 hours. AKI was defined as an increase in serum creatinine level more than 1.5 times baseline during antibiotic therapy. The investigators controlled for severity of illness and concomitant use of other nephrotoxic antibiotics. The incidence of AKI was higher in the vancomycin plus piperacillin-tazobactam group than in the vancomycin-alone group (40.5% vs 9.0%; $P<.001$).

There have since been 7 additional studies published on this topic, including a recent prospective evaluation (**Table 4**). Moenster and colleagues[56] conducted a retrospective cohort study of all diabetic patients with osteomyelitis treated with vancomycin plus either piperacillin-tazobactam or cefepime for at least 72 hours at a Veterans' Affairs Medical Center between January 2006 and December 2011. The primary outcome was development of AKI, defined as an increase in serum creatinine level of 0.5 mg/dL or 50% of baseline. One-hundred and thirty-nine patients met the inclusion criteria: 109 in the piperacillin-tazobactam group and 30 in the cefepime group. AKI developed in 29.3% (32 out of 109) of the patients who received vancomycin plus piperacillin-tazobactam compared with 13.3% (4 out of 30) of those treated

Table 4
Summary of studies evaluating risk of acute kidney injury with piperacillin-tazobactam

Study	Design	Population	AKI Incidence (%)			P Value
			Pip-Tazo + Vanc	Comparator		
Hellwig et al,[54] 2011	Retrospective	Mixed (n = 735)	All: 18.6	All: 4.9 (vanc alone), 11.1 (pip-tazo alone)		All: .0001 (vanc vs combination)
			ICU: 21.2	ICU: 6 (vanc alone), 12.2 (pip-tazo alone)		ICU: .005 (vanc vs combination)
Min et al,[55] 2011	Retrospective	ICU (n = 140)	40.5	9 (vanc alone)		<.001
Moenster et al,[56] 2014	Retrospective	Mixed (n = 139)	29.3	13.3 (vanc + cefepime)		.099
Gomes et al,[57] 2014	Retrospective	Mixed (n = 224)	34.8	12.5 (vanc + cefepime)		.003
Meaney et al,[58] 2014	Retrospective	Internal medicine (n = 125)	22.4	No comparator		NA
Burgess et al,[59] 2014	Retrospective	Mixed (n = 191)	16.3	8.1 (vanc alone)		.041
Peyko et al,[60] 2016	Prospective	Mixed (n = 85)	37.3	7.7 (vanc + cefepime or meropenem)		.005
Karino et al,[61] 2016	Retrospective + case control	Mixed (n = 320)	33	No comparator, but similar for intermittent or extended pip-tazo infusions		NA
Hammond et al,[62] 2016	Retrospective	ICU (n = 122)	32.7	28.8 (vanc + cefepime)		.647

Abbreviations: NA, not available; pip-tazo, piperacillin-tazobactam; vanc, vancomycin.

with vancomycin plus cefepime ($P = .099$). A multiple logistic regression analysis identified weight and average vancomycin trough as the only significant predictors of AKI. The investigators were unable to detect a statistically significant difference in the incidence of AKI between the groups; however, power was not met.

A second retrospective matched cohort examined 224 patients receiving vancomycin plus piperacillin-tazobactam or vancomycin plus cefepime for more than 48 hours.[57] The patients in this study had no preexisting kidney disease. AKI was defined according to the Acute Kidney Injury Network criteria. Its incidence was higher in the piperacillin-tazobactam plus vancomycin group (34.8%) than in the cefepime plus vancomycin group (12.5%) in the unmatched analysis ($P<.0001$). After adjusting for potential sources of bias through propensity score–matched pairs and conditional logistic regression, piperacillin-tazobactam plus vancomycin combination therapy ($P = .003$) was found to be an independent predictor of AKI. There were no significant differences in time to development of AKI or hospital length of stay between the groups.

Meaney and colleagues[58] retrospectively evaluated 125 adult internal medicine patients who received at least 72 hours of vancomycin treatment. Nephrotoxicity, defined as an increase in serum creatinine level of 0.5 mg/dL or 50% more than baseline (whichever was larger), occurred in 17 (13.6%) of the 125 patients. On multivariable logistic regression analysis, after controlling for hypotensive episodes, Charlson Comorbidity Index, and baseline creatinine clearance, concomitant use of piperacillin-tazobactam was associated with an increased incidence of vancomycin-associated nephrotoxicity (adjusted odds ratio, 5.36; 95% confidence interval, 1.41–20.5). Thirteen of the 58 patients (22.4%) receiving the combination developed nephrotoxicity. The investigators concluded that vancomycin-associated nephrotoxicity is prevalent among internal medicine patients, with 5.36-fold higher odds if piperacillin-tazobactam is administered concomitantly.

Burgess and Drew[59] retrospectively reviewed the records of 191 internal medicine and ICU patients, treated at 1 medical center, who received vancomycin or vancomycin plus piperacillin-tazobactam for at least 48 hours. AKI was defined as an increase in serum creatinine level more than 1.5 times baseline during antibiotic therapy. Nephrotoxicity developed in 8 (8.1%) of the 99 patients in the vancomycin group and in 15 (16.3%) of the 92 patients in the combination group (1-sided χ^2 test, $P = .041$). A steady-state vancomycin trough concentration of 15 µg/mL or greater was also associated with an increased risk of the development of nephrotoxicity.

Results of the first prospective study designed to evaluate the incidence of AKI were published recently.[60] The investigators conducted an open-label cohort study at a community academic medical center, which involved adult patients over a 3-month period who received either the combination of piperacillin-tazobactam plus vancomycin or the combination of cefepime or meropenem plus vancomycin for more than 72 hours. AKI was defined using specific criteria introduced by the Kidney Disease: Improving Global Outcomes (KDIGO) AKI Work Group in 2012. Eighty-five patients were enrolled (59 in the piperacillin-tazobactam plus vancomycin group and 26 in the cefepime/meropenem plus vancomycin group). The incidence of AKI was significantly higher in the piperacillin-tazobactam plus vancomycin group (37.3%) (7.7%; $\chi^2 = 7.80, P = .005$). There was no difference in the mean steady-state vancomycin trough levels between groups. The study did not reach the projected sample size of 120 patients and the piperacillin-tazobactam group had disproportionately more patients, both of which decrease the power of the study's findings. Development of AKI was based strictly on the KDIGO definition, and follow-up contact was not made to ascertain the clinical significance of the AKI.

Two additional studies were published in 2016.[61,62] Karino and colleagues[61] performed a combination of retrospective cohort and case-control studies with a primary objective to evaluate the incidence of AKI between intermittent versus extended infusions of piperacillin/tazobactam in combination with vancomycin. Overall, AKI occurred in 105 out of 320 (33%) of the cohort receiving combination therapy. There were similar rates in those receiving intermittent (53 out of 160 [33.1%]) and extended infusions (52 out of 160 [32.5%]) of piperacillin/tazobactam. The investigators identified the following independent risk factors for AKI: having a documented gram-positive infection, the presence of sepsis, receipt of a vancomycin loading dose, and receipt of any concomitant nephrotoxin.

Hammond and colleagues[62] conducted a retrospective cohort study of 122 ICU patients (medical, surgical, and neuroscience) who received at least 48 hours of combination therapy with vancomycin and piperacillin-tazobactam (49 patients) or vancomycin and cefepime (73 patients). The primary outcome was development of AKI as determined by the Acute Kidney Injury Network criteria. Overall, 37 patients (30.3%) developed AKI. The incidence of AKI was similar in the piperacillin-tazobactam group compared with the cefepime group (32.7% vs 28.8%, $P = .647$).

It seems time to acknowledge that there is an association between piperacillin-tazobactam and risk of AKI (with vancomycin). There have been 9 different groups with internal medicine and ICU patients, including a prospective study, showing this adverse effect. In 3 of the retrospective studies, it is difficult to conclude that piperacillin-tazobactam is the primary cause of increased AKI compared with vancomycin alone. If the groups are equally sick, the rationale for using 2 antibiotics rather than 1 is unclear. The prospective study by Peyko and colleagues[60] supports the association, even with vancomycin trough levels the same in each group. Proposed mechanisms for AKI induced by piperacillin-tazobactam include acute interstitial nephritis and toxic effects on the renal tubule. In ICU patients specifically, the results have been conflicting. All 3 ICU studies reported a high rate of AKI with vancomycin plus piperacillin-tazobactam (21.2%–40.5%).[54,55,62] Two of the ICU studies showed a significantly higher rate in the combination group compared with vancomycin alone; the other did not show a difference when piperacillin-tazobactam was replaced with cefepime. A prospective study in ICU patients is needed. The AKI association should be taken into account when developing sepsis order sets and treatment plans.

Dosing Considerations

Critically ill obese patients

Although there is a paucity of data to guide dosing of antimicrobials in critically ill obese patients, some conclusions can be drawn from existing kinetic studies. An increased volume of distribution has been noted in obese patients compared with matched controls.[63] Lean body mass and plasma volume are both increased. Other important pharmacokinetic/pharmacodynamic parameters to consider include the duration the antimicrobial agent binds to the organism and the concentration. Time-dependent antimicrobials, such as penicillins, cephalosporins, carbapenems, aztreonam, macrolides, tetracyclines, vancomycin, and clindamycin, achieve maximum bactericidal effect the longer the drug's concentration is greater than the MIC for a particular bacterial species, which is often quantified as the time greater than the MIC. Concentration-dependent antimicrobials, such as fluoroquinolones and aminoglycosides, achieve maximum bactericidal effect as the serum concentration increases. The peak concentration/MIC is used to evaluate concentration-dependent antimicrobials.

Assuming normal renal and hepatic function, the available data support using the high end of the dosing range for most antimicrobials in critically ill obese patients.[64,65] For penicillins, cephalosporins, carbapenems, and fluoroquinolones, the authors suggest using the high end of the dosing range. For example, if the plan is to use piperacillin/tazobactam, 3.375 g intravenously every 6 hours, for a complicated intra-abdominal infection, the authors suggest using 4.5 g instead. Guideline recommendations for dosing vancomycin in critically ill obese patients suggest a weight-based initial dose of 25 to 30 mg/kg to a maximum of 2 g.[66,67] A recent study provides some guidance on achieving therapeutic vancomycin trough levels quickly with a divided-dose strategy.[68] Obese-specific, divided-load dosing achieved trough concentrations of 10 to 20 g/mL for 89% of obese patients within 12 hours after initial dosing and 97% of obese patients within 24 hours after initial dosing. Subsequent vancomycin dosing should be adjusted based on renal function, trough levels, and possible area under the curve/MIC ratios. Although the nephrotoxicity associated with vancomycin is less than was previously thought, aminoglycosides can still cause nephrotoxicity and ototoxicity even with therapeutic levels. The 2 most-studied dosing strategies are traditional (lower doses more frequently) and once daily. In obese patients weighing more than 30% greater than their ideal body weight (IBW), an adjusted body weight (ABW) is used for dosing:

ABW (kg) = IBW + 0.4 × (actual body weight − IBW)

Levels (including peak, trough, and random) then guide dosing. Renal function (including serum creatinine and urine output) should be monitored along with auditory function.

Pharmacokinetic/pharmacodynamic considerations

Basic pharmacokinetic and pharmacodynamic principles should play a role in the selection and dosing of initial antibiotic therapy. Important distinctions between antibiotic agents include their killing mechanism (concentration vs time) and their character (bacteriostatic vs bactericidal). Time-dependent antibacterial agents (eg, β-lactams) work best when the serum concentration exceeds the organism's MIC for the duration of the dosing interval; therefore, frequency of administration is the most important factor in their dosing. In contrast, concentration-dependent antibacterial drugs (eg, aminoglycosides, fluoroquinolones) work best when the peak serum concentrations are maximized. Therefore, optimizing either the interval for time-dependent antibacterials or the dose for concentration-dependent antibacterials maximizes the likelihood of target attainment. Bactericidal agents cause death by disrupting the bacterial cell and primarily affecting the cell wall or membrane (eg, β-lactams, daptomycin) or the bacterial DNA (eg, fluoroquinolones). Bacteriostatic agents inhibit replication without killing the organism and primarily inhibit protein synthesis. These distinctions are not absolute but, in the case of sepsis, bactericidal agents are preferred.[15,69]

Adequate dosing also depends on the drug's ability to get to the target site of action. Antibiotic concentrations achieved in serum are often not adequate at other sites of infection, such as the cerebrospinal fluid (CSF) or bone. For example, cefazolin, a first-generation cephalosporin, achieves poor CSF concentrations and is not a good agent to use for methicillin-sensitive *S aureus* (MSSA) meningitis, even though it is an excellent agent for MSSA bacteremia.[70] In contrast, tigecycline achieves excellent tissue concentrations but inadequate serum concentrations for use in sepsis.[71] For patients with renal dysfunction, dose reduction to prevent accumulation should be considered. For young septic patients who are hypermetabolic, higher doses may be needed to avoid underdosing.

In the ED, the initial antibiotic dose is important because it is often continued once the patient is admitted.[72] Even patients with renal dysfunction can generally be prescribed a 1-time dose similar to that for a patient with normally functioning kidneys. Subsequent doses should be adjusted based on renal and hepatic parameters. The use of order sets in electronic medical records can serve as a method for implementing evidence-based dose ordering in the ED.[73,74] ED order sets should take into account individual institutional practices with regard to preference for 1-time antibiotic doses versus standing orders. Each approach has advantages and disadvantages. One-time orders allow a loading dose and fewer calculations up front, but antibiotics that need frequent dosing (eg, every 6 hours) might be forgotten if a patient has a long boarding time in the ED while waiting for an inpatient bed to become available. Standing orders solve the problem of overlooking subsequent doses. However, laboratory values (eg, serum creatinine level) measured after the first dose is administered may call for a change in the dose or interval. Without prompts in place, patients could receive supratherapeutic drug doses, possibly increasing the risk of organ injury (eg, AKI). Although there is not a clear best practice for this issue, awareness of the problem is a good first step.

SUMMARY

Antibiotics remain a cornerstone therapy for sepsis syndromes in ED patients. Antibiotics should be given early, and the antimicrobial spectrum should be broad enough to cover the most likely pathogens. Blood and tissue cultures should be obtained before administration of an antibiotic if possible in a timely fashion. Debate remains as to the feasibility of giving antibiotics within a 60-minute time frame and the time point at which outcomes worsen with each additional hour of delay. Patient-specific factors, the presumed site of infection, allergies, and local susceptibility patterns determine what antimicrobials should be prescribed empirically. The routine use of double gram-negative coverage is not supported by evidence. Patient weight and renal comorbidities could alter the dose of antibiotics chosen, and these factors should be evaluated carefully in each patient. Overall, the advice expressed by the German microbiologist Paul Ehrlich[75] in 1913 seems to stand the test of time: "Frapper fort et frapper vite" (Hit hard and hit fast).

REFERENCES

1. Dellinger RP, Levy MM, Rhodes A, et al. Surviving Sepsis Campaign: international guidelines for management of severe sepsis and septic shock: 2012. Crit Care Med 2013;41:580–637.
2. Singer M, Deutschman CS, Seymour CW, et al. The Third International Consensus Definitions for Sepsis and Septic Shock (Sepsis-3). JAMA 2016;315:801–10.
3. Kumar A, Roberts D, Wood KE, et al. Duration of hypotension before initiation of effective antimicrobial therapy is the critical determinant of survival in human septic shock. Crit Care Med 2006;34:1589–96.
4. Ferrer R, Martin-Loeches I, Phillips G, et al. Empiric antibiotic treatment reduces mortality in severe sepsis and septic shock from the first hour: results from a guideline-based performance improvement program. Crit Care Med 2014;42: 1749–55.
5. Weiss SL, Fitzgerald JC, Balamuth F, et al. Delayed antimicrobial therapy increases mortality and organ dysfunction duration in pediatric sepsis. Crit Care Med 2014;42:2409–17.

6. Pines JM. Timing of antibiotics for acute, severe infections. Emerg Med Clin North Am 2008;26:245–57.

7. de Groot B, Ansems A, Gerling DH, et al. The association between time to antibiotics and relevant clinical outcomes in emergency department patients with various stages of sepsis: a prospective multi-center study. Crit Care 2015;19:194.

8. Puskarich MA, Trzeciak S, Shapiro NI, et al. Association between timing of antibiotic administration and mortality from septic shock in patients treated with a quantitative resuscitation protocol. Crit Care Med 2011;39:2066–71.

9. Ryoo SM, Kim WY, Sohn CH, et al. Prognostic value of timing of antibiotic administration in patients with septic shock treated with early quantitative resuscitation. Am J Med Sci 2015;349:328–33.

10. Sterling SA, Miller WR, Pryor J, et al. The impact of timing of antibiotics on outcomes in severe sepsis and septic shock: a systematic review and meta-analysis. Crit Care Med 2015;43:1907–15.

11. Garnacho-Montero J, Garcia-Garmendia JL, Barrero-Almodovar A, et al. Impact of adequate empirical antibiotic therapy on the outcome of patients admitted to the intensive care unit with sepsis. Crit Care Med 2003;31:2742–51.

12. Zilberberg MD, Shorr AF, Micek ST, et al. Multi-drug resistance, inappropriate initial antibiotic therapy and mortality in gram-negative severe sepsis and septic shock: a retrospective cohort study. Crit Care 2014;18:596.

13. Ibrahim EH, Sherman G, Ward S, et al. The influence of inadequate antimicrobial treatment of bloodstream infections on patient outcomes in the ICU setting. Chest 2000;118:146–55.

14. Gaieski DF, Mikkelsen ME, Band RA, et al. Impact of time to antibiotics on survival in patients with severe sepsis or septic shock in whom early goal-directed therapy was initiated in the emergency department. Crit Care Med 2010;38: 1045–53.

15. Leekha S, Terrell CL, Edson RS. General principles of antimicrobial therapy. Mayo Clin Proc 2011;86:156–67.

16. Garnacho-Montero J, Gutiérrez-Pizarraya A, Escoresca-Ortega A, et al. Adequate antibiotic therapy prior to ICU admission in patients with severe sepsis and septic shock reduces hospital mortality. Crit Care 2015;19:302.

17. American Thoracic Society. Infectious Diseases Society of America. Guidelines for the management of adults with hospital-acquired, ventilator-associated, and healthcare-associated pneumonia. Am J Respir Crit Care Med 2005;171: 388–416.

18. Friedman ND, Kaye KS, Stout JE, et al. Health care–associated bloodstream infections in adults: a reason to change the accepted definition of community-acquired infections. Ann Intern Med 2002;137:791–7.

19. Kalil AC, Metersky ML, Lompas M, et al. Management of adults with hospital-acquired and ventilator-associated pneumonia: 2016 clinical practice guidelines by the infectious diseases society of America and the American thoracic society. Clin Infect Dis 2016;63:1–51.

20. Park HK, Song J-U, Um S-W, et al. Clinical characteristics of health care-associated pneumonia in a Korean teaching hospital. Respir Med 2010;104: 1729–35.

21. Micek ST, Kollef KE, Reichley RM, et al. Health care-associated pneumonia and community-acquired pneumonia: a single-center experience. Antimicrob Agents Chemother 2007;51:3568–73.

22. Cardoso T, Ribeiro O, Aragão IC, et al. Additional risk factors for infection by multidrug-resistant pathogens in healthcare-associated infection: a large cohort study. BMC Infect Dis 2012;12:375.
23. Shorr AF, Zilberberg MD, Micek ST, et al. Prediction of infection due to antibiotic-resistant bacteria by select risk factors for health care-associated pneumonia. Arch Intern Med 2008;168:2205–10.
24. Shorr AF, Zilberberg MD, Reichley R, et al. Validation of a clinical score for assessing the risk of resistant pathogens in patients with pneumonia presenting to the emergency department. Clin Infect Dis 2012;54:193–8.
25. Aliberti S, Di Pasquale M, Zanaboni AM, et al. Stratifying risk factors for multidrug-resistant pathogens in hospitalized patients coming from the community with pneumonia. Clin Infect Dis 2012;54:470–8.
26. Lee CE, Zembower TR, Fotis MA, et al. The incidence of antimicrobial allergies in hospitalized patients: implications regarding prescribing patterns and emerging bacterial resistance. Arch Intern Med 2000;160:2819–22.
27. Charneski L, Deshpande G, Smith SW. Impact of an antimicrobial allergy label in the medical record on clinical outcomes in hospitalized patients. Pharmacotherapy 2011;31:742–7.
28. MacLaughlin EJ, Saseen JJ, Malone DC. Costs of beta-lactam allergies: selection and costs of antibiotics for patients with a reported beta-lactam allergy. Arch Fam Med 2000;9:722–6.
29. Campagna JD, Bond MC, Schabelman E, et al. The use of cephalosporins in penicillin-allergic patients: a literature review. J Emerg Med 2012;42:612–20.
30. Sodhi M, Axtell SS, Callahan J, et al. Is it safe to use carbapenems in patients with a history of allergy to penicillin? J Antimicrob Chemother 2004;54:1155–7.
31. Gudlaugsson O, Gillespie S, Lee K, et al. Attributable mortality of nosocomial candidemia, revisited. Clin Infect Dis 2003;37:1172–7.
32. Leroy G, Lambiotte F, Thévenin D, et al. Evaluation of "Candida score" in critically ill patients: a prospective, multicenter, observational, cohort study. Ann Intensive Care 2011;1:50.
33. Kullberg BJ, Arendrup MC. Invasive candidiasis. N Engl J Med 2015;373:1445–56.
34. León C, Ruiz-Santana S, Saavedra P, et al. A bedside scoring system ("Candida score") for early antifungal treatment in nonneutropenic critically ill patients with Candida colonization. Crit Care Med 2006;34:730–7.
35. Flaherty SK, Weber RL, Chase M, et al. Septic shock and adequacy of early empiric antibiotics in the emergency department. J Emerg Med 2014;47:601–7.
36. Zhang D, Micek ST, Kollef MH. Time to appropriate antibiotic therapy is an independent determinant of postinfection ICU and hospital lengths of stay in patients with sepsis. Crit Care Med 2015;43:2133–40.
37. Cullen M, Fogg T, Delaney A. Timing of appropriate antibiotics in patients with septic shock: a retrospective cohort study. Emerg Med Australas 2013;25:308–15.
38. Kalich BA, Maguire JM, Campbell-Bright SL, et al. Impact of an antibiotic-specific sepsis bundle on appropriate and timely antibiotic administration for severe sepsis in the emergency department. J Emerg Med 2016;50:79–88.e1.
39. Lo A, Zhu JN, Richman M, et al. Effect of adding piperacillin-tazobactam to automated dispensing cabinets on promptness of first-dose antibiotics in hospitalized patients. Am J Health Syst Pharm 2014;71:1663–7.
40. Kirn TJ, Weinstein MP. Update on blood cultures: how to obtain, process, report, and interpret. Clin Microbiol Infect 2013;19:513–20.

41. Sendid B, Jouault T, Coudriau R, et al. Increased sensitivity of mannanemia detection tests by joint detection of alpha- and beta-linked oligomannosides during experimental and human systemic candidiasis. J Clin Microbiol 2004;42: 164–71.
42. Cham G, Yan S, Heng BH, et al. Predicting positive blood cultures in patients presenting with pneumonia at an emergency department in Singapore. Ann Acad Med Singapore 2009;38:508–14.
43. Falguera M, Trujillano J, Caro S, et al. A prediction rule for estimating the risk of bacteremia in patients with community-acquired pneumonia. Clin Infect Dis 2009; 49:409–16.
44. Horcajada JP, Shaw E, Padilla B, et al. Healthcare-associated, community-acquired and hospital-acquired bacteraemic urinary tract infections in hospitalized patients: a prospective multicentre cohort study in the era of antimicrobial resistance. Clin Microbiol Infect 2013;19:962–8.
45. Bohr V, Rasmussen N, Hansen B, et al. 875 cases of bacterial meningitis: diagnostic procedures and the impact of preadmission antibiotic therapy. Part III of a three-part series. J Infect 1983;7:193–202.
46. Gunderson CG, Martinello RA. A systematic review of bacteremias in cellulitis and erysipelas. J Infect 2012;64:148–55.
47. Ha YE, Song J-H, Kang WK, et al. Clinical factors predicting bacteremia in low-risk febrile neutropenia after anti-cancer chemotherapy. Support Care Cancer 2011;19:1761–7.
48. Tamma PD, Cosgrove SE, Maragakis LL. Combination therapy for treatment of infections with gram-negative bacteria. Clin Microbiol Rev 2012;25:450–70.
49. Boyd N, Nailor MD. Combination antibiotic therapy for empiric and definitive treatment of gram-negative infections: insights from the Society of Infectious Diseases Pharmacists. Pharmacotherapy 2011;31:1073–84.
50. Kumar A, Safdar N, Kethireddy S, et al. A survival benefit of combination antibiotic therapy for serious infections associated with sepsis and septic shock is contingent only on the risk of death: a meta-analytic/meta-regression study. Crit Care Med 2010;38:1651–64.
51. Peña C, Suarez C, Ocampo-Sosa A, et al. Effect of adequate single-drug vs combination antimicrobial therapy on mortality in *Pseudomonas aeruginosa* bloodstream infections: a post hoc analysis of a prospective cohort. Clin Infect Dis 2013;57:208–16.
52. Mouton JW. Combination therapy as a tool to prevent emergence of bacterial resistance. Infection 1999;27(Suppl 2):S24–8.
53. Schentag JJ, Strenkoski-Nix LC, Nix DE, et al. Pharmacodynamic interactions of antibiotics alone and in combination. Clin Infect Dis 1998;27:40–6.
54. Hellwig T, Hanmmerquist R, Loecker B, et al. Retrospective evaluation of the incidence of vancomycin and/or piperacillin-tazobactam induced acute renal failure. Crit Care Med 2011;39(suppl):301.
55. Min E, Box K, Lane J, et al. Acute kidney injury in patients receiving concomitant vancomycin and piperacillin/tazobactam. Crit Care Med 2011;39(suppl):714.
56. Moenster RP, Linneman TW, Finnegan PM, et al. Acute renal failure associated with vancomycin and β-lactams for the treatment of osteomyelitis in diabetics: piperacillin-tazobactam as compared with cefepime. Clin Microbiol Infect 2014; 20:O384–9.
57. Gomes DM, Smotherman C, Birch A, et al. Comparison of acute kidney injury during treatment with vancomycin in combination with piperacillin-tazobactam or cefepime. Pharmacotherapy 2014;34:662–9.

58. Meaney CJ, Hynicka LM, Tsoukleris MG. Vancomycin-associated nephrotoxicity in adult medicine patients: incidence, outcomes, and risk factors. Pharmacotherapy 2014;34:653–61.
59. Burgess LD, Drew RH. Comparison of the incidence of vancomycin-induced nephrotoxicity in hospitalized patients with and without concomitant piperacillin-tazobactam. Pharmacotherapy 2014;34:670–6.
60. Peyko V, Smalley S, Cohen H. Prospective comparison of acute kidney injury during treatment with the combination of piperacillin-tazobactam and vancomycin versus the combination of cefepime or meropenem and vancomycin. J Pharm Pract 2016. http://dx.doi.org/10.1177/0897190016628960.
61. Karino S, Kaye KS, Navalkele B, et al. Epidemiology of acute kidney injury among patients receiving concomitant vancomycin and piperacillin-tazobactam: opportunities for antimicrobial stewardship. Antimicrob Agents Chemother 2016;60 [pii:AAC.03011–15].
62. Hammond DA, Smith MN, Painter JT, et al. Comparative incidence of acute kidney injury in critically ill patients receiving vancomycin with concomitant piperacillin-tazobactam or cefepime: a retrospective cohort study. Pharmacotherapy 2016. http://dx.doi.org/10.1002/phar.1738.
63. Peck CC, Cross JT. "Getting the dose right": facts, a blueprint, and encouragements. Clin Pharmacol Ther 2007;82:12–4.
64. Erstad BL. Dosing of medications in morbidly obese patients in the intensive care unit setting. Intensive Care Med 2004;30:18–32.
65. Medico CJ, Walsh P. Pharmacotherapy in the critically ill obese patient. Crit Care Clin 2010;26:679–88.
66. Rybak M, Lomaestro B, Rotschafer JC, et al. Therapeutic monitoring of vancomycin in adult patients: a consensus review of the American Society of Health-System Pharmacists, the Infectious Diseases Society of America, and the Society of Infectious Diseases Pharmacists. Am J Health Syst Pharm 2009;66:82–98.
67. Liu C, Bayer A, Cosgrove SE, et al. Clinical practice guidelines by the Infectious Diseases Society of America for the treatment of methicillin-resistant *Staphylococcus aureus* infections in adults and children. Clin Infect Dis 2011;52:e18–55.
68. Denetclaw TH, Yu MK, Moua M, et al. Performance of a divided-load intravenous vancomycin dosing strategy for obese patients. Ann Pharmacother 2015;49: 861–8.
69. Craig WA. Pharmacokinetic/pharmacodynamic parameters: rationale for antibacterial dosing of mice and men. Clin Infect Dis 1998;26:1–102.
70. Dacey RG, Sande MA. Effect of probenecid on cerebrospinal fluid concentrations of penicillin and cephalosporin derivatives. Antimicrob Agents Chemother 1974; 6:437–41.
71. Rodvold KA, Gotfried MH, Cwik M, et al. Serum, tissue and body fluid concentrations of tigecycline after a single 100 mg dose. J Antimicrob Chemother 2006;58: 1221–9.
72. Fuller BM, Mohr N, Skrupky L, et al. Emergency department vancomycin use: dosing practices and associated outcomes. J Emerg Med 2013;44:910–8.
73. Hall AB, Montero J, Cobian J, et al. The effects of an electronic order set on vancomycin dosing in the ED. Am J Emerg Med 2015;33:92–4.
74. Frankel KC, Rosini JM, Levine BJ, et al. Computerized provider order entry improves compliance of vancomycin dosing guidelines in the emergency department. Am J Emerg Med 2013;31:1715–6.
75. Ehrlich P. Address in Pathology, ON CHEMIOTHERAPY. Delivered before the Seventeenth International Congress of Medicine. Br Med J 1913;2:353–9.

Source Identification and Source Control

Zeke P. Oliver, MD*, Jack Perkins, MD

KEYWORDS

- Sepsis • Source identification • Source control • Intra-abdominal infection

KEY POINTS

- Rapid time to antibiotics is important, but they may not themselves provide adequate source control.
- A broad differential is essential in septic patients, because the source of infection may not immediately identifiable.
- Typical workup strategies in sepsis such as the chest radiograph and urinalysis can be inherently misleading.
- Intraabdominal sources of sepsis are difficult to diagnose, treat, and frequently require rapid surgical intervention.

INTRODUCTION

The medical concept of source control as a component of treatment for infection dates back as early as the 17th century BC. The Edwin Smith papyrus of ancient Egypt describes 48 medical cases, one of which details methods at the time to assist with the drainage of a chest wall abscess.[1,2] In modern medicine, the concept of source control continues to be a cornerstone of sepsis management, albeit now far more complex than the astringents and poultices[1] used by the ancient Egyptians to assist with drainage.

Source control in sepsis first requires identification of an infectious source followed by the subsequent interventions used to control specific sites of infection and to modify factors that promote microbial growth or impair host defenses to infection.[3] In the emergency department (ED), this process can be challenging especially because the source of the infection may not be readily apparent. Whereas a chest radiograph, urinalysis (UA), and blood cultures are ubiquitous in the evaluation of sepsis, sometimes further investigation is required as a surgical process (eg, appendicitis, cholecystitis) may be the underlying culprit pathology.

The authors have nothing to disclose.
Emergency Medicine, Department of Emergency Medicine, Carilion Clinic Virginia Tech School of Medicine, 1 Riverside Circle, 4th Floor, Roanoke, VA 24014, USA
* Corresponding author.
E-mail address: zpoliver@carilionclinic.org

The Surviving Sepsis Campaign (2012)[4] provides an update to current sepsis treatment guidelines, including multiple topics pertinent to source control and their level of evidence to support these recommendations. These include recommendations regarding obtaining cultures, starting antibiotic therapy, and performing surgical source control.

GENERAL WORKUP
History

Although obtaining a history is part and parcel of every patient encounter in the ED, unfortunately it may be limited, misleading, or downright unobtainable owing to the patient's illness. If the emergency physician is fortunate, the patient or family member may relate complaints such as fevers and chills that point more toward an infectious etiology. However, sepsis is the most complex disease entity emergency physicians will encounter because the patient complaints are often nonspecific and may simply be dyspnea or abdominal pain, which are associated with a great number of possible differential diagnoses. On the extreme end of the spectrum, a patient may be incapable of providing any history owing to an acute change in mental status or an underlying comorbid condition such as dementia.

Because of the challenges described in trying to arrive at a suspicion of sepsis, it essential that the emergency physician try to gather as much information as possible from all available resources. Information can be garnered from emergency medical services personnel, a long-term care facility, family, friends, and perhaps most important, previous patient encounters. A careful review of the patient's medical record can be invaluable, because it may have previous culture results, recent prior surgeries, significant medications (eg, immunosuppressants), previous and recent antibiotics, or past medical history that changes the evaluation (eg, HIV). Taking the extra time to gather information becomes more important with older patients as they notoriously will have nonspecific presentations of sepsis and may be more likely to harbor surgical disease.

Physical Examination

Some patient complaints such as chest pain allow the emergency physician to direct their physical examination in pursuit of specific disease entities on the differential diagnosis. However, it is not uncommon that a patient may present with vague complaints and the physical examination must be appropriately thorough as no one organ system rises to the top as the potential origin of disease. Sepsis often falls into this category and the astute emergency physician should realize that the physical examination is of tremendous importance in guiding diagnostic inquiry.

The clinical manifestations of inflammation suggestive of infection may or not be apparent on physical examination. These include the *rubor* (redness), *calor* (warmth), *dolor* (pain), and *functio laesa* (loss of function).[3] A thorough examination should be undertaken and any abnormalities noted. General observations such as alertness, distress, and pain are all useful. The examination should take note of any signs of hardware or prior and/or recent surgeries. These could include indwelling venous catheters, port sites, drains, urinary catheters, or any other medical devices. Also consider scars that could be suggestive of underlying hardware, including orthopedic devices.

Although the emergency physician is likely accustomed to considering pulmonary and urinary sources of sepsis, it is important to keep in mind that the skin (eg, cellulitis, abscess), genitourinary (eg, abscess), joints (eg, septic joint), and abdomen (ie, numerous disease processes) may all yield information that suggests further inquiry is required. It is also important to mention that if the initial physical examination is not contributory, consider repeat examinations, especially of the abdomen, because the findings may change over the course of minutes to hours in the ED.

Laboratory Tests

Serum laboratory studies will most certainly be an integral component in the evaluation of sepsis, yet they are fraught with poor sensitivity and a potentially significant time delay. Reasonable laboratory tests to send initially include a complete blood count with differential, a complete metabolic profile, which will include liver functions tests, a UA and a point-of-care lactate (see Brit Long and Alex Koyfman's article, "Ready for Prime Time? Biomarkers in Sepsis," in this issue). Other studies will depend on the patient, current medications (ie, coagulation studies for patient on warfarin), comorbid conditions (ie, B-type natriuretic peptide for patient with congestive heart failure history), and the clinical question the emergency physician desires to explore.

Cultures

Cultures are a vital part of the inpatient management of patients with sepsis. Unfortunately, there remains a large percentage of patients who will have "culture-negative" sepsis. Literature shows rates of negative cultures for septic patients ranging from 40% to 60%; pulmonary infections have the highest rate of culture-negative results.[5-7] The inpatient team is then left to decide which antibiotic to discontinue and when to narrow the antibiotic spectrum without the benefit of a positive culture. This highlights the importance of optimizing the potential to obtain accurate and contributory cultures. Blood cultures should ideally be obtained before the start of antibiotic therapy, as long as this can be done in a timely fashion (<45 minutes). This practice is a bit of a contradiction in sepsis management in that the guidelines and recent evidence strongly suggest that early, broad-spectrum antibiotic therapy is tremendously important for improved patient outcome. However, cultures are essential for the inpatient team to narrow antibiotic therapy and avoid associated consequences of prolonged broad-spectrum antimicrobial therapy (eg, antimicrobial resistance and *Clostridium difficile*). It is incumbent on to the emergency physician to communicate with his patient care team (eg, nurses and techs) about the dual priorities of obtaining blood cultures while not excessively delaying antimicrobial therapy. The emergency physician may have to consider alternative methods for obtaining cultures, such as a radial artery blood draw or perhaps a femoral straight stick to expedite collection.

Blood cultures should always include 2 sets so that both aerobic and anaerobic bottles are obtained. In any patient with an indwelling central venous catheters, one of the culture sets should be drawn through this line to help potential identification of infected devices. Urine cultures should be sent routinely for any patient suspected to have sepsis because interpretation of the UA is notoriously unreliable. If the patient is producing sputum and a pulmonary source is suspected, efforts should be made to induce sputum for gram stain and culture. Consideration should be given to wound cultures as appropriate especially if purulent drainage is evident on examination or able to be expressed. Cerebrospinal fluid should be obtained as appropriate and once again antibiotics should not be significantly delayed to obtain cerebrospinal fluid. Specifically with regard to blood cultures, ideally at least 10 mL of blood should be cultured per tube; this volume has been shown to substantially increase detection rates of bloodstream infections (BSIs).[8] Volumes of blood should also be equal between culture tubes, which may assist with the identification of indwelling devices as a source. For instance, if cultures drawn through an indwelling central line are positive more than 2 hours before those from a fresh peripheral blood draw, this finding suggests that the indwelling device is the source of the infection.[9,10]

Finally, if the patient remains in the ED for a number of hours and has an abrupt onset of fever with or without rigors, this is an ideal time to repeat blood cultures as the patient may be bacteremic. Additional blood cultures will increase the yield of culture results, but also increase the rate of false-positive results, so it is important to consider this when ordering repeat cultures without a change in patient clinical status.

Antibiotics

Antibiotic administration is covered in detail in Michael G. Allison, Emily L. Heil and Bryan D. Hayes's article, "Appropriate Antibiotic Therapy," in this issue. Although narrow spectrum antibiotic therapy is the goal in the inpatient setting when the patient is clinically stable and culture results can be used to guide therapy, in the ED it is "empiric" therapy that guides antimicrobial decision making. The emergency physician needs to use their hospital's antibiogram to determine what is the most appropriate broad-spectrum agent of choice in the initial management of severe sepsis and septic shock (**Fig. 1**). Although this article focuses on source control, it is rare that definitive patient care is achieved without a combined approach between source control and antbimicrobial therapy when a source of sepsis is able to be targeted and amenable to surgical or other invasive management.

Imaging

The ED evaluation of sepsis is very likely to involve imaging, although it is important to keep in mind that the use of imaging should be directed at specific potential sources when clinical suspicion warrants the resource utilization, cost, and potential radiation. Although a chest radiograph is essentially ubiquitous in the sepsis evaluation, ultrasound (US) imaging, computed tomography (CT) scanning, and MRI are less commonly used and associated with more cost, resource allocation, and potential radiation exposure (CT). Perhaps the most important concept to consider when ordering advanced imaging is that the patient will be out of the ED and other important facets of sepsis evaluation and management will be interrupted. For example, if the emergency physician orders a head CT early in the evaluation of a patient with altered mental status potentially owing to sepsis, the patient may quickly be taken out of the ED for this and their antibiotics, blood cultures, and intravenous fluids administration will be delayed. On the other side of the spectrum, it is always good medicine to consider other sources of sepsis beyond the routine sources evaluated by chest radiograph, UA, and blood cultures. The astute emergency physician will pay close attention to the abdominal examination to evaluate for cholecystitis, appendicitis, or noninfectious intraabdominal pathology that may mimic sepsis (eg, hollow viscous perforation, small bowel obstruction). A quick bedside US examination is noninvasive and an easy method to evaluate for biliary pathology. Repeat examinations can be invaluable in guiding the emergency physician toward a decision on advanced imaging, especially if the patient is sick and the chest radiograph and UA do not suggest a clear source of infection. Older patients are especially likely to have more atypical presentations and earlier use of advanced imaging should be considered especially if intraabdominal pathology is suspected.

Surgical Source Control

There are 3 cardinal principles when it comes to obtaining surgical source control. These include drainage of infected fluid collections, debridement of infected tissues

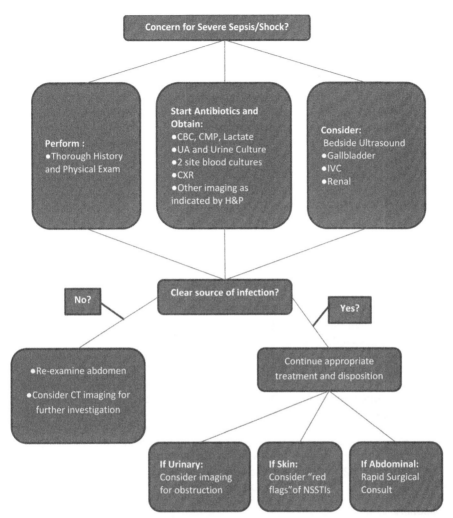

Fig. 1. Determining source in severe sepsis. CBC, complete blood count; CMP, complete metabolic profile; CXR, chest radiograph; CT, computed tomography; H&P, history and physical examination; IVC, inferior vena cava; NSSTIs, necrotizing skin and soft tissue infections; UA, urinalysis.

and/or removal of related foreign bodies, and measures to definitively correct anatomic dysfunctions resulting in ongoing infectious contamination.[2]

Certain specific types of infection may require more urgent mechanical source control than others. These include necrotizing soft tissue infections, peritonitis, and ischemic bowel. Interventions should be undertaken to achieve source control within 12 hours of diagnosing sepsis related to a source that will require an invasive corrective measure. Other specific recommendations regarding source control include using the least invasive procedure possible to achieve source control as well as removal of any vascular devices that are suspected as possible sources of infection. The caveat regarding vascular devices is that if the patient is unstable, the indwelling vascular device may be necessary for resuscitation and this takes priority over source control until hemodynamic stability is achieved.

Further Investigation

Rapid identification in the ED of a specific source of infection can be difficult. Studies have suggested that correct source identification in the ED, even with full diagnostic testing, was accurate in only 85% of pulmonary, 80% of urogenital, and only 68% on of intraabdominal sources.[11] This further reinforces the concept of initiating broad spectrum antibiotics in the ED and allowing the inpatient team to narrow the antibiotic regimen with the benefit of culture results and further investigative workup. Owing to some of the inherent misinformation that can be presented by basic workup of UA and chest radiographs, as discussed, the provider should always keep an open mind regarding the possibility of other sources.

SOURCES
Central Nervous System

The central nervous system (CNS) is a concerning, albeit infrequent source of sepsis. One study found as few as 1% of presenting septic patients had a CNS etiology.[12] Possible sources include meningitis, encephalitis, brain abscess, and epidural abscesses. Although relatively rare, they have high rates of mortality and morbidity. Adult bacterial meningitis has a mortality rate of approximately 25%, and 20% to 30% of survivors will have neurologic sequelae.[13] Typical presenting features include headache, fever, nuchal rigidity, and altered mental status. Although it is unusual for patients to present with all 4 of these classic findings, nearly 95% of patients will present with at least 2 of them.[14]

All patients with clinical suspicion for a CNS source of infection should have a lumbar puncture (LP) performed unless it is contraindicated. A head CT scan before any LP is recommended (by the Infectious Diseases Society of America) for patients who are immunocompromised (eg, AIDS), have a history of prior CNS disease, new-onset seizures, papilledema, abnormal level of consciousness, or a focal neurologic deficit. They also specifically recommend giving empiric antibiotics after obtaining blood cultures, but before proceeding with the LP.[15] That is, do not delay administration of antibiotics at all to obtain the LP. Dexamethasone (10 mg) should be administered intravenously 15 to 20 minutes before giving the antibiotics because it has been shown to reduce morbidity and mortality of bacterial meningitis.[16]

Pulmonary

Respiratory complaints are common presentations in numerous disease entities. In terms of infectious etiologies, these complaints can result from mild upper respiratory infections to severe sepsis or septic shock secondary to pneumonia. The most common presenting symptoms of pneumonia include shortness of breath, chest pain, and cough. One study found at least 96% of patients with pneumonia presented with at least 1 of these complaints.[17]

The chest radiograph is the standard imaging modality used for the diagnosis of pneumonia.[18] Nearly 19% of all visits to an ED include a chest radiograph.[19] It should be noted, however, that these studies can frequently be misleading. Using CT imaging as a standard for comparison, 27% to 43% of patients with an infiltrate on CT imaging will have a negative or nondiagnostic chest radiograph.[17,20] Possible reasons for this include poorly visualized regions on the chest radiograph (eg, lung bases, lingual), very small infiltrates,[17] or early infection that has not yet led to radiographic change. Conversely, a suspected infiltrate on chest radiograph may actually represent pulmonary edema, chronic lung disease, or delay in radiographic resolution of prior infection. Again, using CT imaging as a standard for comparison, one study found 27% of patients with an infiltrate on chest radiography did not have concordant findings on CT scanning.[17] The reasons for false-positive results are also varied and include atelectasis, poor inspiration, or poor positioning.[17]

Abdomen

Abdominal pain is a common chief complaint in the ED and accounts for 5% to 10% visits.[21,22] Intraabdominal infections pose a unique challenge to the emergency physician because they vary in presentation and severity of infection, are frequently polymicrobial, and nearly always require some type of surgical intervention. It is therefore not surprising that mortality rates from intraabdominal infections vary widely from less than 1% to greater than 90%.[23–28] Intraabdominal infections can be divided into 2 major classes, uncomplicated and complicated. Uncomplicated intraabdominal infections are those that are confined to a single organ with no anatomic disruption. Complicated intraabdominal infections occur when an infectious process extends beyond a single organ. These lead to abscesses, peritonitis, and anatomic disruption.[23]

The diagnostic accuracy of a combined history, physical, and laboratory studies in the evaluation of acute abdominal pain is a paltry 43% to 59%.[29] This level of accuracy does not depend on the level of training (ie, resident or attending or even specialist).[30] Thus, it is not unreasonable to have a low threshold for advanced imaging in patients in whom the emergency physician is concerned for an intraabdominal source of sepsis. Conventional radiology (eg, plain films) is of little benefit beyond cases of bowel obstruction.[29] US imaging is a great first option if biliary pathology is suspected. If the emergency physician is proficient, this can be accomplished at bedside. It also avoids the radiation and contrast exposure of CT imaging. CT imaging, however, has the greatest sensitivity and specificity of all imaging modalities, correlating with the correct final diagnosis in 62% to 92% of cases.[29] When ordering CT imaging to evaluate for intraabdominal pathology, it is typically not necessary to use oral contrast. Multiple studies have shown that intravenous contrast is adequate for diagnostic accuracy in abdominal CT imaging and dramatically increases turn around time.[31–33] It is worth mentioning that patients with severe sepsis or septic shock are often hypovolemic and may have acute kidney injury so any consideration of intravenous contrast should be weighed carefully.

In general, intraabdominal infections benefit from rapid source control; delays in definitive management are closely related to increases in morbidity and mortality. Certain intraabdominal infections require rapid surgical source control; these infections include but are not limited to necrotizing soft tissue infections, peritonitis, appendicitis, cholecystitis, and ischemic bowel.[4,34] However, others, specifically pancreatic necrosis, often benefit from delayed surgical intervention.[35,36] Early surgical consultation is of tremendous importance in cases of sepsis owing to an intraabdominal source.

Unfortunately, it is not uncommon to miss an intraabdominal source of sepsis, especially in the elderly. The elderly and those with altered mental status may not always have a history or examination that suggests an intraabdominal infection. These patients may wind up being treated on a medical service and their definitive surgical intervention is significantly delayed, resulting in significant morbidity and mortality. The astute emergency physician will use repeat examinations and appropriate advanced imaging when a source is not readily identified (eg, pneumonia) on the initial patient examination.

Genitourinary

Urinary tract infections (UTIs) are a frequently encountered source of sepsis, also known as urosepsis. The percentage of sepsis presentations attributed to the urinary tract varies widely in the literature, ranging from 8% to 59%,[37,38] with an average compiled from 16 studies (8667 patients) of 13%.[39] Much of this variation has been attributed to the age range of the patients studied. It is a more common source in older patients and is the most common source in patients greater than 65 years of age.[40] The greatest single risk factor is an indwelling urinary catheter, but other risk factors include incontinence or neurologic disorders.[40–42]

Historical factors associated with an increased likelihood of a UTI include fevers, rigors, dysuria, frequency, retention, and physical examination findings of suprapubic or flank tenderness.[43] Other historical factors to consider include frequent prior UTIs, recent urinary tract instrumentation, increased confusion, and falls. All patients presenting with a concern for sepsis should have a UA performed. A urine culture should be sent on all patients admitted for severe sepsis and septic shock.

Urine culture is considered the gold standard for diagnosis of UTI; however, this requires 24 to 48 hours to yield results.[44–47] The emergency physician must rely on the urine dipstick and microanalysis findings when considering an infection. Typically these are nitrite, leukocyte esterase, white blood cells, and bacteria. The sensitivity and specificity of these tests vary widely in the literature and thus they can often be misleading. See **Table 1** for more information.

It is important to realize and consider how misleading bacteriuria can be at times. In the community setting, nearly 20% of both males and females over the age of 70 years old may have asymptomatic bacteriuria.[48] These rates are even higher for elderly patients in long-term care facilities—up to 50% for women and 40% for men.[49] In patients with long-term indwelling urinary catheters the rate approaches 100%.[50] Therefore, providers must leave the differential diagnosis broad when evaluating a septic patient with bacteriuria. Importantly, an unremarkable (ie, completely normal) UA can be useful in ruling out the urinary system as a source; 1 study of nursing home residents found the negative predictive value of leukocyte esterase and nitrite combined (ie, neither detected) was 100%.[51,52]

A final important consideration in cases of urosepsis is the possibility of concomitant obstruction. Approximately 10% of patients with septic shock owing to a urinary tract source will also have urinary tract obstruction.[53] This is an important consideration, because the presence of obstruction requires intervention to achieve source control. The most common cause by far is obstructing calculi. Urinary sepsis with obstruction carries a significantly higher rate of mortality, nearly 30%, as compared with approximately 10% in nonobstructed urinary sepsis.[53]

Imaging is required to diagnose most cases of obstruction because the dual nature of the urinary tract means cases of even complete unilateral ureteral obstruction will still result in urine output. Guidelines are not clear regarding the imaging of choice

Table 1
Sensitivity and specificity of urinalysis

Test (in Setting of Bacteriuria)	Sensitivity (%)	Specificity (%)
+Leukocyte esterase	62–98	41–96
+Nitrite	0–48	48–100
+Leukocyte esterase and +nitrite	0–84	62–100
>5 WBCs per HPF	90–96	47–50
>5 RBCs per HPF	18–44	88–89
Bacteria (any amount)	46–58	89–94

Abbreviations: HPF, high-power field; WBC, white blood cells.

when concerned for obstruction.[54] Noncontrast CT scanning has long been considered the standard for diagnosing calculi, with a sensitivity of 97% and specificity of 95%.[55] However, there is increasing evidence suggesting that bedside US imaging is an appropriate first step in imaging. The use of bedside US imaging in the ED has been shown to decrease the duration of patient stays, decrease overall radiation exposure, and decrease cost, all without increasing risk to the patient.[54] A reasonable approach in cases of suspected urosepsis is to perform a bedside US examination as an initial step and then proceed to noncontrast CT imaging in situations where there is any concern for obstruction.

The astute emergency physician will keep in mind that other sources of infection in the genitourinary system are possible as well and include a tuboovarian abscess, pelvic inflammatory disease, or skin or soft tissue infections of the perineum (eg, Fournier's gangrene).

Skin

Skin and soft tissue infections (SSTIs) are common complaints across all types of care settings. They are estimated to cause nearly 3.5 million ED visits annually and rates of both ED presentation and hospital admission for SSTIs are increasing.[56,57] Although many types of SSTIs are relatively benign, the emergency physician must be aware of the potential for serious SSTIs. Some of these patients have significant comorbid disease (eg, diabetes, peripheral vascular disease, immune compromise).[58] The most ominous SSTI are grouped together under the umbrella term type necrotizing SSTIs (NSSTIs).

NSSTIs have a variety of bacterial etiologies and lead to rapid and extensive tissue destruction and necrosis via secretion of exotoxins. Specific examples include necrotizing fasciitis, Fournier's gangrene, and Ludwig's angina. Physical examination findings (**Box 1**) may include hypotension, altered mental status, pain out of proportion to examination, rapid progression of erythema beyond marked margins, skin fluctuance or crepitus, bullae, and skin necrosis. One retrospective study found that none of these findings individually was sufficiently sensitive to rule in a NSSTI. However, the presence of any 3 of the stated findings together ruled in an NSSTI with 100% specificity and the absence of all nearly ruled out an NSSTI with 97.5% sensitivity.[59]

Box 1
"Red flag" symptoms and signs of necrotizing skin and soft tissue infections

- Hypotension
- Altered mental status
- Pain out of proportion to examination
- Rapid progression of erythema
- Dusky skin color
- Fluctuance/crepitus
- Bullae
- Skin necrosis
- Cutaneous anesthesia
- Tachycardia out of proportion

Plain films have traditionally been used to evaluate for soft tissue gas as evidence of an NSSTI; however, this finding is actually quite infrequent and should not be expected. MRI is considered the gold standard for imaging of NSSTIs owing to its ability to reveal fine details of soft tissues[60]; however, this imaging modality is time consuming and will require a potentially very sick patient to be out of the ED for extended periods of time. CT imaging is often the favored modality because it provides information on intramuscular fluid collections and fascial plane changes, and is much more expeditious than MRI.[61]

An emergency physician may be able to make this diagnosis at the bedside, because necrotic skin from an NSSTI will exhibit cutaneous anesthesia and blunt dissection of the soft tissue will be possible by simply probing with a digit. Necrotizing infections cause local small vessel thrombosis and tissue death locally. The emergency physician may consider incising the area in question (ie, area of fluctuance, maximum discoloration, or cutaneous anesthesia) and trying to use a digit to blunt dissect along tissue planes. Any ability to perform this at bedside secures the diagnosis.

NSSTIs are a surgical emergency and will require surgical debridement in an expeditious fashion. Although broad-spectrum antibiotics to cover gram-positive, gram-negative, and anaerobes (eg, vancomycin, cefepime, and metronidazole) are warranted, mortality approaches 100% without surgical intervention. Clindamycin is often recommended as an adjunctive antibiotic for its antitoxin effect.

An important point to remember for the emergency physician is that a potential NSSTI may be present if a patient has a suspected skin infection and is "sick." Any hypotension, elevation of lactate, or acute end-organ damage (eg, acute kidney injury) should raise immediate concern for an NNSTI and an expeditious search should begin immediately for potential surgical pathology.

Devices

A wide variety of foreign devices can be found in patients presenting with suspected sepsis. These include prosthetic joints, cardiac devices, stimulator units, and a multitude of different vascular access devices. These devices can vary from permanent (eg, joints), to intermediate (eg, peripherally inserted central catheters), to relatively short-term use (eg, central venous catheters). Urinary catheters may be used temporarily or permanently. All of these devices have the potential to become a source of infection. The most common offending device as a source of infection is a vascular access device.[62] An important aspect of device-related infections is the development of a biofilm. Through a combination of mechanical and biological properties, biofilms resist treatment by antibiotics, mechanical cleaning, and natural host defenses.[63,64] This is why in the setting of a device as the source of sepsis, source control typically requires the removal of that device. This tactic is often not prioritized in the ED beyond identifying potential sources and communicating that concern to the inpatient providers.

Bloodstream

Most BSIs are secondary to a primary site of infection. After hematogenous spread from a specific site of infection, the most common cause of BSIs are vascular access devices.[62] Both of these sources require identification and likely removal of the offending infectious source or device. However, primary BSIs (ie, no primary site or device as source) are possible, most commonly with *Staphylococcus aureus* and *Escherichia coli*. Blood cultures from multiple sites, including any suspicious vascular access devices, are paramount for determining BSIs. Although a BSI may not be readily apparent to the emergency physician, there are times when a patient may arrive with a suspicion of sepsis and has a recent known BSI. For example, a nursing home patient is being treated for a BSI and presents with sepsis during the course of treatment. The emergency physician must then focus on secondary infections as a consequence of a BSI, such as endocarditis, epidural abscess, and osteomyelitis.[65]

Viral

Viral etiologies of infection in sepsis should also be considered. Just as in other causes of infection, viral infections can result in sepsis by triggering the inflammatory cascade leading to systemic inflammatory response syndrome, increased vascular permeability, shock, and organ failure.[66] The most widely known and studied viral cause of sepsis is influenza; however, other viral pathogens have been recognized including cytomegalovirus and herpes simplex virus.

Unfortunately, viral infections can lead to increased susceptibility to bacterial infections and bacterial sepsis seems to lead to reactivation of latent viruses. Influenza in particular is known to increase the risk of developing bacterial infections, particularly with S pneumoniae and S aureus. This reactivation occurs through a combination of changes, including impairment of host immune response and changes to the respiratory epithelium.[66] One study found that patients who presented with influenza pneumonia had a 6-fold increase in progression to bacterial sepsis.[67] Recent research has also shown that patients with bacterial sepsis have dramatic rates of reactivation of a wide range of latent viruses, including families of herpes viruses, polyomaviruses, and anellovirus. What is not clear is whether this is simply a sign of the degree of impaired immunity or if it contributes to the morbidity and mortality of bacterial sepsis.[68]

At this time there are no clear guidelines for treatment of viral sepsis. The Centers for Disease Control and Prevention do recommend antivirals be initiated in patients as soon as possible who are hospitalized for influenza. Perhaps most important, a diagnosis of influenza has significant infection control ramifications in the inpatient world. The patients most vulnerable to influenza infection are the ones already in the hospital with another illness. Thus, screening for influenza has ramifications well beyond the patient in the ED.

Finally, unfortunately, it is very difficult to differentiate a viral from bacterial source as a cause of sepsis. As a result, the emergency physician should always err on the side of caution in patients with severe sepsis and septic shock and opt to provide antibiotics empirically and allow the inpatient team to further investigate the source of pathology.

SUMMARY

Identifying the source of infection in presentations of sepsis (**Table 2**) and achieving source control are cornerstones of therapy as highlighted by the Surviving Sepsis Campaign. This requires not only rapid administration of broad spectrum antibiotics, but also a thorough investigation to determine the source. The provider should approach the patient in a methodical manner, including a thorough history and physical examination as well as an appropriate laboratory workup and targeted imaging modalities.

Included with standard workups should be a UA and chest radiograph; however, the emergency physician must be wary of the pitfalls associated with the poor sensitivity and specificity of these examinations in isolation. If a chest radiograph is not diagnostic or leaves room for multiple potential pathologies representing the visualized abnormalities, then CT imaging may be warranted for further clarification. If a urinary

Table 2
Summary of sources and associated key points

Source	Key Points
Central nervous system	• Rare • High morbidity and mortality • Do not delay antibiotics for lumbar puncture
Pulmonary	• Pulmonary complaints are common • Chest radiograph frequently misleading • Most often culture negative
Abdominal	• Difficult diagnosis • Difficult source control • Consider if initial workup does not reveal a source
Genitourinary	• Common • Urinalysis frequently misleading • Maintain concern for obstruction
Skin and soft tissue	• Requires high index of clinical suspicion • Search for "red flags" of necrotizing skin and soft tissue infections • Requires urgent source control
Bloodstream/devices	• Difficult to narrow down to this as a cause • Take note of any devices on physical examination • Consider removing/changing devices
Viral	• Presents similar to bacterial sepsis • Increases risk of bacterial superinfections • Antivirals appropriate in patients in intensive care with influenza

source is suspected, bedside US is a recommended adjunctive investigational tool, but CT imaging should be pursued if any concern remains for obstruction. Additionally, the inherent difficulties in diagnosis and nebulous presentation of intraabdominal infections make this a particularly dangerous pitfall for the emergency physician, especially in the elderly. If the UA or chest radiograph is nondiagnostic, or there is initial concern for an intraabdominal infection, strongly consider early investigation with CT imaging. Overall, both rapid administration of antibiotics and rapid identification of the source of infection are essential components in an effort to improve outcomes in severe sepsis and septic shock.

REFERENCES

1. Vargas A, López M, Lillo C, et al. The Edwin Smith papyrus in the history of medicine. Rev Med Chil 2012;140(10):1357–62 [in Spanish].
2. Marshall JC, al Naqbi A. Principles of source control in the management of sepsis. Crit Care Clin 2009;25(4):753–68, viii–ix.
3. Marshall JC, Maier RV, Jimenez M, et al. Source control in the management of severe sepsis and septic shock: an evidence-based review. Crit Care Med 2004; 32(Supplement):S513–26.
4. Dellinger RP, Levy MM, Rhodes A, et al. Surviving sepsis campaign: international guidelines for management of severe sepsis and septic shock: 2012. Crit Care Med 2013;41(2):580–637.
5. Phua J, Ngerng W, See K, et al. Characteristics and outcomes of culture-negative versus culture-positive severe sepsis. Crit Care 2013;17(5):R202.
6. de Prost N, Razazi K, Brun-Buisson C. Unrevealing culture-negative severe sepsis. Crit Care 2013;17(5):1001.

7. Dark PM, Dean P, Warhurst G. Bench-to-bedside review: the promise of rapid infection diagnosis during sepsis using polymerase chain reaction-based pathogen detection. Crit Care 2009;13(4):217.
8. Mermel LA, Maki DG. Detection of bacteremia in adults: consequences of culturing an inadequate volume of blood. Ann Intern Med 1993;119(4):270–2.
9. Blot F, Schmidt E, Nitenberg G, et al. Earlier positivity of central-venous- versus peripheral-blood cultures is highly predictive of catheter-related sepsis. J Clin Microbiol 1998;36(1):105–9.
10. Weinstein MP, Murphy JR, Reller LB, et al. The clinical significance of positive blood cultures: a comprehensive analysis of 500 episodes of bacteremia and fungemia in adults. II. Clinical observations, with special reference to factors influencing prognosis. Rev Infect Dis 1983;5(1):54–70.
11. Uittenbogaard AJM, de Deckere ERJT, Sandel MH, et al. Impact of the diagnostic process on the accuracy of source identification and time to antibiotics in septic emergency department patients. Eur J Emerg Med 2014;21(3):212–9.
12. Heffner AC, Horton JM, Marchick MR, et al. Etiology of illness in patients with severe sepsis admitted to the hospital from the emergency department. Clin Infect Dis 2010;50(6):814–20.
13. Durand ML, Calderwood SB, Weber DJ, et al. Acute bacterial meningitis in adults. A review of 493 episodes. N Engl J Med 1993;328(1):21–8.
14. van de Beek D, de Gans J, Spanjaard L, et al. Clinical features and prognostic factors in adults with bacterial meningitis. N Engl J Med 2004;351(18):1849–59.
15. Tunkel AR, Hartman BJ, Kaplan SL, et al. Practice guidelines for the management of bacterial meningitis. Clin Infect Dis 2004;39(9):1267–84.
16. de Gans J, van de Beek D, European Dexamethasone in Adulthood Bacterial Meningitis Study Investigators. Dexamethasone in adults with bacterial meningitis. N Engl J Med 2002;347(20):1549–56.
17. Self WH, Courtney DM, McNaughton CD, et al. High discordance of chest x-ray and computed tomography for detection of pulmonary opacities in ED patients: implications for diagnosing pneumonia. Am J Emerg Med 2013;31(2):401–5.
18. Mandell LA, Wunderink RG, Anzueto A, et al. Infectious Diseases Society of America/American Thoracic Society consensus guidelines on the management of community-acquired pneumonia in adults. Clin Infect Dis 2007;44(Suppl 2): S27–72.
19. McCaig LF, Burt CW. National Hospital Ambulatory Medical Care Survey: 2002 emergency department summary. Adv Data 2004;(340):1–34.
20. Hayden GE, Wrenn KW. Chest radiograph vs. computed tomography scan in the evaluation for pneumonia. J Emerg Med 2009;36(3):266–70.
21. Kamin RA, Nowicki TA, Courtney DS, et al. Pearls and pitfalls in the emergency department evaluation of abdominal pain. Emerg Med Clin North Am 2003; 21(1):61–72, vi.
22. Laméris W, van Randen A, van Es HW, et al. Imaging strategies for detection of urgent conditions in patients with acute abdominal pain: diagnostic accuracy study. BMJ 2009;338:b2431.
23. Blot S, De Waele JJ. Critical issues in the clinical management of complicated intra-abdominal infections. Drugs 2005;65(12):1611–20.
24. Bohnen J, Boulanger M, Meakins JL, et al. Prognosis in generalized peritonitis. Relation to cause and risk factors. Arch Surg 1983;118(3):285–90.
25. Nathens AB, Rotstein OD, Marshall JC. Tertiary peritonitis: clinical features of a complex nosocomial infection. World J Surg 1998;22(2):158–63.

26. Pitcher WD, Musher DM. Critical importance of early diagnosis and treatment of intra-abdominal infection. Arch Surg 1982;117(3):328–33.

27. Hartl W, Kuppinger D, Vilsmaier M. Secondary peritonitis. Zentralbl Chir 2011; 136(1):11–7 [in German].

28. Barie PS, Williams MD, McCollam JS, et al. Benefit/risk profile of drotrecogin alfa (activated) in surgical patients with severe sepsis. Am J Surg 2004;188(3): 212–20.

29. Gans SL, Pols MA, Stoker J, et al, Expert Steering Group. Guideline for the diagnostic pathway in patients with acute abdominal pain. Dig Surg 2015;32(1): 23–31.

30. Pines J, Uscher Pines L, Hall A, et al. The interrater variation of ED abdominal examination findings in patients with acute abdominal pain. Am J Emerg Med 2005; 23(4):483–7.

31. Razavi SA, Johnson J-O, Kassin MT, et al. The impact of introducing a no oral contrast abdominopelvic CT examination (NOCAPE) pathway on radiology turn around times, emergency department length of stay, and patient safety. Emerg Radiol 2014;21(6):605–13.

32. Levenson RB, Camacho MA, Horn E, et al. Eliminating routine oral contrast use for CT in the emergency department: impact on patient throughput and diagnosis. Emerg Radiol 2012;19(6):513–7.

33. Schuur JD, Chu G, Sucov A. Effect of oral contrast for abdominal computed tomography on emergency department length of stay. Emerg Radiol 2010;17(4): 267–73.

34. Boyer A, Vargas F, Coste F, et al. Influence of surgical treatment timing on mortality from necrotizing soft tissue infections requiring intensive care management. Intensive Care Med 2009;35(5):847–53.

35. Freeman ML, Werner J, van Santvoort HC, et al. Interventions for necrotizing pancreatitis: summary of a multidisciplinary consensus conference. Pancreas 2012;41(8):1176–94.

36. Tenner S, Baillie J, DeWitt J, et al, American College of Gastroenterology. American College of Gastroenterology guideline: management of acute pancreatitis. Am J Gastroenterol 2013;108(9):1400–15, 1416.

37. Nicolle LE. Urinary tract infection. Crit Care Clin 2013;29(3):699–715.

38. Yahav D, Eliakim-Raz N, Leibovici L, et al. Bloodstream infections in older patients. Virulence 2016;7:341–52.

39. Talan DA, Moran GJ, Abrahamian FM. Severe sepsis and septic shock in the emergency department. Infect Dis Clin North Am 2008;22(1):1–31, v.

40. Gavazzi G, Mallaret M-R, Couturier P, et al. Bloodstream infection: differences between young-old, old, and old-old patients. J Am Geriatr Soc 2002;50(10): 1667–73.

41. van Duin D. Diagnostic challenges and opportunities in older adults with infectious diseases. Clin Infect Dis 2012;54(7):973–8.

42. Leibovici L, Greenshtain S, Cohen O, et al. Toward improved empiric management of moderate to severe urinary tract infections. Arch Intern Med 1992; 152(12):2481–6.

43. Woodford HJ, George J. Diagnosis and management of urinary tract infection in hospitalized older people. J Am Geriatr Soc 2009;57(1):107–14.

44. Gupta K, Sahm DF, Mayfield D, et al. Antimicrobial resistance among uropathogens that cause community-acquired urinary tract infections in women: a nationwide analysis. Clin Infect Dis 2001;33(1):89–94.

45. Bouza E, San Juan R, Muñoz P, et al, Co-operative Group of the European Study Group on Nosocomial Infections. A European perspective on nosocomial urinary tract infections II. Report on incidence, clinical characteristics and outcome (ESGNI-004 study). European Study Group on Nosocomial Infection. Clin Microbiol Infect 2001;7(10):532–42.

46. Wilson ML, Gaido L. Laboratory diagnosis of urinary tract infections in adult patients. Clin Infect Dis 2004;38(8):1150–8.

47. Simerville JA, Maxted WC, Pahira JJ. Urinalysis: a comprehensive review. Am Fam Physician 2005;71(6):1153–62.

48. Nicolle LE. Asymptomatic bacteriuria: when to screen and when to treat. Infect Dis Clin North Am 2003;17(2):367–94.

49. Nicolle LE. Asymptomatic bacteriuria in the elderly. Infect Dis Clin North Am 1997; 11(3):647–62.

50. Warren JW, Tenney JH, Hoopes JM, et al. A prospective microbiologic study of bacteriuria in patients with chronic indwelling urethral catheters. J Infect Dis 1982;146(6):719–23.

51. Juthani-Mehta M, Tinetti M, Perrelli E, et al. Role of dipstick testing in the evaluation of urinary tract infection in nursing home residents. Infect Control Hosp Epidemiol 2007;28(7):889–91.

52. Stovall RT, Haenal JB, Jenkins TC, et al. A negative urinalysis rules out catheter-associated urinary tract infection in trauma patients in the intensive care unit. J Am Coll Surg 2013;217(1):162–6.

53. Reyner K, Heffner AC, Karvetski CH. Urinary obstruction is an important complicating factor in patients with septic shock due to urinary infection. Am J Emerg Med 2016;34(4):694–6.

54. Smith-Bindman R, Aubin C, Bailitz J, et al. Ultrasonography versus computed tomography for suspected nephrolithiasis. N Engl J Med 2014;371(12):1100–10.

55. Coursey CA, Casalino DD, Remer EM, et al. ACR Appropriateness Criteria® acute onset flank pain–suspicion of stone disease. Ultrasound Q 2012;28(3): 227–33.

56. Pallin DJ, Egan DJ, Pelletier AJ, et al. Increased US emergency department visits for skin and soft tissue infections, and changes in antibiotic choices, during the emergence of community-associated methicillin-resistant Staphylococcus aureus. Ann Emerg Med 2008;51(3):291–8.

57. Edelsberg J, Taneja C, Zervos M, et al. Trends in US hospital admissions for skin and soft tissue infections. Emerg Infect Dis 2009;15(9):1516–8.

58. Miller LG, Eisenberg DF, Liu H, et al. Incidence of skin and soft tissue infections in ambulatory and inpatient settings, 2005-2010. BMC Infect Dis 2015;15:362.

59. Alayed KA, Tan C, Daneman N. Red flags for necrotizing fasciitis: a case control study. Int J Infect Dis 2015;36:15–20.

60. Ali SZ, Srinivasan S, Peh WCG. MRI in necrotizing fasciitis of the extremities. Br J Radiol 2014;87(1033):20130560.

61. Fayad LM, Carrino JA, Fishman EK. Musculoskeletal infection: role of CT in the emergency department. Radiographics 2007;27(6):1723–36.

62. Al Mohajer M, Darouiche RO. Sepsis syndrome, bloodstream infections, and device-related infections. Med Clin North Am 2012;96(6):1203–23.

63. Stewart PS. Biophysics of biofilm infection. Pathog Dis 2014;70(3):212–8.

64. Høiby N, Bjarnsholt T, Givskov M, et al. Antibiotic resistance of bacterial biofilms. Int J Antimicrob Agents 2010;35(4):322–32.

65. Watson CM, Al-Hasan MN. Bloodstream infections and central line-associated bloodstream infections. Surg Clin North Am 2014;94(6):1233–44.

66. Florescu DF, Kalil AC. The complex link between influenza and severe sepsis. Virulence 2014;5(1):137–42.
67. Jain S, Benoit SR, Skarbinski J, et al, 2009 Pandemic Influenza A (H1N1) Virus Hospitalizations Investigation Team. Influenza-associated pneumonia among hospitalized patients with 2009 pandemic influenza A (H1N1) virus–United States, 2009. Clin Infect Dis 2012;54(9):1221–9.
68. Walton AH, Muenzer JT, Rasche D, et al. Reactivation of multiple viruses in patients with sepsis. PLoS One 2014;9(2):e98819.

Fluid Resuscitation in Severe Sepsis

Rob Loflin, MD[a], Michael E. Winters, MD[b],*

KEYWORDS

- Fluid resuscitation • Crystalloid • Colloid • Fluid responsiveness • Fluid challenge
- Fluid overload • Acute kidney injury • Hyperchloremia

KEY POINTS

- Fluid resuscitation is the cornerstone of resuscitation in patients with severe sepsis and septic shock.
- Fluids should be considered as medications; it is imperative to consider the type, dose, and duration of intravenous fluid therapy in sepsis.
- Crystalloids remain the intravenous fluid of choice in sepsis resuscitation. Balanced solutions may be preferred to normal saline and colloids.
- It is important to know the difference between empiric fluid loading and a fluid challenge in the assessment of fluid responsiveness.
- Excessive and indiscriminate fluid administration can increase organ dysfunction and mortality in patients with severe sepsis and septic shock.

INTRODUCTION

Intravenous fluid (IVF) therapy began in 1832, when Dr Thomas Latta administered "two drachms of muriate and two scruples of carbonate, of soda, to sixty ounces of water" to 6 patients with hypovolemic shock during the cholera epidemic in London. Dr Latta described an "immediate return of the pulse and improvement in respiration" with the administration of repeated small amounts of his specific fluid.[1] Since the time of Dr Latta's original description, fluid resuscitation has become the cornerstone of early and aggressive treatment of patients with severe sepsis and septic shock.[2] However, fundamental questions still remain about the optimal fluid composition, dose, and rate of fluid administration for critically ill patients.[3]

In 2001, Rivers and colleagues[4] published the landmark Early Goal-directed Therapy (EGDT) trial, which showed a significant mortality benefit in septic patients who received aggressive IVF therapy as a component of resuscitation targeted to

Disclosure: The authors have nothing to disclose.
[a] University of Rochester Medical Center, Rochester, NY, USA; [b] Critical Care Program, Internal Medicine, Emergency Medicine, University of Maryland School of Medicine, 110 South Paca Street, 6th Floor, Suite 200, Baltimore, MD 21201, USA
* Corresponding author.
E-mail address: mwinters@em.umaryland.edu

emed.theclinics.com

specific hemodynamic end points. In the EGDT trial, IVFs were administered to target a predefined value for central venous pressure (CVP). Since the publication of the EGDT trial, there have been significant changes in the approach to fluid resuscitation in patients with sepsis. Specifically, aggressive fluid resuscitation that results in volume overload and organ dysfunction has been associated with increased patient mortality.[5–8] In addition, CVP has been shown to be an unreliable marker of intravascular volume status and fluid responsiveness. The use of CVP to guide IVF therapy did not improve mortality in 3 recent randomized trials designed to compare EGDT with current usual care.[9–11] Furthermore, the administration of IVFs in pursuit of a select CVP goal has been implicated in the development of volume overload.[9–12]

In addition to the potential harm of overzealous fluid administration, the composition of select fluids may affect patient-centered outcomes. Specifically, the supraphysiologic concentration of chloride in 0.9% normal saline has been associated with adverse effects on the pulmonary, circulatory, gastrointestinal, coagulation, and renal organ systems. The recognition of these adverse effects has led to a greater awareness of the phases of sepsis resuscitation and a focus on appropriate fluid administration. Physiology of the circulatory system, the pathogenesis of septic shock, and the phases of sepsis resuscitation is discussed elsewhere in this issue.

PHYSIOLOGY OF THE CIRCULATORY SYSTEM
Frank-Starling Curve

Mean arterial blood pressure (MAP) is determined by cardiac output (CO) and systemic vascular resistance (SVR), and can be calculated according to the following equation:

$$MAP = CO * SVR.$$

The primary determinants of CO are heart rate (HR) and stroke volume (SV). In order to maintain CO, blood ejected from the left ventricle (LV) must traverse the circulatory system, return to the right atrium and right ventricle, and transit the pulmonary circulation. In this way, CO is coupled with venous return (VR). The Frank-Starling curve (**Fig. 1**) illustrates the volume of the LV at the end of diastole (preload) and directly influences SV. Any increases in preload result in an increase in SV, until a plateau is reached. Beyond this point, any additional preload in the form of IVF fails to significantly increase SV and leads to fluid overload, impaired cardiac function, pulmonary edema, and interstitial edema.[13]

Venous Return

Blood is returned to the right atrium via the superior and inferior vena cavae. VR is determined by the gradient between the mean systemic filling pressure (Pms) and the right atrial pressure, which can be approximated by the CVP. VR is also affected by any condition that affects the resistance to return (RVR), such as abdominal ascites. VR can be calculated according to the following equation:

$$VR = (Pms - CVP)/RVR$$

The venous circulation contains approximately 70% of the total blood volume and can be divided into a stressed and unstressed volume. The stressed volume is the main determinant of Pms and directly affects both VR and CO. The unstressed volume

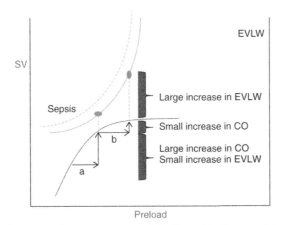

Fig. 1. Frank-Starling curve. Superimposition of the Frank-Starling and Marik-Phillips curves showing the effects of increasing preload on SV and lung water in a patient who is preload responsive (a) and nonresponsive (b). With sepsis, the extravascular lung water (EVLW) curve is shifted to the left. (*From* Marik P, Lemson J. Fluid responsiveness: an evolution of our understanding. Br J Anaesth 2014;112:618; with permission.)

can be converted to the stressed volume either through additional volume expansion (ie, fluid bolus) or venoconstriction with the use of vasopressor medications. As a result of these relationships, IVF administration only augments VR and CO if it increases Pms more than the CVP. In addition to VR and CO, organ blood flow depends on perfusion pressure. Perfusion pressure is determined by subtracting the CVP from the MAP. Under normal conditions, autoregulation maintains constant organ blood flow over a wide range of blood pressures. However, when the patient becomes hypotensive, autoregulation fails and organ blood flow becomes more dependent on CVP. These critical points emphasize why IVF administration can be difficult. For a fluid bolus to increase VR, the Pms must increase more than the CVP. If both Pms and CVP increase with IVF administration, VR and CO remain unchanged. If the CVP increases more than Pms, VR decreases, organ perfusion pressure worsens, and venous congestion and organ injury ensues.[14–16]

Endothelial Glycocalyx

The vascular endothelium plays a critical role in fluid homeostasis and its function is important to understanding fluid administration in patients with severe sepsis and septic shock. In 1896, Ernest Starling described the traditional view that fluid was filtered at the arterial end of capillaries and reabsorbed by the venous system, and that both hydrostatic and colloid oncotic pressures governed this filtration and absorption.[17] In recent years, the discovery of the endothelial glycocalyx later (EGL) has revised the traditional Starling description. The EGL is a complex web of hairlike glycoproteins and proteoglycans that lines the vascular endothelium. The EGL has numerous functions, including the regulation of vascular permeability by limiting tissue edema and modulation of inflammation through the prevention of leukocyte and cytokine adhesion.[18] The EGL has also been shown to hold up to 25% of the intravascular fluid volume.[19,20] Sepsis damages the EGL and results in the loss of vascular integrity, capillary leak, vasodilatation, and hypovolemia.[21] In addition, volume overload results in the release of natriuretic peptides, which have been shown to cause shedding of the EGL and further contribute to interstitial edema and inhibit lymphatic drainage.[22,23]

HEMODYNAMIC INSTABILITY IN SEPTIC SHOCK

In order to understand the goals of fluid resuscitation in sepsis, it is pertinent to review the pathophysiology of sepsis. Sepsis has recently been defined as "life-threatening organ dysfunction caused by a dysregulated host response to infection."[24] Patients with septic shock are defined as those with a lactate value greater than 2 mmol/L who require vasopressor medications to maintain an MAP greater than or equal to 65 mm Hg despite adequate fluid resuscitation.[24] Although dehydration may accompany septic shock, it is not the primary factor that results in hemodynamic instability. The primary mechanisms that cause circulatory compromise in septic shock include systemic vasodilatation, increased vascular permeability, and myocardial dysfunction.

In septic shock, the EGL and vascular endothelium are damaged by inflammation and lose the ability to regulate microvascular blood flow. This loss of regulation results in both arterial and venous dilatation and causes maldistribution of blood flow. The release of nitric oxide and prostacyclin have been implicated in the pathogenesis of vasodilatation. Arterial vasodilatation results in systemic hypotension, whereas venous dilatation increases the unstressed volume and decreases VR. In addition, endothelial and EGL injury result in the activation of the coagulation cascade, leukocyte adhesion, platelet aggregation, reduced red blood cell deformability, disruption of the junctions between cells, alterations in cell-to-cell signaling, and the production of tissue edema. All of these processes can decrease the diffusion of oxygen to cellular mitochondria and increase the accumulation of metabolic waste products.[25] These pathologic changes are summarized in **Fig. 2**.

In addition to pathologic vasodilatation and damaged endothelium, myocardial dysfunction has been shown to be a common occurrence in patients with septic shock. Up to 50% of patients with septic shock have LV systolic dysfunction.[26] Furthermore, up to 62% have LV diastolic dysfunction, whereas as many as 31% of patients have right ventricular dysfunction.[27–30] Diastolic dysfunction is characterized by a stiff, poorly compliant LV. This condition impairs filling and SV and has been shown to be associated with increased mortality in septic shock.[27–29] Excessive fluid administration in the presence of diastolic dysfunction inevitably leads to pulmonary edema, pulmonary hypertension, right ventricular dysfunction, and decreased CO.[31] Adequate preload, maintenance of sinus rhythm, and avoidance of tachycardia are of paramount importance to maximize LV filling and augment SV in these patients.

PHASES OF RESUSCITATION

The complex mechanisms that produce hemodynamic alterations in severe sepsis and septic shock make it difficult to recommend a one-size-fits all approach to fluid resuscitation. Importantly, patients with severe sepsis and septic shock can present along a spectrum of illness and the need for fluid therapy may vary for each patient. A recent conceptual model of circulatory shock has been published that identifies 4 phases of resuscitation: rescue, optimization, stabilization, and de-escalation.[32] These phases are depicted and described in **Fig. 3** and **Table 1**. The goals of fluid therapy depend on the patient's phase of illness at presentation. In general, patients present to the emergency department in the rescue or optimization phase, whereas the stabilization and de-escalation phases typically occur during the inpatient setting.[32]

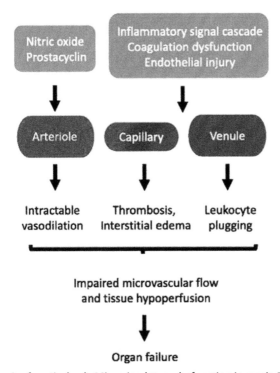

Fig. 2. Pathogenesis of septic shock. Microcirculatory dysfunction in sepsis. The microvascular network undergoes functional and structural changes during inflammatory states such as sepsis and may have a key role in organ dysfunction. Changes include dilatation of arterioles, microvascular thrombosis, increased adhesion of leukocytes in venules, and increased vascular permeability. These alterations result in impaired microcirculatory blood flow and tissue perfusion, ultimately leading to organ failure. Techniques for measuring microcirculatory flow in vivo have been described but these tools have not yet been rigorously tested for use in patients with sepsis. (*Adapted from* Gupta RG, Hartigan SM, Kashiouris MG, et al. Early goal-directed resuscitation of patients with septic shock: current evidence and future directions. Crit Care 2015;19:286; distributed under the terms of the Creative Commons Attribution 4.0 International License (http://creativecommons.org/licenses/by/4.0).)

Rescue Phase

The rescue phase represents the initial minutes to hours of resuscitation and is characterized by profound shock, hypotension, and impaired organ perfusion. Rapid fluid administration is needed to prevent cardiovascular collapse and death. The optimal MAP for sepsis resuscitation has not been established. Current guidelines recommend IVF administration to target a MAP of 65 mm Hg.[2] A recent trial did not find a mortality difference when patients with septic shock were resuscitated to a MAP of 80 to 85 mm Hg compared with a MAP goal of 60 to 65 mm Hg.[33] Of note, the rate of new-onset atrial fibrillation was higher in patients randomized to the higher MAP target. In patients with a history of chronic hypertension, the need for renal replacement therapy was lower in patients randomized to the higher MAP target. However, this finding was not associated with an improvement in mortality.

Because the microcirculation is the site where most derangements occur in sepsis, a targeted approach to microcirculatory resuscitation is appealing. Importantly, perfusion of the microcirculation is regulated by blood flow, not arterial blood

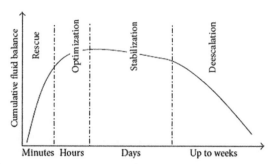

Fig. 3. Phases of resuscitation. (*Adapted from* Goldstein SL. Fluid management in acute kidney injury. J Intensive Care Med 2014;29:184.)

pressure. Microcirculatory impairment may persist despite an MAP greater than 65 mm Hg.[34–36] At present, microcirculatory-guided resuscitation remains primarily investigational.

Although most emergency department patients present in the rescue phase of resuscitation, it is important for emergency providers to be familiar with subsequent phases in the event that the patient has a prolonged length of stay.

Optimization Phase

The optimization phase is characterized by a careful assessment of intravascular volume status and a determination of the need for further fluid administration. For some patients, vasopressor medications are initiated and titrated during this phase. The optimal end points of resuscitation continue to be debated. Notwithstanding, additional IVF administration should be guided by the results of tests to determine fluid responsiveness and the performance of a fluid challenge. Fluid responsiveness and the fluid challenge are discussed in detail later in this article.

Stabilization

The goals of the stabilization phase of resuscitation are to maintain intravascular volume, replace ongoing fluid losses, support organ dysfunction, and avoid iatrogenic harm with unnecessary and indiscriminate IVF administration.

De-escalation

The de-escalation phase is characterized by organ recovery and weaning from mechanical ventilation and vasopressor support. Excess fluid that was accumulated during the previous phases of resuscitation is actively removed with the use of diuretic medications or renal replacement therapy (ie, ultrafiltration). The goal of this phase is to achieve an overall negative fluid balance.

SELECTION OF FLUID

In the past, the selection of which fluid to administer to patients with severe sepsis or septic shock has largely been based on geography, marketing, availability, cost, and even the type of provider training (medical vs surgical).[37] Fluids can largely be separated into crystalloid and colloid solutions. Crystalloid solutions can be further divided into unbalanced and balanced solutions, whereas colloid solutions primarily include albumin, dextran, and hydroxyethyl starch solutions. The compositions of commonly used crystalloid solutions are listed in **Table 2**.

Table 1
Phases of resuscitation

	Rescue	Optimization	Stabilization	De-escalation
Treatment goal	Shock reversal/life salvage	Adequate tissue perfusion	Zero-to-negative daily fluid balance	Fluid accumulation reversal/edema resolution
Time course	Minutes	Hours	Day	Up to weeks
Hemodynamic targets	Autoregulatory thresholds of perfusion pressure	Micro/macrocirculatory blood flow parameters	Weaning of vasopressors with stable hemodynamic conditions	Return to premorbid/chronic values of pressure and flow
Treatment options	Rapid fluid boluses + vasopressors	Repeated fluid challenges + vasopressors + inotropes	Maintenance fluids + decreasing/chronic vasoactive agents	Diuretics or other means of fluid removal

Adapted from Vincent JL, DeBacker D. Circulatory shock. N Engl J Med 2013;369:1732.

Table 2
Composition of common crystalloid solutions

	Plasma	0.9% Saline	Plasma-Lyte 148	Ringer Lactate
Sodium (mmol/L)	136–145	154	140	130
Potassium (mmol/L)	3.5–5.0	0	5	4
Magnesium (mmol/L)	0.8–1.0	0	1.5	0
Calcium (mmol/L)	2.2–2.6	0	0	3
Chloride (mmol/L)	98–106	154	98	109
Acetate (mmol/L)	0	0	27	0
Gluconate (mmol/L)	0	0	23	0
Lactate (mmol/L)	0	0	0	28
Actual Osmolality (mOsmol/kg H_2O)	287	286	271	256
pH	7.35–7.45	4.5–7	4–8	5–7

Data from Reddy S, Weinberg L, Young P. Crystalloid fluid therapy. Crit Care 2016;20:59.

It is important to consider the effect of fluid solutions on the acid-base status of the patient. The final acid-base equilibrium is determined by the strong ion difference (SID) of the IVF, the concentration of nonvolatile weak acids, and the arterial concentration of carbon dioxide. Of these, the SID is the most important determinant of acid-base equilibrium. The SID is calculated as the difference between strong cations (ie, sodium, potassium, calcium, magnesium) and strong anions (ie, chloride, lactate, ketoacids). The normal SID of extracellular fluid is approximately 40 mEq/L.[37]

Normal Saline

The most common fluid used in North America is 0.9% normal saline. Note that 0.9% normal saline is not a true physiologic solution. It contains 154 mEq/L of sodium and 154 mEq/L of chloride. Thus, the SID of 0.9% normal saline is zero. As a result, large volumes of 0.9% normal saline reliably produce a hyperchloremic metabolic acidosis. In addition, the supraphysiologic concentration of chloride in 0.9% normal saline has been associated with adverse effects on the renal, splanchnic, circulatory, pulmonary, and coagulation systems. In a prospective, open-label study of more than 1500 patients from a single center in Australia, Yunos and colleagues[38] showed a lower increase in creatinine level and lower rate of kidney injury through a restriction of the use of IVFs with a high chloride concentration. In a recent retrospective review of more than 109,000 patients, Shaw and colleagues[39] showed an association between chloride load and increased in-hospital mortality among patients with the systemic inflammatory response syndrome who received IVFs with a higher chloride concentration. In another observational study, Shaw and colleagues[40] showed an increased need for renal replacement therapy, transfusions, and a higher mortality in adult patients undergoing major abdominal surgery who received 0.9% normal saline compared with patients who received the balanced solution Plasma-Lyte. As a result of these and other observational studies, many emergency and critical care providers have decreased the use of 0.9% normal saline in favor of a balanced fluid solution.

Balanced Solutions

Balanced solutions (ie, Plasma-Lyte, Ringer lactate, Hartmann solution) have less of an effect on acid-base equilibrium than 0.9% normal saline. The SID of many balanced solutions more closely approximates that of plasma. In addition, balanced solutions have significantly lower concentrations of chloride compared with 0.9% normal saline. These solutions contain organic anions (ie, lactate, acetate, gluconate, citrate) that act as buffers to generate bicarbonate.[37] Balanced solutions also contain varying concentrations of cations (ie, potassium, calcium). The physiologic benefit of these added cations remains unclear.

Recent trials suggest that balanced solutions may be superior to 0.9% normal saline for fluid resuscitation in sepsis. In a retrospective cohort of a large database from more than 360 hospitals, Raghunathan and colleagues[41] showed lower in-hospital mortality among patients with sepsis who received a balanced solution compared with patients who exclusively received saline. In a recent systematic review and network meta-analysis, Rochwerg and colleagues[42] reported that balanced solutions may be superior to 0.9% normal saline for fluid resuscitation in sepsis.

Young and colleagues[43] recently published the only prospective, randomized trial comparing the effect of a balanced crystalloid solution (Plasma-Lyte 148) with saline among intensive care unit patients. In this large study of almost 2300 patients, the investigators sought to determine the effect of fluid solutions on renal complications in intensive care unit patients. Overall, the investigators found no difference in the proportion of patients who developed acute kidney injury. Furthermore, there was no difference in the need for renal replacement therapy, intensive care unit and hospital length of stay, the need for mechanical ventilation, or mortality between patients who received the balanced solution and those who received saline. Although the study was well performed, several limitations should be noted. More than 70% of patients included in this trial were postsurgical patients, not critically ill emergency department patients. The volume of IVF administered during the trial period was small, averaging just 2 L for both groups. In addition, the study was a feasibility study. Therefore, sample size and power calculations were not possible.

There is currently no perfectly balanced crystalloid solution. Notwithstanding, the potential negative effects of 0.9% normal saline must be considered when resuscitating patients with severe sepsis and septic shock. Although current evidence remains primarily limited to observational studies, balanced solutions may be superior to saline in sepsis resuscitation.

Colloids

Current guidelines for the management of severe sepsis and septic shock recommend consideration of albumin in patients who continue to require substantial amounts of crystalloid to maintain MAP.[2] This recommendation is primarily based on a subgroup analysis of the SAFE (Saline versus Albumin Fluid Evaluation) trial, in which 1218 patients with severe sepsis who received 4% albumin had lower odds of death compared with patients who received 0.9% normal saline.[44] More recently, Caironi and colleagues[45] failed to show a difference in mortality in more than 1800 patients with severe sepsis or septic shock who were randomized to receive crystalloids alone or crystalloids with the addition of a 20% albumin solution. However, the objective of this study was to correct hypoalbuminemia and not to resuscitate patients with a hyperoncotic albumin solution. Patel and colleagues[46] performed a systematic review and meta-analysis to determine the effect on all-cause mortality of albumin as part of the resuscitation of patients with sepsis of any severity. However, the investigators were unable to find a statistically significant survival benefit for albumin in any subgroup of sepsis severity. Based on these recent studies, albumin should not be part of the routine resuscitation of emergency department patients with severe sepsis or septic shock.

Hydroxyethyl starch (HES) solutions are still administered to millions of patients each year around the world. HES solutions are characterized by their molecular weight and the degree of hydroxyethylation. New generations of HES solutions use lower molecular weights and lower substitution ratios. Despite the popularity of these products, numerous studies in recent years have shown increased mortality and a trend toward a higher need for renal replacement therapy in patients who have received these fluid solutions.[47–49] Many critical care providers think that HES products should no longer be used in critically ill patients.

FLUID ADMINISTRATION
Empiric Fluid Loading

Empiric fluid loading is the administration of a predetermined volume of fluid with the intent to ensure adequate organ perfusion. In the EGDT by Rivers and colleagues,[4] refractory hypotension was defined as a systolic blood pressure less than 90 mm Hg after a 20 to 30 mL/kg fluid bolus. Largely based on the EGDT trial, the Surviving Sepsis Campaign guidelines recommend an initial 30-mL/kg bolus of crystalloids for patients with severe sepsis and septic shock.[2] In the 3 most recent studies that evaluated EGDT, patients received an average of 30 to 35 mL/kg as an empiric fluid bolus before study enrollment.[9–11] Note that the recommendation to administer 30 mL/kg as an initial fluid bolus is based on limited evidence. Best practice is to individualize fluid therapy and administer enough fluid to rectify hypovolemia.

Fluid Responsiveness

Fluid responsiveness is defined as the state of preload reserve in which an increase in VR results in an increase in CO, which corresponds with the ascending portion of the Frank-Starling curve. An increase in SV or CO by approximately 15% in response to an increase in preload suggests that the patient is fluid responsive and will tolerate additional fluid administration. A change in SV or CO less than 10% to 15% suggests that the patient is not likely to benefit from additional fluid administration. In these patients, the emergency provider should consider initiation of vasopressor medications in order to achieve resuscitation targets.

However, only 50% of critically ill adult patients are fluid responsive.[50,51] Physical examination findings have been shown to be poor indicators of fluid responsiveness.[52–54] As a result of the limitations of the physical examination and traditional vital sign measurement, numerous methods and devices have been developed to better assess fluid responsiveness. These methods and devices can be divided into invasive and noninvasive techniques and produce measurements that are described as static or dynamic. Static measurements of fluid responsiveness are measured intermittently, whereas dynamic measurements are measured continuously. Two traditional static measurements of fluid responsiveness are CVP and the pulmonary artery occlusion pressure (PAOP) obtained via pulmonary artery catheter. Importantly, CVP and PAOP do not accurately determine fluid responsiveness and should not be used in the most critically ill patients.[55] Furthermore, the 3 recent sepsis trials that compared EGDT with usual care found no difference in outcome with the use of CVP to guide fluid administration.[9–11] Dynamic indices of fluid responsiveness have been consistently shown to be superior to static measurements.[56] Current dynamic measures to assess fluid responsiveness are listed in **Table 3**.

Fluid Challenge

To accurately measure fluid responsiveness a test of the circulatory system must be performed. This test can be accomplished with a fluid challenge or a passive leg raise

Table 3
Dynamic indices of fluid responsiveness

Test/Parameter	Mechanism	Advantages	Limitations
Fluid challenge	Infusion of 250–500 mL of crystalloids over 5–10 min	Small amount of fluid	Requires fluid administration
Mini–fluid challenge	Infusion of 100 mL of crystalloids over 1 min	Small amount of fluid	Requires fluid administration
PPV, SVV, dVTI, IVC variability	Heart-lung interaction in mechanically ventilated patients	No fluid infusion necessary	Spontaneous breathing efforts Vt <8 mL/kg Cr <30 mL/cm H_2O HR/RR >3.6 Arrhythmias RV failure
EEO test	Heart-lung interaction in mechanically ventilated patients	No fluid infusion Independent of arrhythmias Independent of respiratory compliance	Strong spontaneous breathing efforts
PLR	Self-volume challenge	No fluid infusion Reversible effect	IAH ICH

Abbreviations: Cr, creatinine; dVTI, velocity time integral; EEO, end-expiratory occlusion; IAH, intra-abdominal hypertension; ICH, intracranial hemorrhage; IVC, inferior vena cava; PLR, passive leg raise; PPV, pulse pressure variation; RR, respiratory rate; RV, right ventricle; SVV, stroke volume variation; Vt, tidal volume.

Adapted from Carsetti A, Cecconi M, Rhodes A. Fluid bolus therapy: monitoring and predicting fluid responsiveness. Curr Opin Crit Care 2015;21:389; with permission.

(PLR) test. In contrast with empiric fluid loading (previously described), a fluid challenge is characterized by the administration of a smaller volume of fluid combined with an objective hemodynamic measurement. Performance of a fluid challenge to assess fluid responsiveness may prevent the harm of excessive fluid administration.[57,58] To perform a fluid challenge an initial set of hemodynamic measurements should be obtained. Next, administer 100 mL to 500 mL of crystalloid over 5 to 10 minutes. The hemodynamic response to this fluid challenge is then measured using a dynamic method of fluid responsiveness. Patients showing a positive response to the fluid challenge are considered to be fluid responsive.

A PLR maneuver can be performed in lieu of the administration of a fluid challenge. The PLR maneuver is noninvasive and can be performed repeatedly to assess fluid responsiveness without the administration of additional volume.

ADVERSE EFFECTS OF FLUID RESUSCITATION

Excessive and indiscriminate fluid administration can lead to a positive cumulative fluid balance and the potential for patient harm. Fluid overload is a state of excess total body water that is caused by both increased fluid administration and decreased renal elimination in critical illness. Patients with severe sepsis and septic shock are susceptible to fluid overload because of the pathogenesis of sepsis described earlier. It has been traditionally taught that approximately one-third of the crystalloid volume infused remains in the intravascular space. More recent evidence suggests that the percentage is likely to be much lower, with as little as 5% of infused volume remaining in the intravascular space of septic patients.[59] Fluid overload may lead to acute kidney injury as a result of increased venous congestion, interstitial edema, and extrarenal compression from increases in intra-abdominal pressure.[60] The adverse effects of fluid overload on other organ systems are shown in **Fig. 4**.

Numerous studies have shown the potential harm of fluid overload. In a prospective survey of European intensive care units, Vincent and colleagues[8] found a positive fluid balance to be an independent predictor of mortality in septic patients. Similarly,

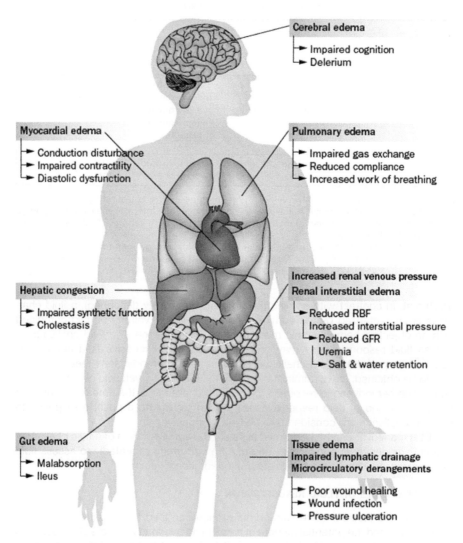

Fig. 4. Adverse effects of fluid overload. GFR, glomerular filtration rate; RBF, renal blood flow. (*From* Prowle JR, Echeverri JE, Ligabo EV, et al. Fluid balance and acute kidney injury. Nat Rev Nephrol 2010;6:110; with permission.)

a retrospective review of almost 800 septic patients showed that a positive fluid balance at 12 hours and 4 days was associated with an increased 28-day mortality.[5] These studies highlight the importance of an accurate determination of fluid responsiveness during the optimization and stabilization phases of resuscitation. Methods to minimize additional fluid administration for patients who are not fluid responsive during these phases should be considered. These methods include discontinuation of maintenance fluids, minimization of carrier solutions, and removal of fluid with diuretic medications or ultrafiltration.

SUMMARY

Fluid therapy is a cornerstone of the resuscitation and management of patients with severe sepsis and septic shock. The complex pathophysiologic processes of sepsis and the various phases of resuscitation make a one-size-fits-all approach to fluid resuscitation impractical. Early fluid administration is necessary in the rescue phase of resuscitation, whereas fluid administration should be guided by dynamic measurements of fluid responsiveness in later stages of resuscitation. Based on current literature, balanced crystalloids may be superior to 0.9% normal saline for most septic patients. It is important to avoid overly aggressive and indiscriminate administration of fluids, because an overall positive fluid balance has been associated with increased patient morbidity and mortality in sepsis.

REFERENCES

1. Awad S, Allison SP, Lobo DN. The history of 0.9% saline. Clin Nutr 2008;27: 179–88.
2. Dellinger RP, Levy MM, Rhodes A, et al. Surviving sepsis campaign: international guidelines for management of severe sepsis and septic shock. Crit Care Med 2013;41:580–637.
3. McDermid RC. Controversies in fluid therapy: type, dose, and toxicity. World J Crit Care Med 2014;3:24.
4. Rivers EP, Nguyen B, Havstad S, et al. Early goal-directed therapy in the treatment of severe sepsis and septic shock. N Engl J Med 2001;345:1368–77.
5. Boyd JH, Forbes J, Nakada T, et al. Fluid resuscitation in septic shock: a positive fluid balance and elevated central venous pressure are associated with increased mortality. Crit Care Med 2011;39:259–65.
6. Kelm DJ, Perrin JT, Cartin-Ceba R, et al. Fluid overload in patients with severe sepsis and septic shock treated with early goal-directed therapy is associated with increased acute need for fluid-related medical interventions and hospital death. Shock 2015;43:68–73.
7. Sadaka F, Juarez M, Naydenov S, et al. Fluid resuscitation in septic shock: the effect of increasing fluid balance on mortality. J Intensive Care Med 2014;29: 213–7.
8. Vincent JL, Sakr Y, Sprung CL, et al. Sepsis in European intensive care units: results of the SOAP study. Crit Care Med 2006;34:344–53.
9. Mouncey PR, Osborn TM, Power GS, et al. Trial of early, goal-directed resuscitation for septic shock. N Engl J Med 2015;372:1301–11.
10. ProCESS Investigators, Yealy DM, Kellum JA, Huang DT, et al. A randomized trial of protocol-based care for early septic shock. N Engl J Med 2014;370:1683–93.
11. ANZICS Clinical Trials Group, Peake SL, Delaney A, Bailey M, et al. Goal-directed resuscitation for patients with early septic shock. N Engl J Med 2014;371: 1496–506.

12. Marik P, Bellomo R. A rational approach to fluid therapy in sepsis. Br J Anaesth 2016;116:339–49.

13. Marik P, Lemson J. Fluid responsiveness: an evolution of our understanding. Br J Anaesth 2014;112:617–20.

14. Berlin DA, Bakker J. Starling curves and central venous pressure. Crit Care 2015; 19:55.

15. Sondergaard S, Parkin G, Aneman A. Central venous pressure: we need to bring clinical use into physiological context: applied physiology of central venous pressure. Acta Anaesthesiol Scand 2015;59:552–60.

16. Story AP. Venous function and central venous pressure. Anesthesiology 2008; 108:735–48.

17. Starling EH. On the absorption of fluids from the connective tissue spaces. J Physiol 1896;19:312–26.

18. Becker BF, Chappell D, Bruegger D, et al. Therapeutic strategies targeting the endothelial glycocalyx: acute deficits, but great potential. Cardiovasc Res 2010;87:300–10.

19. Michel CC, Curry FRE. Glycocalyx volume: a critical review of tracer dilution methods for its measurement. Microcirculation 2009;16:213–9.

20. Rehm M, Haller M, Orth V, et al. Changes in blood volume and hematocrit during acute preoperative volume loading with 5% albumin or 6% hetastarch solutions in patients before radical hysterectomy. Anesthesiology 2001;95:849–56.

21. Steppan J, Hofer S, Funke B, et al. Sepsis and major abdominal surgery lead to flaking of the endothelial glycocalix. J Surg Res 2011;165:136–41.

22. Bruegger D, Schwartz L, Chappell D, et al. Release of atrial natriuretic peptide precedes shedding of the endothelial glycocalyx equally in patients undergoing on- and off-pump coronary artery bypass surgery. Basic Res Cardiol 2011;106: 1111–21.

23. Bruegger D, Jacob M, Rehm M, et al. Atrial natriuretic peptide induces shedding of endothelial glycocalyx in coronary vascular bed of guinea pig hearts. Am J Physiol Heart Circ Physiol 2005;289:H1993–9.

24. Singer M, Deutschman CS, Seymour C, et al. The third international consensus definitions for sepsis and septic shock (Sepsis-3). JAMA 2016;315:801–10.

25. Lundy DJ, Trzeciak S. Microcirculatory dysfunction in sepsis. Crit Care Clin 2009; 25:721–31.

26. Parker MM, Shelhamer J, Bacharach SL, et al. Profound but reversible myocardial depression in patients with septic shock. Ann Intern Med 1984;100:483–90.

27. Landesberg G, Gilon D, Meroz Y, et al. Diastolic dysfunction and mortality in severe sepsis and septic shock. Eur Heart J 2012;33:895–903.

28. Brown SM, Pittman JE, Hirshberg EL, et al. Diastolic dysfunction and mortality in early severe sepsis and septic shock: a prospective, observational echocardiography study. Crit Ultrasound J 2012;4:8.

29. Sanfilippo F, Corredor C, Fletcher N, et al. Diastolic dysfunction and mortality in septic patients: a systematic review and meta-analysis. Intensive Care Med 2015;41:1004–13.

30. Pulido JN, Afessa B, Masaki M, et al. Clinical spectrum, frequency, and significant of myocardial dysfunction in severe sepsis and septic shock. Mayo Clin Proc 2012;87:620–8.

31. Schneider AJ, Teule GJ, Groeneveld AB, et al. Biventricular performance during volume loading in patients with early septic shock, with emphasis on the right ventricle: a combined hemodynamic and radionuclide study. Am Heart J 1988; 116:103–22.

32. Vincent JL, DeBacker D. Circulatory shock. N Engl J Med 2013;369:1726–34.
33. Asfar P, Meziani F, Hamel JF, et al. High versus low blood-pressure target in patients with septic shock. N Engl J Med 2014;370:1583–93.
34. Segal SS. Regulation of blood flow in the microcirculation. Microcirculation 2005; 12:33–45.
35. Leone M, Blidi S, Antonini F, et al. Oxygen tissue saturation is lower in nonsurvivors than in survivors after early resuscitation of septic shock. Anesthesiology 2009;111:366–71.
36. Payen D, Luengo C, Heyer L, et al. Is thenar tissue hemoglobin oxygen saturation in septic shock related to macrohemodynamic variables and outcome? Crit Care 2009;13:S6.
37. Reddy S, Weinberg L, Young P. Crystalloid fluid therapy. Crit Care 2016;20:59.
38. Yunos NM, Bellomo R, Hegarty C, et al. Association between a chloride-liberal vs chloride-restrictive intravenous fluid administration strategy and kidney injury in critically ill adults. JAMA 2012;308:1566–72.
39. Shaw AD, Raghunathan K, Peyerl FW, et al. Association between intravenous chloride load during resuscitation and in-hospital mortality among patients with SIRS. Intensive Care Med 2014;40:1897–905.
40. Shaw AD, Bagshaw SM, Goldstein SL, et al. Major complications, mortality, and resource utilization after open abdominal surgery: 0.9% compared to Plasma-Lyte. Ann Surg 2012;255:821–9.
41. Raghunathan K, Shaw AD, Nathanson B, et al. Association between the choice of IV crystalloid and in-hospital mortality among critically ill adults with sepsis. Crit Care Med 2014;42:1585–91.
42. Rochwerg B, Alhazzani W, Sindi A, et al. Fluid resuscitation in sepsis: a systematic review and network meta-analysis. Ann Intern Med 2014;161:347–55.
43. Young P, Bailey M, Beasley R, et al. Effect of a buffered crystalloid solution vs saline on acute kidney injury among patients in the intensive care unit. The SPLIT randomized clinical trial. JAMA 2015;314:1701–10.
44. Finfer S, Bellomo R, Boyce N, et al. A comparison of albumin and saline for fluid resuscitation in the intensive care unit. N Engl J Med 2004;350:2247–56.
45. Caironi P, Tognoni G, Masson S, et al. Albumin replacement in patients with severe sepsis or septic shock. N Engl J Med 2014;370:1412–21.
46. Patel A, Laffan MA, Waheed U, et al. Randomised trials of human albumin for adults with sepsis: systematic review and meta-analysis with trial sequential analysis of all-cause mortality. BMJ 2014;349:g4561.
47. Perner A, Haase N. Hydroxyethyl starch 130/0.42 versus Ringer's acetate in severe sepsis. N Engl J Med 2012;367:124–34.
48. Guidet B, Martinet O, Boulain T, et al. Assessment of hemodynamic efficacy and safety of 6% hydroxyethylstarch 130/0.4 vs. 0.9% NaCl fluid replacement in patients with severe sepsis: the CRYSTMAS study. Crit Care 2012;16:R94.
49. Myburgh JA, Finfer S, Bellomo R, et al. Hydroxyethyl starch or saline for fluid resuscitation in intensive care. N Engl J Med 2012;367:1901–11.
50. Marik PE, Baram M, Vahid B. Does central venous pressure predict fluid responsiveness? A systematic review of the literature and the tale of seven mares. Chest 2008;134:172–8.
51. Michard F, Teboul JL. Predicting fluid responsiveness in ICU patients: a critical analysis of the evidence. Chest 2002;121:2000–8.
52. Pierrakos C, Velissaris D, Scolletta S, et al. Can changes in arterial pressure be used to detect changes in cardiac index during fluid challenge in patients with septic shock? Intensive Care Med 2012;38:422–8.

53. Rady MY, Rivers EP, Martin G, et al. Continuous central venous oximetry and shock index in the emergency department: use in the evaluation of clinical shock. Am J Emerg Med 1992;10:538–41.
54. Rady MY, Rivers EP, Nowak RM. Resuscitation of the critically ill in the ED: responses of blood pressure, heart rate, shock index, central venous oxygen saturation, and lactate. Am J Emerg Med 1996;14:218–25.
55. Osman D, Ridel C, Ray P, et al. Cardiac filling pressures are not appropriate to predict hemodynamic response to volume challenge. Crit Care Med 2007; 35:64–8.
56. Marik PE, Cavallazzi R, Vasu T, et al. Dynamic changes in arterial waveform derived variables and fluid responsiveness in mechanically ventilated patients: a systematic review of the literature. Crit Care Med 2009;37:2642–7.
57. Vincent JL, Weil MH. Fluid challenge revisited. Crit Care Med 2006;34:1333–7.
58. Carsetti A, Cecconi M, Rhodes A. Fluid bolus therapy: monitoring and predicting fluid responsiveness. Curr Opin Crit Care 2015;21:388–94.
59. Chowdury AH, Cox EF, Francis ST, et al. A randomized, controlled, double-blind crossover study on the effects of 2-L infusions of 0.9% normal saline and Plasma-Lyte 148 on renal blood flow velocity and renal cortical tissue perfusion in healthy volunteers. Ann Surg 2012;256:18–24.
60. Prowle JR, Kirwan CJ, Bellomo R. Fluid management for the prevention and attenuation of acute kidney injury. Nat Rev Nephrol 2014;10:37–47.

Vasopressors and Inotropes in Sepsis

Leeanne Stratton, MD[a], David A. Berlin, MD[b], John E. Arbo, MD[a,b],*

KEYWORDS

- Vasopressors • Inotropes • Sepsis • Septic shock • Cardiac contractility
- Norepinephrine • Epinephrine • Dopamine

KEY POINTS

- Vasopressors and inotropes are beneficial in shock states when they increase the systemic arterial pressure to allow autoregulation, increase venous return, augment abnormal cardiac contractility, or increase the coronary perfusion gradient.
- Norepinephrine should be administered within 6 hours in patients with sepsis-associated hypotension that does not correct with an initial 30 mL/kg crystalloid fluid bolus.
- Dobutamine should be considered in septic patients with evidence of myocardial dysfunction or signs of hypoperfusion despite restoration of adequate intravascular volume and mean arterial pressure with fluid and vasopressor therapy.

INTRODUCTION

The British physician George Oliver was among the first to investigate the vasoactive properties of the adrenal gland. In 1893, using his son as a research subject, Dr Oliver observed that ingestion of sheep adrenal extract produced narrowing of the radial artery diameter.[1] Over the next 2 years, Dr Oliver, working with the physiologist Edward A. Schäfer from the University of London, described both the lethal effects of large amounts of the substance and the ability of lower doses to increase arteriolar blood pressure in animal models.[2] Efforts to isolate a pure form of the active constituent of the adrenal gland extract, generically referred to as 'epinephrine,' would not be achieved until 1901, when the Japanese chemist Jokichi Takamine successfully marketed the substance under the proprietary name *adrenalin*.[2] George Crile, the cardiovascular surgeon and Cleveland Clinic cofounder, would be among the first to

Authorship Criteria: All authors provided equal contribution to this article.
Financial Disclosures: None of the authors have any financial arrangements to disclose.
[a] Division of Emergency Medicine, New York Presbyterian Hospital/Weill Cornell Medical Center, New York, NY, USA; [b] Division of Pulmonary and Critical Care Medicine, New York Presbyterian Hospital/Weill Cornell Medical Center, New York, NY, USA
* Corresponding author. Division of Emergency Medicine, 525 East 68th Street, Suite M-130, New York, NY 10016.
E-mail address: jea9030@med.cornell.edu

demonstrate the clinical applications of synthetic adrenaline and its power to restore arterial blood pressure in surgical patients with various forms of shock.[3] He would go on to describe adrenaline's resuscitative effects in dogs with induced cardiac arrest. There would not, however, be a definitive thesis of the adrenoreceptor mechanism until Raymond Ahlquist published his seminal paper in 1948 proposing the existence of alpha- and beta-receptors.[4]

PHYSIOLOGIC RATIONALE FOR VASOACTIVE MEDICATIONS IN PATIENTS WITH SEVERE SEPSIS

Vasopressor and inotrope medications are vasoactive agents used in shock states to assist in the restoration of impaired perfusion. The physiologic effects these agents in sepsis-associated hypoperfusion are diverse and, often, overlap (**Table 1**). Before reviewing the clinical application of individual vasoactive medications, it is useful to consider the primary therapeutic effects of each agent on the arterial, venous, and cardiac systems of patients in shock.

Effect of Vasopressors and Inotropes on the Systemic Arterial System

In general, vasopressors induce vasoconstriction within the arterial system, whereas inotropes increase cardiac contractility. In reality, most vasoactive agents produce both effects. The most commonly used vasopressor and inotrope medications are synthetic catecholamines that stimulate alpha, beta, and dopaminergic receptors in the arteries and arterioles. Typically, the alpha effects predominate in these vessels, especially at standard doses. Specifically, stimulation of alpha-1 receptors on vascular smooth muscle cells leads to an increase in intracellular calcium, and, consequently, intense vasoconstriction and increased systemic blood pressure.[4,5]

The small arterioles supply most of the resistance in the high-pressure systemic arterial circulation. This is essential for autoregulation, the process by which tissues control their own blood flow. Tissues that require increased perfusion can dilate their arterioles and admit additional blood flow into their capillary beds. Autoregulation, therefore, improves the distribution of blood flow within the arterial system. Importantly, autoregulation requires that the pressure in systemic arteries exceed a minimum threshold.[6] If systemic arterial blood pressure falls below this minimum threshold, there can be an insufficient pressure gradient for perfusion.[7] Agents with vasoconstrictive activity can therefore help to increase the resistance and pressure in the systemic arteries and arterioles above the threshold required to enable autoregulation, restoring critical perfusion to regional vascular beds.

Effect of Vasopressors and Inotropes on the Systemic Venous System

Normally, the compliant systemic venous system contains two-thirds of the total blood volume. Smooth muscle in the walls of systemic veins constrict in response to activation of alpha and vasopressin (a noncatecholamine vasoconstrictor) receptors.[8–10] This feature allows the systemic veins to serve as an adjustable blood reservoir that is under autonomic control. The venous reservoir has an average pressure that is independent of the pressure generated by the heart's pumping, and is determined by both the circulating volume of blood and the intrinsic stiffness of the vessel walls. This pressure, called the mean systemic filling pressure (MSFP), is normally around 7 mm Hg. For blood to return to the heart, the MSFP must be greater than the right atrial pressure, which is normally 0 mm Hg in early diastole. The rate of venous return to the heart depends on the pressure gradient between the MSFP and the right atrium. Endogenous vasopressors play an essential role in regulating venous return through

Table 1
Summary of vasopressor and inotropic agents

Agent	Indication	Activity in Sepsis and Septic Shock	Receptor Binding		Typical Dose	Adverse Effects
Norepinephrine	Shock (septic, cardiogenic)	Inoconstriction, mobilizes unstressed venous blood volume; provides some direct inotropic support	Heart β_1: +++	Vasculature α_1: +++++ β_2: ++	0.02–0.3 μg/kg/min	Tachyarrhythmias, cardiac myocyte apoptosis, limb ischemia
Epinephrine	Shock (septic, cardiogenic), cardiac arrest, symptomatic bradycardia, anaphylaxis	Inoconstriction, mostly β_1 effects at doses up to 0.1 μg/kg/min; α_1 effects predominate at higher doses	Heart β_1: ++++	Vasculature α_1: +++++ β_2: +++	0.01–0.20 μg/kg/min	Ventricular arrhythmias, severe hypertension leading to cerebrovascular events, limb ischemia, metabolic acidemia, and lactic acidosis
Vasopressin	Shock (septic, vasoplegic), ± cardiac arrest	Vasoconstriction of the pulmonary and systemic vasculature, adjunctive	Vasculature V_1: vascular smooth muscle V_2: renal collecting ducts		0.01–0.04 U/min	Tachyarrhythmias, digital ischemia
Dopamine	Symptomatic bradycardia, shock (septic, cardiogenic)	Inoconstriction, vasodilatory via DA receptors at doses <2 μg/kg/min; β_1 effects from 2–5 μg/kg/min; α_1 predominate at higher doses	Heart β_1: ++++	Vasculature α_1: +++ β_2: ++ DA: +++++	2–20 μg/kg/min	Tachyarrhythmias, cardiac ischemia, severe hypertension

(continued on next page)

Table 1
(continued)

Agent	Indication	Activity in Sepsis and Septic Shock	Receptor Binding		Typical Dose	Adverse Effects
Phenylephrine	Acute hypotension (vagal, medication related), aortic stenosis w/hypotension, HCM with LVOT gradient	Vasoconstriction, adjunctive	Heart β₁: 0	Vasculature α₁: +++++ β₂: 0	100–180 μg/min initial, 40–60 μg/min maintenance; boluses 50–200 μg q20 min	Worsening cardiac function, baroreflex bradycardia
Dobutamine	Shock (cardiogenic, septic cardiomyopathy), ADHF/low CO states	Inodilatation, mostly β₁ and β₂ effects <15 μg/kg/min; mild α₁ at higher doses but offset by β₂	Heart β₁: +++++	Vasculature α₁: + β₂: +++	5–15 μg/kg/min	Ventricular arrhythmias, cardiac ischemia, hypotension as a known β₂ effect
Milrinone	Low CO states refractory to dobutamine and/or in chronically β-blocked patients, or in RV failure with pHTN	Inodilatation, decreases pulmonary vascular resistance	Heart Blocks PDE3 degradation of cAMP, equivalent to β₁: +++++	Vasculature Blocks PDE3 degradation of cAMP, equivalent to β₂: ++++	0.25–0.75 μg/kg/min	Profound vasodilatory effects mediated through PDE3 inhibition, torsades and other ventricular arrhythmias

Abbreviations: ADHF, acute decompensated heart failure; CO, cardiac output; HCM, hypertrophic cardiomyopathy; LVOT, left ventricular outflow tract; MAPs, mean arterial pressures; PDE3, phosphodiesterase 3; pHTN, pulmonary hypertension; RV, right ventricle.

their ability to increase MSFP, increase this pressure gradient, and drive blood into the heart. A normal heart responds to increased venous return by increasing its output by the Frank–Starling mechanism and autonomic reflexes.[11,12] Importantly, this mechanism of increasing cardiac output occurs independent of direct cardiac stimulation, and is similar to the effect of a fluid bolus.[13–16]

Effect of Vasopressors and Inotropes on the Heart

Vasoactive agents that stimulate beta-receptors, specifically beta-1 receptors, increase cardiac myocyte contractility; an effect mediated by an increase in intracellular cyclic adenosine monophosphate (cAMP) and intracellular calcium. The enhanced contractility that results can increase stroke volume and reduce ventricular end-diastolic volume and filling pressures.[17] Beta agonists, however, typically cause only a modest increase in cardiac output because the unstimulated heart is normally able to eject almost all of the blood that has returned to it. Significant increases in cardiac output will only occur if the end-diastolic volume is abnormally increased, as occurs in the setting of myocardial dysfunction. Beta agonists may also improve cardiac performance through increased chronotropy (beta-1) and enhanced lusitropy (beta-2).[18] Activation of beta-2 receptors also results in relaxation of vascular smooth muscle and, consequently, peripheral arterial vasodilation. In certain clinical scenarios, this can offset the work imposed on the heart by the vasculature and improve cardiac performance.

Vasopressors also improve cardiac performance by augmenting coronary artery perfusion. The coronary arteries carry nutrient blood flow from the aorta to the myocardium. During systole, the high pressure generated by ventricular contraction compresses the coronary arteries within the walls of the myocardium, resulting in both anterograde and retrograde flow. The relative proportion of anterograde and retrograde flow depends on the pressure gradient between the aorta and the ventricles. Coronary perfusion to either ventricle can decrease precipitously if intraventricular pressures increase at the same time systemic arterial pressure decreases. A vicious and potentially rapidly fatal cycle of low cardiac output reducing coronary perfusion ensues, which further reduces cardiac performance. This can occur in multiple clinical scenarios (**Box 1**). In these settings, vasopressors can serve to increase vascular tone, restore systemic arterial pressure, and preserve the coronary perfusion gradient, thereby minimizing myocardial ischemia. This approach has been shown to be effective in experimental models of pulmonary embolism, tamponade, and cardiogenic shock from left ventricular ischemia.[19–22]

Box 1
Conditions in which vasopressors may improve coronary perfusion

- Cardiac tamponade
- Aortic stenosis
- Hypertrophic obstructive cardiomyopathy
- Pulmonary embolism
- Pulmonary hypertension
- Systolic heart failure
- Cardiopulmonary resuscitation

Vasopressors and inotropes have multiple effects on cardiac performance and perfusion in shock states. The net effect will vary depending on the clinical situation. In general, benefit will be realized when use of vasoactive agents (1) increases the systemic arterial pressure to greater than the threshold to allow autoregulation, (2) increases venous return, (3) augments abnormal cardiac contractility, or (4) increases the coronary perfusion gradient.

Other Physiologic Effects of Vasopressors and Inotropes

Vasoactive agents exert a multitude of other significant physiologic effects. Select agents result in pulmonary artery constriction and increased pulmonary vascular resistance.[23] However, the right ventricular strain this effect can produce is typically offset by a simultaneous improvement in both cardiac contractility and the coronary perfusion gradient.[24] Vasoactive agents also have important metabolic effects.[25] Beta agonists, particularly epinephrine, can increase blood glucose and lactate concentrations. Both epinephrine and norepinephrine increase kaliuresis and urine output independent of their effect on blood pressure and cardiac output.[26]

INITIATING VASOPRESSOR THERAPY IN SEVERE SEPSIS

The Surviving Sepsis Campaign (SSC) recommends vasopressor therapy in patients with severe sepsis within 6 hours if hypotension, defined as a mean arterial blood pressure (MAP) of less than 65 mm Hg, persists after a 30 mL/kg crystalloid fluid bolus. In practice, many patients whose hemodynamics and physical examination findings improve with appropriate initial volume resuscitation will, nevertheless, receive additional volume before vasopressor therapy is started. Accurate estimation of intravascular volume status is challenging in an emergency department setting. What is considered 'adequate' volume resuscitation is often determined at the point of volume unresponsiveness, or the failure of additional fluid boluses to further augment indices of cardiac output. This approach, however, can lead to overresuscitation with large volumes of crystalloid and the sequelae of acute renal insufficiency, cardiac insufficiency, pulmonary edema, and prolonged ventilator dependency.[24,27]

Time to initiation of vasopressors may prove to be an independent predictor of mortality. A recent retrospective cohort study in patients with septic shock found that mortality rates increased with increasing time to norepinephrine initiation; this was true even when vasopressors were begun within the SSC's recommended 6-hour window.[28] Patients who received norepinephrine within 2 hours of onset of septic shock had significantly lower 28-day mortality rates compared with patients who received vasopressors after 2 hours of shock (30% vs 43%). In this study, mortality rates increased by 5.3% for every hour delay in vasopressor initiation once shock was recognized. Earlier administration of norepinephrine also led to shorter duration of vasopressor use and lower total doses of the drug administered. Patients in whom norepinephrine was started after 2 hours also took significantly longer to achieve goal MAPs than patients in the early initiation group (6.1 vs 4.6 hours; $P<.001$). Importantly, both groups received similar volumes of fluid within the first 6 hours, and there were no differences in time to antibiotic initiation or corticosteroid use.

Vasopressor use typically requires a central venous catheter. The time and effort required for catheter insertion, as well as the known complications of the procedure, may contribute to provider delay in initiating vasopressor therapy. Central venous catheter placement and use is associated with infectious, thrombotic, and mechanical complications.[29] The safety of peripherally administered vasopressors, however, remains a subject of debate, with tissue necrosis, gangrene, or limb ischemia resulting from vasopressor extravasation being primary concerns. The first randomized controlled trial comparing mechanical, infectious, and thrombotic complication rates in patients in the intensive care unit (ICU) receiving vasopressor therapy via peripheral or central venous catheters demonstrated a trend toward increased complications in the peripheral catheter group.[30] The majority of complications were attributed to difficulty with peripheral catheter insertion, insertion-site erythema, and subcutaneous extravasation with subsequent blistering, or local tissue necrosis. There were no differences in mortality between the central and peripheral catheter groups; however, more than one-half of the peripheral catheter group eventually required central venous catheter placement because of increasing vasopressor requirements or because peripheral access could not be obtained.

A more recent single-arm study in 734 ICU patients who received peripheral norepinephrine, dopamine, or phenylephrine for a median of 49 hours demonstrated the safety of administering these agents peripherally when local phentolamine and nitroglycerin paste were used in combination to treat incidences of peripheral extravasation.[31] No cases of tissue injury resulted. Importantly, the study protocol mandated the use of at least 20-G catheters placed in vessels with diameters of greater than 4 mm, as determined on bedside ultrasonography. Importantly, the integrity of the catheters was assessed every 2 hours by nursing staff.

A recent systematic review composed of mostly case reviews and case studies concluded that the peripheral administration of vasopressors is safe for short durations (<2 hours) via larger bore catheters that are placed proximal to the antecubital and popliteal fossae.[32] This review recommended the use of peripherally administered vasopressors only as a temporizing measure while central access is obtained.

When using vasopressors, it is important to remember that local derangements of the microcirculation (ie, perfusion of regional capillary beds) may persist despite optimization of surrogate macrocirculatory variables. Boerma and Ince[33] cite in vitro studies demonstrating that capillary hematocrits vary dynamically, from 6.8% to 38%, despite a systemic hematocrit of 50%, depending on whether there is upstream vasoconstriction or dilatation of the contributing arterioles. Vasoconstriction also increases the diffusion distance of oxygen, which is inversely proportional to oxygen delivery at the cellular level. Various imaging and detection modalities have been used to capture the state of the microcirculation in severe sepsis and have underscored the heterogeneity of flow to different microvascular beds despite optimization of macrocirculatory variables.[33] Although it is clear that a functioning microcirculation requires a minimum MAP, it is not always the case that meeting threshold MAPs will be sufficient to normalize flow to these low-pressure vascular beds.

Norepinephrine

Norepinephrine is the first-line vasopressor in patients with sepsis or septic shock. It is a hydroxylated derivative of dopamine and stimulates both alpha and beta receptors. Its alpha-1 effects predominate at therapeutic doses. As noted, the venous effects of norepinephrine (augmentation of MSFP) act similarly to a fluid bolus, and can provide preload support during simultaneous fluid resuscitation. Norepinephrine also provides moderate inotropic support via its beta-1 activity.

At therapeutic doses, norepinephrine carries a lesser risk of serious adverse events than dopamine in the treatment of septic shock, with an absolute risk reduction of 11% in mortality compared with dopamine in a recent systematic review.[34] Dopamine also doubled the risk of cardiac arrhythmias in this analysis and in an earlier metaanalysis by De Backer and colleagues,[35] who reported a relative risk of arrhythmias of 2.34 when dopamine was used instead of norepinephrine in patients with septic shock.

Prolonged use of norepinephrine, however, can be directly toxic to cardiac myocytes and may result in reflex bradycardia, cardiac arrhythmia, and tissue ischemia as a result of profound vasoconstriction.

Epinephrine

Epinephrine is a potent nonselective alpha and beta agonist recommended by the SSC for use in sepsis-associated hypotension as either a first alternative or in addition to norepinephrine when norepinephrine fails to achieve hemodynamic goals. It is also the first-line vasopressor in cardiac arrest and, like dopamine, is recommended for use in symptomatic bradycardia that does not respond to atropine.

Epinephrine is typically administered at doses of 0.01 to 0.20 µg/kg/min. Its beta effects predominate at lower doses, up to 0.1 µg/kg/min, and it has powerful effects on cardiac contractility and heart rate in this range.[36] At higher doses, epinephrine's alpha-1–mediated vasoconstrictive effects predominate, and its inoconstricting properties begin to approximate those of combined norepinephrine and dobutamine. A multicenter, randomized, controlled, double-blind study of 330 patients with septic shock showed no differences in the duration of vasopressor dependency, ICU or hospital duration of stay, or 28- and 90-day mortality when vasopressor therapy with epinephrine plus placebo was compared with combined norepinephrine and dobutamine.[37] There was no increase in adverse events in the epinephrine group; however, the epinephrine group did have significantly lower arterial pH values over the first 4 days, with significantly higher arterial lactate values on day one. Although these findings had no effect on the primary outcomes of interest, epinephrine's acid–base and metabolic effects are well-documented, and may reflect local ischemia from alpha-1–mediated vasoconstriction,[38] although it is increasingly believed that these effects result from the beta-2–mediated activation of the aerobic glycolytic pathway.[39]

Vasopressin

Vasopressin is an endogenous peptide hormone that produces contraction of vascular smooth muscle via V_1 receptors, which are ubiquitous in the systemic circulation, especially the skin and splanchnic vessels.[40] It is considered a nonadrenergic vasopressor adjunct in the treatment of sepsis-associated hypotension. Under normal physiologic conditions, vasopressin is primarily responsible for free water homeostasis. In healthy subjects, it is associated with only moderate vasoconstriction in the pulmonary and renal arterial systems and, at very low doses, can actually lead to pulmonary vasodilatation via release of endothelial nitric oxide.[41] The latter effect may be helpful in specific instances of acute right ventricular failure.[42] Vasopressin's effects on arterial tone becomes more significant in instances of acute hypotension, when it is released from the neurohypophysis in concentrations that are tens to hundreds of times greater than basal levels.[43] Endogenous vasopressin stores can become depleted within hours of shock onset. In this setting, normalization of circulating concentrations with exogenous administration can result in marked peripheral vasoconstriction and increased systolic and diastolic pressures.[44]

At the standard therapeutic dose, vasopressin is considered a "catecholamine-sparing" agent in severe sepsis, and is used most often in conjunction with norepinephrine. The SSC does not recommended its use as a single agent. The VASST (Vasopressin and Septic Shock Trial) study was a multicenter, randomized controlled, double-blind study of 778 septic patients who were dependent on vasopressor therapy to maintain goal MAPs. The study was designed to evaluate the use of the combination of vasopressin and norepinephrine compared with norepinephrine alone. Patients were stratified by disease severity based on their vasopressor requirements

1 hour before randomization; patients requiring 5 to 14 μg/min and greater than or equal to 15 μg/min of norepinephrine (or the equivalent) were considered to have less and more severe forms of septic shock, respectively. The use of low-dose vasopressin (0.03 U/min) significantly decreased the requirement for norepinephrine over the first 4 days of treatment, although this did not result in fewer adverse events. The study authors did report a trend toward improved 28- and 90-day mortality among patients with less severe shock in the combined therapy group, although the vasopressin group also demonstrated a trend toward higher incidence of digit ischemia (P = .11). Importantly, the study was neither powered to detect a mortality difference between combination vasopressin and norepinephrine therapy and single-agent norepinephrine, nor was it a study of vasopressor-refractory shock.[45]

Dopamine

Dopamine is no longer considered first-line treatment for hypotension in sepsis or septic shock. Its recommended use in sepsis is limited to a subset of patients at low risk for tachyarrhythmias or with bradycardia.[46] In the 2013 American Heart Association guidelines, dopamine was also no longer recommended as the first-line vasoactive medication in cardiogenic shock.[47] Dopamine remains an important component of the Advanced Cardiac Life Support protocol for the treatment of symptomatic bradycardia.

At low doses, dopamine acts primarily through presynaptic and postsynaptic dopaminergic DA2 and DA1 receptors, respectively. These receptors are scattered throughout the coronary, cerebral, renal, and splanchnic vascular beds. In healthy subjects, dopamine has been shown to directly increase effective renal plasma flow and natriuresis in a dose-dependent fashion, via a noncatecholaminergic pathway and independent of any changes in cardiac output.[48,49] For this reason, 'renal dose' dopamine was once thought to restore renal perfusion and protect septic patients from risk of acute kidney injury. However, one of the first randomized controlled trials on the subject demonstrated no benefit for progression to severe kidney injury or need for renal replacement therapy when low-dose dopamine was compared with placebo.[50] Similarly, Marik and Iglesias[51] showed no difference in progression to acute renal failure, the need for renal replacement therapy, or 28-day survival when low-dose dopamine, high-dose dopamine, and no dopamine strategies were compared in 395 oliguric patients with septic shock. The study authors postulated that renal afferent arteriolar dilatation is already maximized under septic conditions, thus limiting low-dose dopamine's potential renovascular protective effects.[52] In another prospective, double-blind, randomized controlled study of 40 ICU patients, low-dose dopamine resulted in decreased renal vascular resistance in patients with preserved renal function; the same doses, however, worsened resistive indices and renal perfusion in patients greater than 55 years of age with preexisting renal insufficiency.[53] The physiologic basis for this finding is not clear, but the study authors suggest that increased levels of endogenous dopamine in older patients with underlying renal insufficiency may predispose to higher tissue-specific concentrations of dopamine when the drug is administered exogenously. As a result of these and other studies, the use of low-dose dopamine for renal protection in sepsis is no longer recommended.

At doses of 2 to 10 μg/kg/min, dopamine's beta-1 effects become more apparent, and its effects on inotropy, dromotropy, and chronotropy predominate.[54] In chronically beta-blocked patients, however, dopamine's DA1- and DA2-mediated effects may continue to have significant effect even at these doses, and vasodilatation of the renal and splanchnic vasculature can precipitate worsening hypotension.[55]

At doses between 10 and 20 μg/kg/min, dopamine's alpha-1 effects predominate, increasing peripheral vascular resistance and MAP. Administration of doses of greater than 20 μg/kg/min can result in profound vasoconstriction, lead to limb ischemia, and worsen end-organ perfusion. Doses in this range are not recommended.

In a predefined subgroup analysis of the SOAP (Sepsis Occurrence in Acutely Ill Patients) II trial, a 2010 randomized controlled trial comparing dopamine and norepinephrine use in all forms of shock, there were no apparent differences in 28-day mortality in patients with septic shock; dopamine use was, however, associated with worse survival curves in patients with cardiogenic shock.[55] The reason for the increased mortality risk in these patients is unclear, but study investigators surmised that dopamine-mediated increases in heart rate were contributory. Notably, the median dopamine doses for all patients over the first 7 days fell within the medium to high dose range, but did not exceed 17 μg/kg/min.[55]

Phenylephrine

Phenylephrine is a pure alpha-1 agonist whose use in sepsis is not recommended except in very circumscribed conditions that include when norepinephrine use leads to or can be expected to exacerbate serious cardiac arrhythmias, when cardiac output is known to be high despite persistent hypotension, or as a vasopressor adjunct in refractory hypotension. Its use is more ideally suited to the purpose of rapidly correcting vasodilatory hypotension (eg, medication related or vagally mediated). Phenylephrine increases both arterial and venous tone at therapeutic doses and leads to rapid changes in MAP and a baroreflex-mediated bradycardia.

Randomized, controlled trials comparing the use of phenylephrine with norepinephrine in septic shock have explicitly excluded patients with underlying cardiac dysfunction,[56,57] or only included patients with baseline normal-to-high cardiac indices.[58] These studies failed to demonstrate any worsening of cardiac output when phenylephrine was used for hemodynamic support in septic shock. A study using animal models of septic shock with sepsis-induced cardiomyopathy, however, demonstrated worsening ventricular performance when phenylephrine was used.[59] A study of 18 nonseptic patients with underlying cardiac insufficiency demonstrated that single dose phenylephrine, in boluses of 50 to 200 μg, increased the MAP within 20 to 40 seconds of the infusion, with a concurrent and predictable worsening of cardiac output.[60] Negative effects on cardiac output were greatest in the patients with the poorest baseline cardiac function. Given the prevalence of sepsis-associated cardiomyopathy[61,62] and the challenges of appreciating the full complexity of an acutely ill patient's medical history in an emergency department setting, phenylephrine should be used rarely and with extreme caution.

INITIATING INOTROPIC THERAPY IN SEPSIS

Septic shock is a hyperdynamic process characterized by increased cardiac output and low systemic vascular resistance. Prolonged peripheral vasodilation and increased cardiac indices in sepsis can lead to high-output failure, or may mask an underlying myocardial depression.[63] Myocardial dysfunction is, in fact, common in sepsis and is thought to be explained by to a nonischemic phenomenon of myocardial depression and, possibly, even a self-protective 'hibernation' of the myocardium.[64] Although coronary artery blood flow has been shown to increase in sepsis, the measured difference between coronary artery and coronary sinus oxygen tensions is smaller than expected.[27] This finding suggests that a combination of altered cellular metabolism and autoregulatory changes in the microvasculature of the heart underlie the observed impairment in cardiac contractility in sepsis.

The use of inotropes in sepsis should be considered when there is evidence of myocardial dysfunction, as suggested by low cardiac output, increased filling pressures, or ongoing signs of hypoperfusion despite the restoration of adequate intravascular volume and adequate MAP with fluid and vasopressor therapy. Depending on the presence or absence of fixed valvular insufficiency, diastolic dysfunction, impaired venous return, or increased systemic vascular resistance, selective inotropy may have variable effects on intraventricular filling pressures. Ideally, the use of inotrope therapy augments cardiac contractility while offsetting increases in myocardial oxygen demand (owing to increased contractility and heart rate) with lower filling pressures.[65] Concurrent vasopressor use is often required to achieve this goal.

Dobutamine

Dobutamine is a dehydroxylated derivative of isoproterenol, with predominantly beta-1 and, to a lesser extent, beta-2 agonism.[66] Dobutamine is also a mild alpha-1 agonist, which is apparent at doses of greater than 15 μg/kg/min, but is more likely to lower systemic vascular resistance via its beta-2 effect at more clinically relevant doses of 5 to 15 μg/kg/min. Dobutamine is the SSCs first-line recommendation for inotropic support in septic patients with high filling pressures or other evidence of impaired cardiac output.

Dobutamine's inotropic effects are more prominent than its chronotropic effects; nevertheless, even at low doses it may increase myocardial oxygen demand and can precipitate malignant arrhythmias. In a 2007 multicenter, randomized controlled trial of 330 ICU patients in septic shock, the combination of dobutamine and norepinephrine had similar efficacy when compared with monotherapy epinephrine.[37] The 2 treatment groups also demonstrated similar side effect profiles and comparable frequencies of adverse events. The majority of adverse events in both the dobutamine plus norepinephrine and monotherapy epinephrine groups were supraventricular tachycardias (13% vs 12%, respectively) and ventricular arrhythmias (5% vs 7%, respectively). Lower frequencies of coronary events, central nervous system bleeding, ischemic strokes, and limb ischemia occurred in both groups (0.9%–2% overall). Vasopressor requirements were also comparable in the groups, and the median daily requirements for dobutamine did not exceed 6 μg/kg/min.

Milrinone

Milrinone is a nonadrenergic inodilator that exerts its effects via the inhibition of phosphodiesterase 3 and augmentation of cAMP. Cyclic AMP is a critical second messenger in cardiac cell signaling, and is degraded by phosphodiesterase 3. Cyclic AMP triggers the release of calcium from the sarcoplasmic reticulum, and increased cytosolic concentrations of calcium augment cardiac contractility. In the periphery, cAMP inhibits myosin light chain kinase, which binds and activates smooth muscle myosin. Milrinone's potentiation of cAMP's activity in the peripheral vasculature accounts for its vasodilatory effects. These effects may be welcome in cases of cardiogenic shock owing to right ventricular failure, because milrinone also decreases pulmonary vascular resistance. Administration of milrinone for its inotropic properties, however, frequently necessitates the concurrent use of a vasopressor if the phosphodiesterase 3 inhibitor's vasodilatory effects predominate. Milrinone, and inotropes in general, should be used very cautiously, if at all, in patients who are intravascularly volume depleted.

Because milrinone does not exert its effects through the catecholaminergic pathway, its use is specifically recommended in chronically beta-blocked patients, as well as in patients with longstanding heart failure who demonstrate downregulated expression and desensitization of adrenergic receptors.[66] Importantly, milrinone has a notably long half-life (2–4 hours) when compared with dobutamine (2 minutes), and is further prolonged in patients with renal failure. It is also significantly more expensive than dobutamine, and the 2 drugs have demonstrated similar clinical efficacy and mortality outcomes in patients with decompensated heart failure.[67]

Levosimendan

Levosimendan is currently not approved for use in the United States, but is used throughout Europe to provide inotropic support in acute decompensated heart failure. Levosimendan is a cardiac myofilament calcium-sensitizing inodilator. Its vasodilatory effects, which are active in the pulmonary, coronary, and peripheral vasculature, are thought to be mediated through various potassium channels in the smooth muscle. Levosimendan is believed to produce its inotropic effects through stabilization and prolongation of the binding of intracellular calcium to cardiac troponin C, thereby augmenting myofilament contractile forces without increasing the amplitude of intracellular calcium transit (ie, the rapid inward current of calcium that occurs during an action potential).[68] Cardiac dysfunction and electrical instability in patients with heart failure reflect, in part, a pattern of abnormal calcium cycling in and out of the cell and sarcoplasmic reticulum. This abnormal calcium cycling ultimately leads to cytoplasmic calcium overload, which is proarrhythmogenic[69]; in these circumstances, the desire for an inotropic agent that avoids beta-adrenergic stimulation is understandable.

Cardiac myocyte calcium homeostasis may, however, become altered in sepsis for a variety of reasons. Animal studies investigating calcium homeostasis in cardiac myocytes in the setting of endotoxemia have reported conflicting findings on the effects of lipopolysaccharide (an endotoxin) exposure, both in terms of myocyte calcium cycling and the myofilament force–calcium relationship.[70,71] It is clear that cardiac myocytes exposed to lipopolysaccharide demonstrate worsening contractility; it is less clear whether this phenomenon reflects abnormally rapid calcium cycling (which increases myocardial oxygen demand) and decreased myofilament sensitivity to calcium (with subsequent worsening of the myofilament force–calcium relationship) or, simply, sluggish intracellular calcium cycling. Pending the outcome of further investigation, future recommendations for inotropic support in sepsis may favor calcium-sensitizing agents over currently used inotropic agents, all of which increase cytoplasmic calcium concentrations.

VASOPRESSOR AND INOTROPE THERAPY IN PATIENTS WITH BASELINE HYPERTENSION

Higher MAP targets may be warranted in septic patients who have a history of chronic hypertension, and whose autoregulatory thresholds for end-organ perfusion are shifted rightward. The 2014 SEPSISPAM (Sepsis and Mean Arterial Pressure) study, although not adequately powered to detect a mortality benefit, showed no increased incidence of serious adverse events when higher MAPs of 80 to 85 mm Hg were targeted in septic patients with a history of hypertension.[72] The study was pragmatic in nature and allowed for provider discretion; the low target group ultimately achieved average MAPs of 70 to 75 mm Hg, compared with average MAPs of 85 to 90 mm Hg in the high target group. Among the significant subgroup of patients with chronic hypertension the high target group had a significantly lesser incidence of acute renal insufficiency (38.9% compared with 52.0%; $P = .02$), and a significantly decreased need for renal replacement within the first week (31.7% vs 42.2%; $P = .046$). Importantly, the time delay to achieving a minimum MAP of 65 mm Hg may be an independent predictor of mortality in chronically hypertensive patients.[73] Targeting MAPs of greater than 75 mm Hg in this patient population reflects a reasonable balance of the known risks and benefits.

SUMMARY

Evidence suggests that, once reasonable fluid resuscitation goals have been achieved, if hypotension persists, providers should promptly initiate vasopressor support with norepinephrine. If, after achieving adequate intravascular volume and adequate MAPs with fluid and vasopressor therapy, there is evidence of myocardial dysfunction or ongoing hypoperfusion, inotropic support with dobutamine should be considered. Vasopressor and inotrope therapy has complex effects that are often difficult to predict, and providers should consider both the physiology of these agents and clinical trial data when contemplating their use. As with any such intervention, it is essential to continually reevaluate the patient to determine if the selected treatment is having the intended result.

REFERENCES

1. Zarychanski R, Ariano RE, Paunovic B, et al. Historical perspectives in critical care medicine: blood transfusion, intravenous fluids, inotropes/vasopressors, and antibiotics. Crit Care Clin 2009;25:201–20.
2. Davenport HW. Epinephrin(e). Physiologist 1982;25(2):76–82. Available at: http://www.the-aps.org/mm/Publications/Journals/Physiologist/1980-1989/1982/April.pdf. Accessed February 22, 2016.
3. Hoffman BF. Adrenaline zips from bench to bedside. In: Hoffman BF, editor. Adrenaline. Cambridge (MA): Harvard University Press; 2013.
4. Ahlquist RP. A study of the adrenotropic receptors. Am J Physiol 1948;153: 586–600.
5. Glick G, Epstein SE, Wechsler AS, et al. Physiological differences between the effects of neuronally released and bloodborne norepinephrine on beta adrenergic receptors in the arterial bed of the dog. Circ Res 1967;21: 217–27.
6. Shepherd AP, Granger HJ, Smith EE, et al. Local control of tissue oxygen delivery and its contribution to the regulation of cardiac output. Am J Physiol 1973;225: 747–55.
7. Guyton AC, Jones CE, Coleman TG. Cardiac output and its regulation. 2nd edition. Philadelphia: Saunders; 1973.
8. Guimaraes S, Osswald W. Adrenergic receptors in the veins of the dog. Eur J Pharmacol 1969;5:133–40.
9. Medina P, Acuna A, Martinez-Leon JB, et al. Arginine vasopressin enhances sympathetic constriction through the V1 vasopressin receptor in human saphenous vein. Circulation 1998;97:865–70.
10. Kaiser GA, Ross J Jr, Braunwald E. Alpha and beta adrenergic receptor mechanisms in the systemic venous bed. J Pharmacol Exp Ther 1964;144: 156–62.
11. Guyton AC, Lindsey AW, Abernathy B, et al. Mechanism of the increased venous return and cardiac output caused by epinephrine. Am J Physiol 1957;192: 126–30.
12. Cannesson M, Jian Z, Chen G, et al. Effects of phenylephrine on cardiac output and venous return depend on the position of the heart on the Frank-Starling relationship. J Appl Physiol (1985) 2012;113:281–9.

13. Maas J, Pinsky MR, de Wilde RB, et al. Cardiac output response to norepineph-rine in postoperative cardiac surgery patients: interpretation with venous return and cardiac function curves. Crit Care Med 2013;41:143–50.
14. Persichini R, Silva S, Teboul JL, et al. Effects of norepinephrine on mean systemic pressure and venous return in human septic shock. Crit Care Med 2012;40:3146–53.
15. Cecconi M, Aya HD, Geisen M, et al. Changes in the mean systemic filling pres-sure during a fluid challenge in postsurgical intensive care patients. Intensive Care Med 2013;39:1299–305.
16. Berlin DA, Bakker J. Understanding venous return. Intensive Care Med 2014;40: 1564–6.
17. Goldberg LI, Bloodwell RD, Braunwald E, et al. The direct effects of norepineph-rine, epinephrine, and methoxamine on myocardial contractile force in man. Cir-culation 1960;22:1125–32.
18. Zausig YA, Geilfus D, Missler G, et al. Direct cardiac effects of dobutamine, dopa-mine, epinephrine, and levosimendan in isolated septic rat hearts. Shock 2010; 34:269–74.
19. Binion JT, Morgan WJ, Welch GH, et al. Effect of sympathomimetic drugs in acute experimental cardiac tamponade. Circ Res 1956;4:705–9.
20. Mueller H, Ayres SM, Gregory JJ, et al. Hemodynamics, coronary blood flow, and myocardial metabolism in coronary shock; response of 1-norepinephrine and isoproterenol. J Clin Invest 1970;49:1885–902.
21. Guyton AC, Lindsey AW, Gilluly JJ. The limits of right ventricular compensation following acute increase in pulmonary circulatory resistance. Circ Res 1954;2: 326–32.
22. Gould KL. Why angina pectoris in aortic stenosis. Circulation 1997;95:790–2.
23. Aviado DM Jr, Schmidt CF. Effects of sympathomimetic drugs on pulmonary cir-culation: with special reference to a new pulmonary vasodilator. J Pharmacol Exp Ther 1957;120:512–27.
24. Micek ST, McEvoy C, McKenzie M, et al. Fluid balance and cardiac function in septic shock as predictors of hospital mortality. Crit Care 2013;17:R246.
25. Bangash MN, Kong ML, Pearse RM. Use of inotropes and vasopressor agents in critically ill patients. Br J Pharmacol 2012;165:2015–33.
26. Langston JB, Guyton AC. Effect of epinephrine on the rate of urine formation. Am J Physiol 1958;192:131–4.
27. Hunter JD, Doddi M. Sepsis and the heart. Br J Anaesth 2010;104(1):3–11.
28. Bai X, Yu W, Ji W. Early versus delayed administration of norepinephrine in pa-tients with septic shock. Crit Care 2014;18:532. Available at: http://www.ncbi. nlm.nih.gov/pmc/articles/PMC4194405/. Accessed February 10, 2016.
29. McGee DC, Gould MK. Preventing complications of central venous catheteriza-tion. N Engl J Med 2003;348:1123–33.
30. Ricard JD, Salomon L, Boyer A, et al. Central or peripheral catheters for initial venous access of ICU patients: a randomized controlled trial. Crit Care Med 2013;41(9):2108–15.
31. Cardenas-Garcia J, Schaub K, Belchikov Y, et al. Safety of peripheral administra-tion of vasoactive medication. J Hosp Med 2015;10(9):581–5.
32. Loubani OM, Green RS. A systematic review of extravasation and local tissue injury from administration of vasopressors through peripheral intravenous cathe-ters and central venous catheters. J Crit Care 2015;30(3):653.e9-17.
33. Boerma EC, Ince C. The role of vasoactive agents in the resuscitation of micro-vascular perfusion and tissue oxygenation in critically ill patients. Intensive Care Med 2010;36:2004–18.

34. Avni T, Lador A, Lev S, et al. Vasopressors for the treatment of septic shock: systematic review and meta-analysis. PLoS One 2015;10(8):e0129305. Available at: http://www.ncbi.nlm.nih.gov/pmc/articles/PMC4523170/?report=reader.   Accessed March 10, 2016.

35. De Backer D, Aldecoa C, Nijmi H, et al. Dopamine versus norepinephrine in the treatment of septic shock: a meta-analysis. Crit Care Med 2012;40(3):725–30.

36. Jentzer JC, Coons JC, Link CB, et al. Pharmacotherapy update on the use of vasopressors and inotropes in the intensive care unit. J Cardiovasc Pharmacol Ther 2015;20(3):249–60.

37. Annane D, Vignon P, Renault A, et al, CATS Study Group. Norepinephrine plus dobutamine versus epinephrine alone for management of septic shock: a randomised trial. Lancet 2007;370:676–84.

38. Mahmoud KM, Ammar AS. Norepinephrine supplemented with dobutamine or epinephrine for the cardiovascular support of patients with septic shock. Indian J Crit Care Med 2012;16(2):75.

39. Levy B. Lactate and shock: the metabolic view. Curr Opin Crit Care 2006;12(4):315–21.

40. Barr JW, Lakin RC, Rosch J. Similarity of arterial and intravenous vasopressin on portal and systemic hemodynamics. Gastroenterology 1975;69:13–9.

41. Holmes CL, Landry DW, Granton JT. Science review: vasopressin and the cardiovascular system part 1–receptor physiology. Crit Care 2003;7:427–34.

42. Ventetuolo CE, Klinger JR. Management of acute right ventricular failure in the intensive care unit. Ann Am Thorac Soc 2014;11(5):811–22.

43. Landry DW, Oliver JA. The pathogenesis of vasodilatory shock. N Engl J Med 2001;345(8):588–95.

44. Landry DW, Levin HR, Gallant EM, et al. Vasopressin deficiency contributes to the vasodilation of septic shock. Circulation 1997;95(5):1122–5.

45. Russell JA, Walley KR, Singer J, et al. Vasopressin versus norepinephrine infusion in patients with septic shock. N Engl J Med 2008;358(9):877–87.

46. Dellinger RP, Levy MM, Rhodes A, et al. Surviving Sepsis Campaign: international guidelines for management of severe sepsis and septic shock: 2012. Crit Care Med 2013;41(2):580–637.

47. O'Gara PT, Kushner FG, Ascheim DD, et al. 2013 ACCF/AHA guideline for the management of ST-elevation myocardial infarction: a report of the American College of Cardiology Foundation/American Heart Association Task Force on Practice Guidelines. Circulation 2013;127:e362–425. Available at: https://www.heart.org/idc/groups/heart-public/@wcm/@mwa/documents/downloadable/ucm_453635.pdf. Accessed March 14, 2016.

48. Olsen NV. Effects of dopamine on renal haemodynamics, tubular function and sodium excretion in normal humans. Dan Med Bull 1998;45(3):282–97.

49. McDonald RH, Goldberg LI, McNay JL, et al. Effect of dopamine in man: augmentation of sodium excretion, glomerular filtration rate, and renal plasma flow. J Clin Invest 1964;43(6):1116–24.

50. Bellomo R, Chapman M, Finfer S, et al, ANZICS Clinical Trials Group. Low-dose dopamine in patients with early renal dysfunction: a placebo-controlled randomised trial. Lancet 2000;356(9248):2139–43.

51. Marik PE, Iglesias J, NORASEPT II. Low-dose dopamine does not prevent acute renal failure in patients with septic shock and oliguria. Am J Med 1999;107(4):392–5.

52. Bersten AD, Rutten AJ. Renovascular interaction of epinephrine, dopamine and intraperitoneal sepsis. Crit Care Med 1995;23(3):537–44.

53. Lauschke A, Teichgräber UK, Frei U, et al. 'Low-dose' dopamine worsens renal perfusion in patients with acute renal failure. Kidney Int 2006;69:1669–74.

54. Strehlow MC. Vasopressors and inotropes. In: Arbo JE, editor. Decision making in emergency critical care. Philadelphia: Wolters Kluwer; 2015.

55. De Backer D, Biston P, Devriendt J, et al. Comparison of dopamine and norepinephrine in the treatment of shock. N Engl J Med 2010;362(9):779–89. Available at: http://www.nejm.org/doi/suppl/10.1056/NEJMoa0907118/suppl_file/nejm_de_backer_779sa1.pdf. Accessed March 11, 2016.

56. Morelli A, Ertmer C, Rehberg S, et al. Phenylephrine versus norepinephrine for initial hemodynamic support of patients with septic shock: a randomized, controlled trial. Crit Care 2008;12(6):R143. Available at: http://www.ncbi.nlm.nih.gov/pmc/articles/PMC2646303/. Accessed February 10, 2015.

57. Jain G, Singh DK. Comparison of phenylephrine and norepinephrine in the management of dopamine-resistant septic shock. Indian J Crit Care Med 2010;14(1):29–34.

58. Gregory JS, Bonfiglio MF, Dasta JF, et al. Experience with phenylephrine as a component of the pharmacologic support of septic shock. Crit Care Med 1991;19(11):1396–400.

59. Ducrocq N, Kimmoun N, Furmaniuk A, et al. Comparison of equipressor doses of norepinephrine, epinephrine, and phenylephrine on septic myocardial dysfunction. Anesthesiology 2012;116(5):1083–91.

60. Schwinn DA, Reevs JG. Time course and hemodynamic effects of alpha-1-adrenergic bolus administration in anesthetized patients with myocardial disease. Anesth Analg 1989;68(5):571–8.

61. Vieillard-Baron A. Septic cardiomyopathy. Ann Intensive Care 2011;1:6. Available at: http://www.ncbi.nlm.nih.gov/pmc/articles/PMC3159902/pdf/2110-5820-1-6.pdf. Accessed March 15, 2016.

62. Romero-Bermejo FJ, Ruiz-Bailen M, Gil-Cebrian J, et al. Sepsis-induced cardiomyopathy. Curr Cardiol Rev 2011;7(3):163–83. Available at: http://www.ncbi.nlm.nih.gov/pmc/articles/PMC3263481/. Accessed March 15, 2016.

63. Merx MW, Weber C. Cardiovascular involvement in general medicine conditions: sepsis and the heart. Circulation 2007;116:793–802.

64. Levy RJ, Piel DA, Acton PD, et al. Evidence of myocardial hibernation in the septic heart. Crit Care Med 2005;33(12):2752–6.

65. Stevenson LW. Clinical use of inotropic therapy for heart failure: looking backward or forward? Part I: inotropic infusions during hospitalization. Circulation 2003;108:367–72.

66. Overgaard CB, Džavík V. Inotropes and vasopressors: review of physiology and clinical use in cardiovascular disease. Circulation 2008;118:1047–56.

67. Yamani MH, Haji SA, Starling HC, et al. Comparison of dobutamine-based and milrinone-based therapy for advanced decompensated congestive heart failure: hemodynamic efficacy, clinical outcome, and economic impact. Am Heart J 2001;142(6):998–1002.

68. Papp Z, Édes I, Fruhwald S, et al. Levosimendan: molecular mechanisms and clinical implications: consensus of experts on the mechanisms of action of levosimendan. Int J Cardiol 2012;159(2):82–7.

69. Wang Y, Goldhaber JI. Return of calcium: manipulating intracellular calcium to prevent cardiac pathologies. Proc Natl Acad Sci U S A 2004;101(16):5697–8.

70. Stamm C, Cowan DB, Friehs I, et al. Rapid endotoxin-induced alterations in myocardial calcium handling. Anesthesiology 2001;95(6):1396–405.

71. Takeuchi K, del Nido PJ, Ibrahim AE, et al. Increased myocardial calcium cycling and reduced myofilament calcium sensitivity in early endotoxemia. Surgery 1999; 126(2):231–8.
72. Asfar P, Meziani F, Hamel J, et al. High versus low blood-pressure targets in patients with septic shock. N Engl J Med 2014;370(17):1583–93.
73. Leone M, Asfar P, Radermacher P, et al. Optimizing mean arterial pressure in septic shock: a critical reappraisal of the literature. Crit Care 2015;19:101. Available at: http://www.ncbi.nlm.nih.gov/pmc/articles/PMC4355573/pdf/13054_2015_Article_794.pdf. Accessed March 8, 2016.

End Points of Sepsis Resuscitation

John C. Greenwood, MD[a,b],*, Clinton J. Orloski, MD[c]

KEYWORDS

- Resuscitation end points • Resuscitation • Sepsis • Septic shock • Critical care
- Lactate • Capillary refill time

KEY POINTS

- Using the CVP as an initial resuscitation end point and estimate of preload adequacy in the patient with sepsis is fraught with error; dynamic indices are preferred.
- Peripheral vasoactive infusions are acceptable in the short-term while assessing response to additional fluid challenges or central venous access is being secured.
- Targeting a supranormal cardiac index to provide higher levels of tissue oxygen delivery has not been shown to improve clinical outcomes.
- A peripheral lactate level of greater than 2 mmol/L is now recommended as a threshold that indicates sepsis-induced organ dysfunction.
- Serial assessment of capillary refill time, with normalization at 6 hours, is independently associated with successful resuscitation when compared with traditional microcirculatory resuscitation targets, such as $ScvO_2$, Pcv-aCO_2 gap, and lactate normalization.

INTRODUCTION

Sepsis is defined as a syndrome of life-threatening organ dysfunction caused by a dysregulated host response to infection.[1] If unrecognized and left untreated, patients with sepsis can quickly deteriorate, develop multisystem organ failure, and die. Physiologic changes that occur include peripheral vasodilation, myocardial depression, systemic microcapillary injury, coagulopathy, and end-organ malperfusion.[2–4]

Resuscitation goals for the patient with sepsis and septic shock attempt to return the patient to a physiologic state that promotes adequate organ perfusion along

Funding Sources: Nothing to disclose.
Conflict of Interest: Nothing to disclose.
[a] Department of Emergency Medicine, Perelman School of Medicine, University of Pennsylvania, 3400 Spruce Street, Ground Ravdin, Philadelphia, PA 19014, USA; [b] Department of Anesthesiology & Critical Care, Perelman School of Medicine, University of Pennsylvania, 3400 Spruce Street, Ground Ravdin, Philadelphia, PA 19014, USA; [c] Department of Emergency Medicine, Hospital of the University of Pennsylvania, 3400 Spruce Street, Ground Ravdin, Philadelphia, PA 19104, USA
* Corresponding author. Department of Emergency Medicine, Perelman School of Medicine, University of Pennsylvania, 3400 Spruce Street, Ground Ravdin, Philadelphia, PA 19014.
E-mail address: john.greenwood@uphs.upenn.edu

with matching metabolic supply and demand. Ideal resuscitation end points should assess the adequacy of tissue oxygen delivery (DO_2), oxygen consumption (VO_2), and should be quantifiable and reproducible. Despite years of research, a single resuscitation end point to assess the adequacy of sepsis resuscitation has yet to be found. As a result, the clinician must rely on multiple end points to determine the patient's overall response to therapy. This article discusses the roles and limitations of currently recommended resuscitation end points, and identifies novel resuscitation targets that may help guide therapeutic interventions in the patient with sepsis and septic shock.

CURRENT RESUSCITATION TARGETS FOR SEPSIS AND SEPTIC SHOCK

To address the many physiologic derangements that occur in patients with sepsis, and also provide objective resuscitation triggers to guide clinical intervention, several organizations have developed treatment "bundles" that include hemodynamic and physiologic markers used to assess physiologic status of the patient with sepsis. The Surviving Sepsis Campaign has become one of the international leaders of bundled or protocolized sepsis care, and has made a significant impact on the mortality attributed to sepsis and septic shock.[5,6] The most recent iteration of the Surviving Sepsis Campaign guidelines focuses on several resuscitation targets identified by the original early goal-directed therapy (EGDT) protocol, with an emphasis on macrocirculatory and microcirculatory end points (**Box 1**).[7,8]

Protocolized sepsis resuscitation is not without controversy. To test the current paradigm of sepsis care, three separate multicenter randomized control trials compared the EGDT protocol with contemporary care and found no difference in clinical outcomes.[9–11] The results of ProCESS, ARISE, and ProMISe trials have generated a significant debate about the value of a "one size fits all" approach in sepsis resuscitation.[5,12]

MACROCIRCULATORY RESUSCITATION END POINTS

In the initial phase of sepsis resuscitation, it is important to first target macrocirculatory resuscitation end points. Macrocirculatory targets can usually be measured rapidly at the bedside and address intravascular volume status, mean arterial pressure (MAP), and cardiac output. Early recognition of macrocirculatory derangements often prevents early cardiovascular collapse and is a good initial step in the resuscitation of the patient with sepsis or septic shock.

Box 1
Surviving Sepsis Campaign resuscitation goals within the first 6 hours

1. Protocolized, quantitative resuscitation of patients with sepsis-induced tissue hypoperfusion (defined as hypotension persisting after initial fluid challenge or blood lactate concentration ≥4 mmol/L).
   a. Central venous pressure
      i. Spontaneously breathing patients: 8 to 12 mm Hg
      ii. Mechanically ventilated patients: 12 to 15 mm Hg
   b. Mean arterial pressure ≥65 mm Hg
   c. Urine output ≥0.5 mL/kg/h
   d. Central venous oxygen saturation 70% or mixed venous oxygen saturation ≥65%

2. In patients with elevated lactate levels targeting resuscitation to normalize lactate as rapidly as possible.

Intravascular Volume Status

Intravenous fluid administration is a cornerstone of sepsis resuscitation. Rapid fluid administration in the setting of hypovolemia or significant vasoplegia often restores visceral blood flow and tissue DO_2 by improving cardiac output and consequently MAP. An initial, empiric fluid challenge of 500 mL of intravenous crystalloid solution up to a maximum of 30 mL/kg is a reasonable first approach to improve a patient's hemodynamic status.[9,10,13]

Additional crystalloid administration should be driven by objective clinical findings that suggest additional fluid therapy would improve cardiac output and organ perfusion. The utility of intravascular fluid resuscitation is limited by the amount of time resuscitative fluids remain within the intravascular space.[14,15] Overresuscitation can lead to significant downstream complications, which include significant third spacing and reduced delivery of oxygen to end-organ tissues.[16]

Static measures of volume responsiveness are defined as pressure or volumetric hemodynamic indices that are measured at a single point in time for preload assessment (ie, central venous pressure [CVP], pulmonary artery occlusion pressure). Static measures of preload assessment have largely been replaced with dynamic indices that take advantage of heart-lung interactions to predict volume responsiveness. Stroke volume variation, pulse pressure variation, and inferior vena cava variability all have a better positive predictive value, sensitivity, and specificity than static measures.[17–19] Direct measurement tests of volume responsiveness include the end-expiratory occlusion test and passive leg raise and may be preferred over dynamic measures, because these tests can be used in patients who are spontaneously breathing, have arrhythmias, and can help avoid unnecessary fluid administration.[20–22]

Central Venous Pressure

The CVP is a static, barometric measurement that requires a central venous catheter for measurement, and describes the pressure generated by the intravascular blood volume present in the superior vena cava. It is a directly measured estimate of right atrial and right ventricular end-diastolic pressure. Traditionally, the CVP has been used as an estimate of intravascular volume status and a predictor of volume responsiveness. In a healthy, nonintubated patient, the CVP is approximately 2 mm Hg to 4 mm Hg.

Current recommendations suggest that CVP in the patient with sepsis should be increased with intravenous fluids to a goal of 8 mm Hg to 12 mm Hg in spontaneously breathing patients, or 12 mm Hg to 15 mm Hg in mechanically ventilated patients, to ensure adequate preload to optimize cardiac output.[23] Unfortunately, several patient-related and physiologic changes can impact the CVP and make it an unreliable tool for preload optimization.[24–26] Even traditional teaching, that a low CVP is often a reliable measure of volume responsiveness, has been found to have a positive predictive value of only 47% in patients with sepsis.[24]

Using the CVP as an initial resuscitation target and estimate of preload adequacy is fraught with error, because there are several confounding factors that can impact the CVP outside of intravascular volume status (**Box 2**). In general, initial fluid resuscitation should be actively guided by dynamic measures of volume responsiveness to improve cardiac output and end-organ perfusion.

Mean Arterial Pressure

One of the hallmark hemodynamic derangements that can lead to organ dysfunction in sepsis is hypotension. Diagnostic criteria for sepsis-related arterial hypotension

---

Box 2
Potential factors impacting central venous pressure

1. Central venous blood volume
   a. Venous return/cardiac output
   b. Total blood volume
   c. Regional vascular tone

2. Thoracic, cardiac, and vascular compliance
   a. Pulmonary hypertension
   b. Right ventricular compliance, diastolic dysfunction
   c. Pericardial disease
   d. Tamponade

3. Valvular disease
   a. Tricuspid stenosis
   b. Tricuspid regurgitation

4. Cardiac rhythm
   a. Junctional rhythm
   b. Atrial fibrillation
   c. Nonsinus rhythm

5. Intrathoracic pressure
   a. Spontaneous or noncontrolled respiration
   b. Intermittent positive pressure ventilation
   c. Positive end-expiratory pressure

6. Reference level of pressure transducer and patient positioning

---

include a systolic blood pressure of less than 100 mm Hg (recently increased from 90 mm Hg),[1] MAP less than 70 mm Hg, or an systolic blood pressure decrease of more than 40 mm Hg in adults or less than two standard deviations below normal for a given age.[8]

An initial MAP target of 65 mm Hg during the acute phases of sepsis resuscitation is generally recommended, with individualized MAP titration after stabilization.[8] The threshold target of 65 mm Hg is largely based off of a small set of retrospective, prospective, and observational studies that found adequate perfusion measures and a reduction in associated mortality with MAP threshold of 65 mm Hg.[27,28] Targeting a higher MAP has not been found to reduce organ dysfunction or improve global outcomes, but may improve microvascular perfusion on an individualized basis.[28,29]

In 2014, the multicenter Sepsis and Mean Arterial Pressure (SEPSISPAM) randomized controlled trial was conducted to look specifically at outcomes related to higher MAP compared with standard goals (target of 80–85 mm Hg vs 65–70 mm Hg) and found no significant difference in 28- or 90-day mortality. A predefined subset of patients with chronic hypertension required less renal-replacement therapy than those in the low-target group.[30] The SEPSISPAM trial reinforced the need for clinicians to recognize the potential benefit of individualized blood pressure titration, especially in patients with chronic disease.

Interventions to achieve a MAP greater than 65 mm Hg in the patient presenting with sepsis or septic shock should begin with an assessment of intravascular volume status to determine the clinical utility of intravascular fluid loading to improve cardiac output and mean blood pressure. Once adequate intravascular volume status has been achieved, early administration of vasopressors should be initiated if the patient remains hypotensive. Norepinephrine is generally the initial vasopressor of choice in septic shock, starting at a dose of 0.05 μg/kg/min.[31]

Rapid initiation of vasopressor therapy in the setting of fluid-refractory shock is a time-critical intervention. Delayed initiation of vasopressor therapy can lead to excessive fluid resuscitation and increased morbidity and mortality. A mortality increase of 5.3% has been estimated to occur for every 1-hour delay in vasopressor initiation during the first 6 hours of septic shock.[32] In patients who are not responding to escalating doses of norepinephrine, early administration of adjunctive therapies should also be considered. The addition of stress-dose hydrocortisone, along with vasopressin-replacement therapy, or an epinephrine infusion is generally recommended as second-line agents.

Traditionally, vasoactive administration required a central venous catheter out of fear of complications related to extravasation and soft tissue necrosis; however, more recent literature suggests that this complication is rare.[33,34] Delays in vasoactive support are avoided safely by administering vasopressors through a proximal, large-bore peripheral intravenous access line. Peripheral vasoactive infusions are acceptable in the short-term while assessing response to additional fluid challenges or central venous access is being secured.

Cardiac Output and Cardiac Index

The early phase of septic shock is often characterized by a low systemic vascular resistance and a high cardiac output or cardiac index. Most patients with sepsis present with "warm shock," a term used to describe a hypotensive patient with flushed skin, bounding peripheral pulse, yet a significant mismatch between DO_2 and metabolic demand. The patient with sepsis with "cold shock," presenting with poor peripheral perfusion and cool extremities, suggesting poor cardiac output, is less common. An abnormally low cardiac output presenting as cold shock is associated with inadequate volume resuscitation, but can occur in the setting of acute sepsis-induced cardiac dysfunction or during the late phases of septic shock.[35]

Sepsis-induced cardiac dysfunction is a well-described phenomenon that leads to a reduction in left ventricular stroke volume and impaired myocardial performance. The incidence of myocardial depression is estimated to occur in up to 60% of patients with septic shock.[3] The exact cause of cardiac dysfunction in sepsis is unclear, but is believed to be a multifactorial cellular insult on myocardial tissues that includes decreased β-adrenergic receptor sensitivity, calcium sensitivity, increased nitric oxide production, mitochondrial dysfunction, and cell death.[35]

Assessing cardiac output in patients with septic shock is performed by several minimally invasive and noninvasive methods, including pulse wave contour analysis devices, such as the LiDCO (LiDCO Ltd, London, UK); PiCCO (Pulsion Maquet, Munich, Germany); FloTrac/Vigileo system (Edwards Lifesciences Corp, Irvine, CA); bioreactance measurement systems, such as the NICOM (Cheetah Medical, Boston, MA); or bedside echocardiography. The routine use of invasive cardiac output monitoring devices, such as the pulmonary artery catheter, has been associated with increased patient risks without significant benefit, and as a result their use has fallen out of favor.[36]

Despite the increased recognition of sepsis-induced cardiac dysfunction, not all patients with a reduced left ventricular ejection fraction require inotropic therapy. Using equipment that is generally available in most acute care settings, a general assessment of cardiac function is acquired with minimal training. Calculating a patient's cardiac output is performed by obtaining two, simple echocardiographic measurements (**Fig. 1**). Stroke volume is estimated by calculating the product of the patient's left ventricular outflow tract (LVOT) velocity-time integral and the patient's aortic valve area measured with bedside echocardiography. The LVOT velocity-time integral is

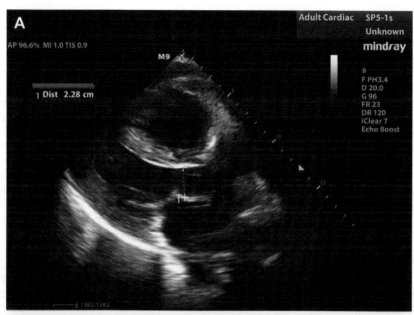

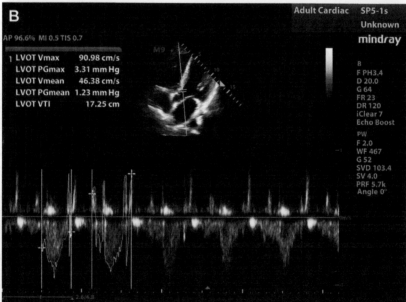

Fig. 1. (*A*) Measurement of the left ventricular outflow tract (LVOT) diameter during systole, which can be used to estimate the aortic valve area using transthoracic echocardiography (TTE). (*B*) Measurement of the LVOT velocity time integral (VTI) in the apical five-chamber view.

measured in the apical five-chamber view using the pulsed-wave Doppler function, with the marker placed within the LVOT. The aortic valve area is estimated by measuring the diameter of the patient's LVOT approximately 1 cm below the aortic valve in the parasternal long axis. Multiplying the patient's estimated stroke volume by their current heart rate yields the cardiac output. Cardiac index is calculated by dividing the patient's cardiac output by their body surface area. Note that cardiac dysrhythmias and inaccurate LVOT diameter measurements can significantly impact the accuracy of cardiac output measurement.

After adequate volume resuscitation and initiation of vasopressor support, if a patient continues to have poor cardiac output (cardiac index of <2.2 L/min/m^2) with evidence of poor perfusion, it is reasonable to add inotropic therapy. Dobutamine is recommended as the first-line inotropic infusion, at a starting dose of 2.5 mg/kg/min in patients with adequate ventricular filling and MAP.[8] Alternatively, epinephrine may provide adequate inotropic support if given at lower infusion doses (up to 0.1 μg/kg/min) without the vasodilatory effects caused by dobutamine's β$_2$ activity.[37] If choosing epinephrine, it is important to recognize that the ability to monitor lactate clearance may be negatively impacted because of increased aerobic glycolysis and lactate production.[38]

In patients with adequate volume resuscitation and an escalating norepinephrine requirement, the decision algorithm in **Fig. 2** may be considered. A specific cardiac index goal is not currently recommended; however, a reasonable approach is to initially target a cardiac index of 2.2 L/min/m^2 to 2.5 L/min/m^2. Targeting a supranormal cardiac index to provide higher levels of tissue DO$_2$ has not been shown to improve clinical outcomes.[39]

MICROCIRCULATORY RESUSCITATION END POINTS

After achieving the macrocirculatory targets during the initial phase of sepsis resuscitation it is important to assess whether these end points have established adequate organ perfusion. Some patients who achieved macrocirculatory thresholds may

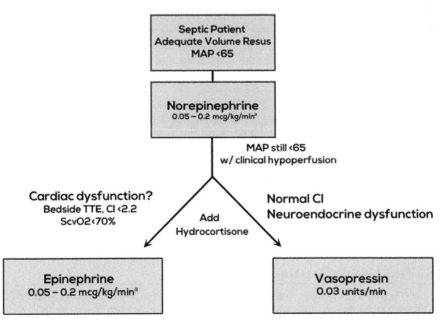

Fig. 2. Potential decision algorithm for second-line vasoactive therapy in the management of septic shock. [a] There is no maximum dose for norepinephrine or epinephrine. CI, cardiac index; ScvO$_2$, central venous oxygen saturation; TTE, transthoracic echocardiography.

require continued resuscitative efforts to reverse their occult, or "cryptic," shock, whereas others may not need to be maintained at the established macrocirculatory thresholds.[40,41]

The next step of resuscitation is to assess the adequacy of organ perfusion by way of microcirculatory resuscitation targets. Microcirculation is defined by a network of arterioles, capillaries, and postcapillary venules that are responsible for the delivery of red blood cells and plasma to organs so that cellular exchange of oxygen, carbon dioxide, nutrients, cytokines, and metabolic waste removal can occur. Sepsis-induced inflammation, coagulopathy, leukocyte dysfunction, and overproduction of nitric oxide can lead to significant changes in microvascular blood flow, cytotoxic stress, and an imbalance between oxygen delivery and demand.[2,42–44]

There are several clinical and laboratory values used to assess microvascular perfusion, the most common being peripheral lactate and central venous oxygen saturation ($ScvO_2$). Clinical assessment of microcirculation can also be performed by way of capillary refill time (CRT), and in some cases urine output.

Lactate

Peripheral lactate, also referred to as lactic acid, has become one of the most widely used biomarkers to diagnose sepsis-induced organ dysfunction. It is drawn from a peripheral intravenous line and has been shown to correlate with venous, arterial, and capillary blood samples.[45,46] Traditionally, a venous lactate greater than or equal to 4 mmol/L has been used as an initial screen for sepsis-induced organ dysfunction, but more recently, a lactate threshold of 2 mmol/L has been recommended.[1,8,47–49]

In a healthy individual at rest, peripheral lactate concentrations are usually between 0.5 mmol/L and 2 mmol/L. During periods of physiologic stress, lactate generation often occurs. An elevated lactate in the patient with sepsis has been associated with a significantly increased risk of mortality.[50] Unfortunately, a rise in lactate is not always associated with obvious hemodynamic abnormalities.[51] "Cryptic shock" is a term used to describe the patient with apparently normal vital signs but a significant elevation in peripheral lactate. Despite reassuring vital signs, the patient with sepsis with cryptic shock has a mortality risk similar to those with overt shock, and should receive careful resuscitation.[41]

A significant debate regarding the utility of lactate as a resuscitation end point remains in the academic community.[52] Traditional theory is that increased lactate production occurs in sepsis as a result of global tissue hypoxia, where oxygen supply (DO_2) fails to meet oxygen demand (VO_2). The resulting DO_2/VO_2 mismatch leads to increased anaerobic metabolism and a rise in the patient's lactate level.

Unfortunately, this simplistic explanation for a rise in lactate fails to consider multiple other physiologic and nonphysiologic contributors to an elevated lactate (**Box 3**). Despite the nuances of lactate generation and metabolism, the use of lactate as a marker of microcirculatory perfusion adequacy and resuscitation response seems to be the best option to date, but clinicians should be aware of its limitations and potential confounders.[53,54]

Mixed and Central Venous Oxygen Saturation

Achieving adequate tissue oxygenation along with avoiding tissue dysoxia is essential to prevent cell injury, oxygen debt, organ dysfunction, and death. Both mixed venous oxygen saturation (SvO_2) and $ScvO_2$ have been proposed as important resuscitation targets in the patient with sepsis, because they can be used to estimate a global balance of cellular oxygen delivery and demand. A low $ScvO_2$ (<70%) indicates an

---

Box 3
Causes of lactate elevation in sepsis

1. Anaerobic glycolysis: caused by tissue hypoxemia

2. Aerobic glycolysis: increased stress response, endogenous catecholamine release, and stimulation of β_2 receptors

3. Mitochondrial dysfunction: limited pyruvate metabolism

4. Acute lung injury: metabolic adaptation to inflammatory mediators

5. Decreased lactate clearance
   a. Liver failure or dysfunction
   b. Renal failure or dysfunction

6. Drugs and toxins: patient medications (eg, metformin), vasoactive agents, toxic ingestions (eg, ethanol)

7. Other causes: metabolic alkalosis

---

inadequate DO_2 to tissues, an increased extraction at the cellular level (Vo_2), or a combination of these two factors.

To obtain an SvO_2/$ScvO_2$ measurement, the sampling location is an important consideration. A true SvO_2 measurement requires a pulmonary artery catheter, and an $ScvO_2$ measurement must be obtained through a central venous catheter where the tip is appropriately placed at the junction of the superior vena cava and right atrium. Femoral-based $ScvO_2$ is not a reliable substitute for an $ScvO_2$ measurement taken from the superior vena cava–right atrium junction.[55]

If measured from the appropriate location, an $ScvO_2$ between 70% and 89% would suggest an adequate Vo_2/DO_2 balance, and seems to correlate well with a normal SvO2 value between 60% and 70%.[56] A supranormal $ScvO_2$ value equal or greater than 90% suggests poor oxygen utilization, tissue dysoxia, or significant microcirculatory shunting and is associated with a high mortality.[57]

Since the original EGDT trial was published in 2001, several studies have examined the use of peripheral lactate versus $ScvO_2$ optimization and have found no difference in patient-centered outcomes.[9,10,13,48] Outside of the EGDT trial, the incidence of an abnormally low $ScvO_2$ in patients with sepsis that present to the emergency department and at intensive care unit admission seems to be low.[9,58] Currently, the routine use of $ScvO_2$ should not be incorporated into current sepsis resuscitation protocols. However, there may be a role for $ScvO_2$ monitoring in specific sepsis phenotypes (eg, sepsis-induced cardiac dysfunction) and future research should attempt to determine its utility.[59]

Central Venous-Arterial CO₂ Gradient

The inability of a normal or high $ScvO_2$ to regularly determine adequate organ perfusion has led clinicians to look for other markers of tissue hypoxia and metabolic disequilibrium. The venous-to-arterial carbon dioxide gradient has been proposed as one of these adjunctive tests to determine if the patient has achieved adequate cardiac output along with adequate microcirculatory flow and perfusion. It is calculated by subtracting the arterial Pco_2 from the central venous Pco_2 ($ScvO_2$).

The Pcv-aCO₂ gap has become more popular in recent years as a resuscitation end point largely because CO_2 is more soluble than O_2 in the blood and may be able to more accurately detect microcirculatory dysfunction, even in the setting of heterogeneous or poor microcirculatory flow. In multiple studies, a $Pcv-aCO_2$ gap that is less than 6 mm Hg has been found to be associated with a higher cardiac index, better lactate clearance, and improved microcirculatory perfusion.[60–62] Conversely, a $Pcv-aCO_2$ gap that is greater than 6 mm Hg can reliably reflect critical hypoperfusion and the need for further resuscitation.[63]

CLINICAL ASSESSMENTS OF PERFUSION

Interventions during the resuscitation of the patient with sepsis or shock should be performed in tandem with regular reassessment of clinical response. Laboratory testing is often relied on to determine improvements in end-organ perfusion, but in some cases advanced laboratory testing may not be readily available. It is important for the clinician to also have an array bedside tools that can help assess resuscitation adequacy if necessary.

Capillary Refill Time

The assessment of CRT in the patient with sepsis may seem counterintuitive, because pathophysiologic derangements often lead to peripheral vasodilation resulting in warm, flushed extremities. However, emerging literature suggests CRT may be a valuable bedside tool to assess the adequacy of not only regional, but also global tissue perfusion during the resuscitation phase of septic shock.[64]

CRT is a simple, low cost, and reliable evaluation of microvascular perfusion that is performed rapidly at the bedside.[65,66] It is defined as the duration of time needed for the patient's fingertip to regain color after direct pressure is applied to cause blanching. In a healthy patient, the CRT should be less than 3.5 seconds. Skin temperature, ambient room temperature, age, and vasoactive medications can significantly impact CRT and should be considered during each assessment.

In the patient with sepsis, assuming the patient's extremities are normothermic, delayed CRT of more than 5 seconds suggests abnormal microcirculatory flow and need for further intervention (**Fig. 3**).[67] Serial assessment of CRT with normalization at 6 hours is independently associated with successful resuscitation when compared against traditional resuscitation targets, such as $ScvO_2$, $Pcv-aCO_2$ gap, and lactate normalization.[68] In the postresuscitation phase of critical illness, delayed CRT may also be a predictor of worsening organ failure and shock.[69]

Urine Output and Oliguria

Acute kidney injury (AKI) is defined by a relative increase in serum creatinine, reduction in glomerular filtration rate, or reduced urine output and is the most common organ dysfunction associated with sepsis in critically ill patients.[70,71] Traditional resuscitation

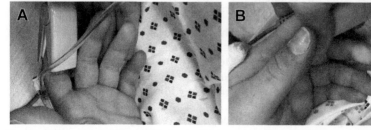

Fig. 3. (A) Normal capillary refill time of less than 3.5 seconds. (B) Abnormal capillary refill time of greater than 5 seconds.

end points, including those from the most recent Surviving Sepsis Campaign, recommend a patient's urine output be greater than 0.5 mL/kg/min to suggest adequate renal perfusion in the early stages of resuscitation.[8]

Urine output is largely a function of glomerular filtration, tubular secretion, and reabsorption. Glomerular filtration is particularly dependent on renal blood flow (RBF), which is dependent on circulating blood volume, cardiac output, and renal perfusion pressure. In a healthy state, RBF is stable over a wide range of MAPs because of local autoregulation.[72] In periods of shock, or specifically the patient with sepsis, mechanisms responsible for blood flow autoregulation become impaired.

Unfortunately, the pathophysiologic process leading to oliguria and AKI is far more complex than addressing macrocirculatory resuscitation targets alone. Clinicians have attempted to pharmacologically increase urine output in high-risk patients by increasing RBF with low-dose dopamine and decrease tubular Vo_2 with diuretics, but neither of these interventions has been shown to reduce the incidence of AKI, and is not recommended.[73,74]

During the resuscitation phase of sepsis and shock, interventions to improve urine output should focus on intravascular fluid optimization, achieving macrohemodynamic goals, and avoiding unnecessary nephrotoxic agents. Choice of intravenous crystalloid, at least for the first 2 to 3 L, does not seem to have an impact on the development of AKI.[75] For large-volume resuscitations, it is reasonable to switch to a balanced crystalloid solution (eg, lactated Ringer) to avoid the development of a worsening hyperchloremic metabolic acidosis, which has been associated with the development of AKI and need for renal-replacement therapy.[76]

SUMMARY

Early, aggressive resuscitation of the acutely ill patient with sepsis and septic shock is a fundamental concept in emergency medicine and critical care. Initial resuscitative efforts should focus on achieving established macrocirculatory goals, including adequate intravascular volume status, MAP, and cardiac output. The patient's global response to resuscitative interventions is assessed with the evaluation of microcirculatory end points including peripheral lactate, $ScvO_2$, and carbon dioxide gradients ($Pcv\text{-}aCO_2$). Further attention to clinical findings, such as CRT and urine output, may help the clinician recognize subtle microvascular perfusion abnormalities, but have important limitations to consider.

REFERENCES

1. Singer M, Deutschman CS, Seymour C, et al. The third international consensus definitions for sepsis and septic shock (SEPSIS-3). JAMA 2016;315(8):801–10.
2. De Backer D, Creteur J, Preiser J-C, et al. Microvascular blood flow is altered in patients with sepsis. Am J Respir Crit Care Med 2002;166(1):98–104.
3. Vieillard-Baron A, Caille V, Charron C, et al. Actual incidence of global left ventricular hypokinesia in adult septic shock. Crit Care Med 2008;36(6):1701–6.
4. King EG, Bauzá GJ, Mella JR, et al. Pathophysiologic mechanisms in septic shock. Lab Invest 2014;94(1):4–12.
5. Levy MM, Rhodes A, Phillips GS, et al. Surviving Sepsis Campaign: association between performance metrics and outcomes in a 7.5-year study. Crit Care Med 2015;43(1):3–12.
6. Levy MM, Dellinger RP, Townsend SR, et al. The Surviving Sepsis Campaign: results of an international guideline-based performance improvement program targeting severe sepsis. Crit Care Med 2010;38(2):367–74.

7. Rivers E, Nguyen B, Havstad S, et al. Early goal-directed therapy in the treatment of severe sepsis and septic shock. N Engl J Med 2001;345(19):1368–77.

8. Dellinger RP, Levy MM, Rhodes A, et al. Surviving Sepsis Campaign: international guidelines for management of severe sepsis and septic shock: 2012. Crit Care Med 2013;41(2):580–637.

9. ProCESS Investigators, Yealy DM, Kellum JA, et al. A randomized trial of protocol-based care for early septic shock. N Engl J Med 2014;370(18):1683–93.

10. ARISE Investigators, ANZICS Clinical Trials Group, Delaney A, Bailey M, Peake SL, et al. Goal-directed resuscitation for patients with early septic shock. N Engl J Med 2014;371(16):1496–506.

11. Mouncey PR, Osborn TM, Power GS, et al. Protocolised Management In Sepsis (ProMISe): a multicentre randomised controlled trial of the clinical effectiveness and cost-effectiveness of early, goal-directed, protocolised resuscitation for emerging septic shock. Health Technol Assess 2015;19(97):1–150.

12. Girbes ARJ, Robert R, Marik PE. Protocols: help for improvement but beware of regression to the mean and mediocrity. Intensive Care Med 2015;41(12): 2218–20.

13. Mouncey PR, Osborn TM, Power GS, et al. Trial of early, goal-directed resuscitation for septic shock. N Engl J Med 2015;372(14):1301–11.

14. Gondos T, Marjanek Z, Ulakcsai Z, et al. Short-term effectiveness of different volume replacement therapies in postoperative hypovolaemic patients. Eur J Anaesthesiol 2010;27(9):794–800.

15. Lobo DN, Stanga Z, Aloysius MM, et al. Effect of volume loading with 1 liter intravenous infusions of 0.9% saline, 4% succinylated gelatine (Gelofusine) and 6% hydroxyethyl starch (Voluven) on blood volume and endocrine responses: a randomized, three-way crossover study in healthy volunteers. Crit Care Med 2010; 38(2):464–70.

16. Monnet X, Julien F, Ait-Hamou N, et al. Lactate and venoarterial carbon dioxide difference/arterial-venous oxygen difference ratio, but not central venous oxygen saturation, predict increase in oxygen consumption in fluid responders. Crit Care Med 2013;41(6):1412–20.

17. Feissel M, Michard F, Faller J-P, et al. The respiratory variation in inferior vena cava diameter as a guide to fluid therapy. Intensive Care Med 2004;30(9):1834–7.

18. Reuter DA, Bayerlein J, Goepfert MSG, et al. Influence of tidal volume on left ventricular stroke volume variation measured by pulse contour analysis in mechanically ventilated patients. Intensive Care Med 2003;29(3):476–80.

19. Michard F, Boussat S, Chemla D, et al. Relation between respiratory changes in arterial pulse pressure and fluid responsiveness in septic patients with acute circulatory failure. Am J Respir Crit Care Med 2000;162(1):134–8.

20. Monnet X, Bataille A, Magalhaes E, et al. End-tidal carbon dioxide is better than arterial pressure for predicting volume responsiveness by the passive leg raising test. Intensive Care Med 2013;39(1):93–100.

21. Monnet X, Bleibtreu A, Ferré A, et al. Passive leg-raising and end-expiratory occlusion tests perform better than pulse pressure variation in patients with low respiratory system compliance. Crit Care Med 2012;40(1):152–7.

22. Monnet X, Rienzo M, Osman D, et al. Passive leg raising predicts fluid responsiveness in the critically ill. Crit Care Med 2006;34(5):1402–7.

23. Packman MI, Rackow EC. Optimum left heart filling pressure during fluid resuscitation of patients with hypovolemic and septic shock. Crit Care Med 1983; 11(3):165–9.

24. Osman D, Ridel C, Ray P, et al. Cardiac filling pressures are not appropriate to predict hemodynamic response to volume challenge. Crit Care Med 2007; 35(1):64–8.

25. Vincent J-L, Weil MH. Fluid challenge revisited. Crit Care Med 2006;34(5): 1333–7.

26. Marik PE, Cavallazzi R. Does the central venous pressure predict fluid responsiveness? An updated meta-analysis and a plea for some common sense. Crit Care Med 2013;41(7):1774–81.

27. Varpula M, Tallgren M, Saukkonen K, et al. Hemodynamic variables related to outcome in septic shock. Intensive Care Med 2005;31(8):1066–71.

28. LeDoux D, Astiz ME, Carpati CM, et al. Effects of perfusion pressure on tissue perfusion in septic shock. Crit Care Med 2000;28(8):2729–32.

29. Wo CC, Shoemaker WC, Appel PL, et al. Unreliability of blood pressure and heart rate to evaluate cardiac output in emergency resuscitation and critical illness. Crit Care Med 1993;21(2):218–23.

30. Asfar P, Meziani F, Hamel J-F, et al. High versus low blood-pressure target in patients with septic shock. N Engl J Med 2014;370(17):1583–93.

31. De Backer D, Aldecoa C, Njimi H, et al. Dopamine versus norepinephrine in the treatment of septic shock: a meta-analysis. Crit Care Med 2012;40(3):725–30.

32. Bai X, Yu W, Ji W, et al. Early versus delayed administration of norepinephrine in patients with septic shock. Crit Care 2014;18(5):532.

33. Cardenas-Garcia J, Schaub KF, Belchikov YG, et al. Safety of peripheral intravenous administration of vasoactive medication. J Hosp Med 2015;10(9):581–5.

34. Loubani OM, Green RS. A systematic review of extravasation and local tissue injury from administration of vasopressors through peripheral intravenous catheters and central venous catheters. J Crit Care 2015;30(3):653.e9–e17.

35. Rabuel C, Mebazaa A. Septic shock: a heart story since the 1960s. Intensive Care Med 2006;32(6):799–807.

36. Harvey S, Harrison DA, Singer M, et al. Assessment of the clinical effectiveness of pulmonary artery catheters in management of patients in intensive care (PAC-Man): a randomised controlled trial. Lancet 2005;366(9484):472–7.

37. Le Tulzo Y, Seguin P, Gacouin A, et al. Effects of epinephrine on right ventricular function in patients with severe septic shock and right ventricular failure: a preliminary descriptive study. Intensive Care Med 1997;23(6):664–70.

38. Levy B, Desebbe O, Montemont C, et al. Increased aerobic glycolysis through beta2 stimulation is a common mechanism involved in lactate formation during shock states. Shock 2008;30(4):417–21.

39. Hayes MA, Timmins AC, Yau EH, et al. Elevation of systemic oxygen delivery in the treatment of critically ill patients. N Engl J Med 1994;330(24):1717–22.

40. Howell MD, Donnino M, Clardy P, et al. Occult hypoperfusion and mortality in patients with suspected infection. Intensive Care Med 2007;33(11):1892–9.

41. Puskarich MA, Trzeciak S, Shapiro NI, et al. Outcomes of patients undergoing early sepsis resuscitation for cryptic shock compared with overt shock. Resuscitation 2011;82(10):1289–93.

42. Sato Y, Walley KR, Klut ME, et al. Nitric oxide reduces the sequestration of polymorphonuclear leukocytes in lung by changing deformability and CD18 expression. Am J Respir Crit Care Med 1999;159(5 Pt 1):1469–76.

43. Díaz NL, Finol HJ, Torres SH, et al. Histochemical and ultrastructural study of skeletal muscle in patients with sepsis and multiple organ failure syndrome (MOFS). Histol Histopathol 1998;13(1):121–8.

44. Ellis CG, Bateman RM, Sharpe MD, et al. Effect of a maldistribution of microvascular blood flow on capillary O(2) extraction in sepsis. Am J Physiol Heart Circ Physiol 2002;282(1):H156–64.

45. Weil MH, Michaels S, Rackow EC. Comparison of blood lactate concentrations in central venous, pulmonary artery, and arterial blood. Crit Care Med 1987;15(5): 489–90.

46. Younger JG, Falk JL, Rothrock SG. Relationship between arterial and peripheral venous lactate levels. Acad Emerg Med 1996;3(7):730–4.

47. Nguyen HB, Rivers EP, Knoblich BP, et al. Early lactate clearance is associated with improved outcome in severe sepsis and septic shock. Crit Care Med 2004;32(8):1637–42.

48. Jones AE, Shapiro NI, Trzeciak S, et al. Lactate clearance vs central venous oxygen saturation as goals of early sepsis therapy: a randomized clinical trial. JAMA 2010;303(8):739–46.

49. Puskarich MA, Trzeciak S, Shapiro NI, et al. Whole blood lactate kinetics in patients undergoing quantitative resuscitation for severe sepsis and septic shock. Chest 2013;143(6):1548–53.

50. Shapiro NI, Howell MD, Talmor D, et al. Serum lactate as a predictor of mortality in emergency department patients with infection. Ann Emerg Med 2005;45(5): 524–8.

51. Mikkelsen ME, Miltiades AN, Gaieski DF, et al. Serum lactate is associated with mortality in severe sepsis independent of organ failure and shock. Crit Care Med 2009;37(5):1670–7.

52. Garcia-Alvarez M, Marik P, Bellomo R. Sepsis-associated hyperlactatemia. Crit Care 2014;18(5):503.

53. Jansen TC, van Bommel J, Schoonderbeek FJ, et al. Early lactate-guided therapy in intensive care unit patients: a multicenter, open-label, randomized controlled trial. Am J Respir Crit Care Med 2010;182(6):752–61.

54. Hernandez G, Boerma EC, Dubin A, et al. Severe abnormalities in microvascular perfused vessel density are associated to organ dysfunctions and mortality and can be predicted by hyperlactatemia and norepinephrine requirements in septic shock patients. J Crit Care 2013;28(4):538.e9-e14.

55. Davison DL, Chawla LS, Selassie L, et al. Femoral-based central venous oxygen saturation is not a reliable substitute for subclavian/internal jugular-based central venous oxygen saturation in patients who are critically ill. Chest 2010;138(1): 76–83.

56. Ladakis C, Myrianthefs P, Karabinis A, et al. Central venous and mixed venous oxygen saturation in critically ill patients. Respiration 2001;68(3):279–85.

57. Pope JV, Jones AE, Gaieski DF, et al. Multicenter study of central venous oxygen saturation (ScvO(2)) as a predictor of mortality in patients with sepsis. Ann Emerg Med 2010;55(1):40–6.e1.

58. van Beest PA, Hofstra JJ, Schultz MJ, et al. The incidence of low venous oxygen saturation on admission to the intensive care unit: a multi-center observational study in The Netherlands. Crit Care 2008;12(2):R33.

59. Rivers EP, Yataco AC, Jaehne AK, et al. Oxygen extraction and perfusion markers in severe sepsis and septic shock: diagnostic, therapeutic and outcome implications. Curr Opin Crit Care 2015;21(5):381–7.

60. Bakker J, Vincent JL, Gris P, et al. Veno-arterial carbon dioxide gradient in human septic shock. Chest 1992;101(2):509–15.

61. Vallée F, Vallet B, Mathe O, et al. Central venous-to-arterial carbon dioxide difference: an additional target for goal-directed therapy in septic shock? Intensive Care Med 2008;34(12):2218–25.

62. Ospina-Tascón GA, Umaña M, Bermúdez WF, et al. Can venous-to-arterial carbon dioxide differences reflect microcirculatory alterations in patients with septic shock? Intensive Care Med 2016;42(2):211–21.

63. Zhang H, Vincent JL. Arteriovenous differences in PCO2 and pH are good indicators of critical hypoperfusion. Am Rev Respir Dis 1993;148(4 Pt 1):867–71.

64. van Genderen ME, Engels N, van der Valk RJP, et al. Early peripheral perfusion-guided fluid therapy in patients with septic shock. Am J Respir Crit Care Med 2015;191(4):477–80.

65. Ait-Oufella H, Bige N, Boelle PY, et al. Capillary refill time exploration during septic shock. Intensive Care Med 2014;40(7):958–64.

66. van Genderen ME, Paauwe J, de Jonge J, et al. Clinical assessment of peripheral perfusion to predict postoperative complications after major abdominal surgery early: a prospective observational study in adults. Crit Care 2014;18(3):R114.

67. Lima A, van Bommel J, Sikorska K, et al. The relation of near-infrared spectroscopy with changes in peripheral circulation in critically ill patients. Crit Care Med 2011;39(7):1649–54.

68. Hernandez G, Pedreros C, Veas E, et al. Evolution of peripheral vs metabolic perfusion parameters during septic shock resuscitation. A clinical-physiologic study. J Crit Care 2012;27(3):283–8.

69. Lima A, Jansen TC, van Bommel J, et al. The prognostic value of the subjective assessment of peripheral perfusion in critically ill patients. Crit Care Med 2009; 37(3):934–8.

70. Summary of Recommendation Statements. Kidney Int Suppl 2012;2(1):8–12.

71. Uchino S, Kellum JA, Bellomo R, et al. Acute renal failure in critically ill patients: a multinational, multicenter study. JAMA 2005;294(7):813–8.

72. Bullivant M. Autoregulation of plasma flow in the isolated perfused rat kidney. J Physiol 1978;280:141–53.

73. Bellomo R, Chapman M, Finfer S, et al. Low-dose dopamine in patients with early renal dysfunction: a placebo-controlled randomised trial. Australian and New Zealand Intensive Care Society (ANZICS) Clinical Trials Group. Lancet 2000; 356(9248):2139–43.

74. Lassnigg A, Donner E, Grubhofer G, et al. Lack of renoprotective effects of dopamine and furosemide during cardiac surgery. J Am Soc Nephrol 2000;11(1): 97–104.

75. Young P, Bailey M, Beasley R, et al. Effect of a buffered crystalloid solution vs saline on acute kidney injury among patients in the intensive care unit: the SPLIT randomized clinical trial. JAMA 2015;314(16):1701–10.

76. Yunos NM, Bellomo R, Hegarty C, et al. Association between a chloride-liberal vs chloride-restrictive intravenous fluid administration strategy and kidney injury in critically ill adults. JAMA 2012;308(15):1566–72.

Ready for Prime Time? Biomarkers in Sepsis

Brit Long, MD[a],*, Alex Koyfman, MD[b]

KEYWORDS

- Biomarkers • Lactate • Procalcitonin • Troponin • Proadrenomedullin • Sepsis

KEY POINTS

- Clinical biomarkers should be used in association with clinical gestalt, but they cannot replace the bedside clinician.
- Lactate has many uses in sepsis including assessment of severity, screening for disease, and as a marker for resuscitation but it is not always elevated in sepsis and can be elevated for other reasons.
- Procalcitonin is a marker used to distinguish bacterial from viral infection and has been studied in de-escalation of antibiotics in intensive care unit populations; however, its use in the emergency department for antibiotic use and resuscitation monitoring requires further study.
- Besides myocardial infarction, troponin can be elevated in many other conditions and is associated with worse prognosis in sepsis.
- New biomarkers include endothelial activators, acute-phase reactants, B-type natriuretic peptide/N-terminal B-type natriuretic peptide, and proadrenomedullin.

INTRODUCTION

Sepsis is a common cause of death in patients presenting to the emergency department (ED), and the condition results from the host response to the presence of infection.[1] Current diagnosis relies on physiologic criteria and suspicion of a source of infection using history, physical examination, laboratory studies, and imaging studies. Diagnostic uncertainty often results with the patient who presents with systemic inflammatory response syndrome (SIRS) criteria and suspected sepsis, but a source of infection has not been discovered.[1–4]

The authors have no disclosures related to this article.
[a] Department of Emergency Medicine, San Antonio Uniformed Services Health Education Consortium (SAUSHEC) Emergency Medicine, San Antonio Military Medical Center, 3841 Roger Brooke Drive, Fort Sam Houston, TX 78234, USA; [b] Department of Emergency Medicine, Parkland Memorial Hospital, UT Southwestern Medical Center, 5323 Harry Hines Boulevard, Dallas, TX 75390, USA
* Corresponding author.
E-mail address: brit.long@yahoo.com

Biomarkers are laboratory assessments used to detect and characterize diseases and improve clinical decision making. Numerous laboratory markers have been used to assist decision making, including complete blood cell count, troponin, creatine kinase, lactate, C-reactive protein, and myoglobin. Some have argued the use of these biomarkers shows a lack of history and examination skills, whereas others have argued these tests have the potential to supplant physical examination and history taking. A reliable biomarker for sepsis should assist with earlier diagnosis, improve risk stratification, or improve decision making for care in sepsis patients.[4–8]

LACTATE
Causes of Elevated Lactate Level

Lactate has numerous uses in sepsis, particularly in resuscitation and categorization of illness severity. Lactate is produced from all body tissue with the metabolism of pyruvate and Nicotinamide adenine dinucleotide (NADH), with normal production of 20 mmol/kg/d. Traditionally, lactate production with acidosis was thought to be caused by anaerobic metabolism or impaired hepatic metabolism. Elevated lactate can be broken into several categories, shown in **Table 1**. Of note, lactate elevation may be caused by endogenous epinephrine-stimulating β-2 receptors, which produce excess pyruvate during aerobic glycolysis and circulation of inflammatory mediators and liver disease.[8–12]

Screening

Serum lactate measurement is recommended as a screen for severe sepsis by the Surviving Sepsis Campaign.[1] Many studies evaluating lactate in sepsis support its use to evaluate and prognosticate for sepsis, with an initial elevated lactate

Table 1
Lactate elevation

Type A	Type B1 Associated with Disease	Type B2 Drugs and Toxins	Type B3 Associated with Inborn Errors of Metabolism
Tissue Hypoperfusion	Leukemia	Phenformin	Pyruvate carboxylase deficiency
Anaerobic muscular activity	Lymphoma	Metformin	Glucose-6-phosphatase deficiency
Reduced tissue oxygen delivery	Thiamine deficiency	Epinephrine	Fructose-1,6-bisphosphatase deficiencies
	Pancreatitis	Norepinephrine	
	Hepatic or renal failure	Xylitol	Oxidative phosphorylation enzyme defects
	Short bowel syndrome	Sorbitol	
		Lactate-based dialysate fluid	
		Cyanide	
		β-agonist	
		Alcohols: methanol, ethylene glycol	
		Salicylates	
		Nitroprusside	
		Isoniazid	
		Fructose	
		Paracetamol	
		Biguanides	
		Antiretroviral agents	

Adapted from Anderson LW, Mackenhauer J, Roberts JC, et al. Etiology and therapeutic approach to elevated lactate. Mayo Clin Proc 2013;88(10):1127–40.

concentration associated with suspected infection and severity of illness.[11–16] Point of care lactate is useful for sepsis screening, with a specificity of 82% for patients with confirmed sepsis for lactate levels ≥2 mmol/L. However, sensitivies of approximately 30% do warrant caution, and emergency providers should take the clinical picture into account rather than relying on one laboratory value. As lactate levels increase, illness severity, intensive care unit (ICU) admission, and vasopressor requirements increase.[16]

This screening can be conducted through peripheral venous blood and does not necessitate arterial blood draw. Point of care and laboratory levels are equivalent if samples are run on a blood gas machine, and arterial and venous levels strongly correlate.[16] Studies have evaluated the effect of tourniquet and temperature on lactate levels. No effect from tourniquet time or room temperature has been found if analysis occurs within 15 minutes of obtaining the sample.[17] Samples obtained after this period, especially after 30 minutes, should likely be redrawn to minimize error. Other laboratory evaluations, including an electrolyte panel, should not be used as a substitute for lactate levels. Bicarbonate and anion gap levels do not correlate with lactate, as a normal bicarbonate level is found in 22.2% and normal anion gap in 25% of patients with lactate level greater than 4.0 mmol/L.[18,19]

Prognostication

An association between lactate level and mortality has been established in several studies. Puskarich and colleagues[20] found that with lactate levels of 2.1 mmol/L, the mortality rate was 14.4%, but at levels approaching 20 mmol/L, the mortality rate was 39%. Irrespective of other variables such as blood pressure and illness severity, lactate is an independent predictor of mortality. Levels greater than 2 mmol/L are correlated with increased mortality and meet criteria for severe sepsis, whereas levels greater than 4 mmol/L correlate with mortalities of septic shock even if the patient is normotensive.[1,21,22]

Lactate levels greater than 4 mmol/L are strongly associated with increased mortality, no matter the etiology.[23–25] Patients lacking other criteria for sepsis with a lactate level ≥4.0 should be regarded with caution and given careful consideration for sepsis. Evaluation for other etiologies of elevated lactate levels, including gastrointestinal bleeding, any shock state (eg, cardiogenic, anaphylactic), mesenteric ischemia, and toxicologic etiologies (eg, salicylate overdose), should be conducted.[23–25] These patients should be admitted for trending of lactate levels to ensure normalization, as these levels are associated with significant mortality regardless of ultimate etiology.[23–35]

Cryptic Shock

Lactate can also be used to screen for sepsis in the patient with normal vital signs, otherwise known as cryptic septic shock. The hemodynamically stable patient with elevated lactate level (especially ≥4.0 mmol/L) is at risk for increased mortality. As the body begins to undergo inflammation and increased glycolysis, lactate production increases before clinically apparent end-organ damage and patient decompensation. Thus, lactate serves well as an early marker of sepsis and severe sepsis, with elevated levels associated with increased mortality.[9,11,20,21]

Intermediate Levels

Intermediate lactate levels of 2.0 to 3.9 mmol/L present a quandary, particularly in the setting of hemodynamic stability. Lactate levels between 2 and 4 mmol/L meet Centers for Medicare and Medicaid Services criteria for severe sepsis following Surviving

Sepsis Campaign guidelines.[1] Recent literature supports increased morbidity and mortality with lactate levels in this range, with mortality rates ranging from 3.2% to 16.4% in patients with no hypotension.[22] Close to one-quarter of these patients progress to having septic shock.[22] Thus, lactate levels in this range warrant close monitoring and aggressive treatment with early fluid administration and antimicrobials. **Table 2** describes resuscitation measures based on lactate level.

Lactate Clearance

Resuscitation of the septic patient can be evaluated with lactate clearance, with a target of 10% clearance in lactate from the initial level. Delayed clearance of lactate in patients with septic shock is correlated with poor outcome.[22,26–29] Early lactate clearance is associated with improved outcomes, with targeting lactate normalization as a resuscitation goal.[26–29] Arnold and colleagues[28] found a lactate clearance of 10% to be a strong predictor of improved survival, with 60% of those in the nonclearance arm suffering death.

Lactate parameters may be a better reflection of body homeostasis compared with oxygen-derived variables, which may not reflect actual clinical status of patients. The advantage of using lactate clearance is that no specialized, invasive equipment is needed, such as in continuous central venous oxygen monitoring (ScvO2), which was used in the original Early Goal-Directed Therapy trial.[4,28–30] Jones and colleagues used lactate clearance in place of ScvO2 in the final endpoint of resuscitation and found lactate clearance of 10% to be noninferior to the measurement of ScvO2 as a resuscitation measure for mortality.[31]

Lactate Pitfalls

As discussed earlier, lactate levels may not always be elevated in patients with septic shock. One study found that 45% of patients with vasopressor-dependent septic shock had a lactate level of less than 2.4 mmol/L but a mortality rate of 20%.[32] Patients with elevated lactate had higher rates of prior liver disease, acute liver injury, and acute bacteremia.[32] Hernandez and colleagues[33] found that 34% of patients with septic shock did not have elevated lactate levels, but these patients had a low mortality rate of 7.7% when compared with those with elevated lactate levels (42.9%).

There are also states in which lactate may be elevated but sepsis is not present. These states include hepatic disease, shock states (eg, cardiogenic, obstructive),

Table 2		
Resuscitation measures based on lactate		
Lactate Level	**Centers for Medicare and Medicaid Services Measure**	**Resuscitation Recommendation**
<2 mmol/L	None	Lactate levels may be negative in more than half of patients with sepsis. Clinical gestalt takes precedence over markers.
2–4 mmol/L	Severe sepsis	Resuscitation with intravenous fluids and antimicrobials and reassessment of lactate within 60 min
≥4 mmol/L	Septic shock	Aggressive resuscitation warranted regardless of vital signs.

From Dellinger RP, Levy MM, Rhodes A, et al. Surviving sepsis campaign: international guidelines for management of severe sepsis and septic shock, 2012. Intensive Care Med 2013;39:171–5; with permission.

trauma, seizure, medications and toxins (eg, acetaminophen, metformin, β agonists, epinephrine, propofol, alcohol, cocaine, carbon monoxide, linezolid, cyanide), excessive muscle activity, smoke inhalation, burns, regional ischemia such as mesenteric ischemia, thiamine deficiency, diabetic ketoacidosis, malignancy, and inborn errors of metabolism.[13] Lactate should not be used in isolation for resuscitation but rather in association with other resuscitation measures.[5–7,11]

PROCALCITONIN

Procalcitonin (PCT) is a propeptide of calcitonin produced by endocrine tissue in the thyroid, gastrointestinal tract, and lungs, normally in low concentrations. In bacterial infections, production is upregulated by toxins and proinflammatory mediators, resulting in PCT production. Viral infections increase interferon-γ, which inhibits PCT. Initial levels begin to increase within 3 to 6 hours and peak at 6 to 22 hours with bacterial infection. With infection resolution, levels typically decrease by 50% per day, as opposed to other biomarkers such as white blood cell count and C-reactive protein.[5–7,34–40]

Procalcitonin has several advantages, including specificity for bacterial infection, rapid increase with bacterial infection, rapid decrease with treatment of infection, and no impairment in the presence of neutropenia or immunosuppressive states. Other inflammatory states may cause an increase, however. These states include surgery, paraneoplastic states, autoimmune diseases, prolonged shock states, chronic parasitic diseases (such as malaria), certain immunomodulatory medications, and major trauma.[34–37]

Antibiotic Stewardship

Most evidence for PCT has been published in ICU patients with lower respiratory tract infections and sepsis. These studies, including meta-analyses, found that PCT-guided algorithms can reduce antibiotic exposure and costs of treatment and hospitalization with no effect on patient outcomes.[37–49]

In lower respiratory tract infections, especially chronic obstructive pulmonary disease and bronchitis, the clinical picture is not always clear as to whether the patient is experiencing a viral infection or bacterial pneumonia. The ProResp trial randomly assigned patients to standard antibiotic therapy versus PCT-guided therapy whereby if the PCT was less than 0.25 µg/L, antibiotics were discouraged. If PCT was greater than 0.25 µg/L, antibiotics were used. No difference in mortality or length of stay was found, although a significant decrease in antibiotic use was observed in the PCT-guided group (83% vs 44%).[40] A second trial, ProHOSP, evaluated patients with lower respiratory tract infections in an ED using a PCT-guided algorithm with similar cutoff levels. Similar results were found with a reduction in antibiotic use (**Table 3**).[41]

Diagnosis

PCT levels can also be useful in diagnosing sepsis.[43–47] However, the clinical context and patient scenario including possible source of infection, severity of illness, and likelihood of bacterial infection should take precedence over PCT. A laboratory sample drawn for PCT testing will likely not return while the patient is in the ED. Thus, if severe sepsis or septic shock is suspected, it is imperative the emergency provider treat the patient with broad-spectrum coverage for bacterial etiologies. A PCT can benefit the ICU team, but its use in the ED is controversial.

PCT has potential in identification of culture-positive sepsis, as levels correlate with bacterial load and may have prognostic implications.[34–47] Differentiating culture-negative sepsis and noninfectious SIRS can be assisted with PCT, with 92% sensitivity for culture-negative sepsis.[43,44] PCT levels of less than 0.25 μg/L are unlikely to have bacterial infection (<1%).[38] Several meta-analyses have been conducted on PCT diagnostic accuracy in sepsis, with one finding a sensitivity and specificity of 77% and 79%, respectively.[45] Most of these studies state PCT is helpful in diagnosis of documented infection.[45–49]

The prospective PRORATA trial evaluated septic patients admitted to the ICU in which one study arm had antibiotic initiation dependent on initial PCT level. A PCT level of 0.5 μg/L was used to trigger antibiotic administration. No difference in mortality or length of stay was found between patients in the PCT-guided group versus standard group. A decrease in antimicrobial use was found in the group using PCT to initiate antibiotics (see **Table 3**).[48] A 2015 meta-analysis found the most optimal cutoff value to be 0.5 μg/L for ruling out bacteremia.[49]

Table 3
Antibiotic use based on procalcitonin levels in ProHOSP and PRORATA trials

Study Antibiotic Use	PCT Level				
	<0.1 μg/L	0.1–0.25 μg/L	0.25–0.5 μg/L	0.5–1 μg/L	>1.0 μg/L
ProHOSP antibiotic use (respiratory infection only)	No	No	Yes	Yes	Yes
PRORATA antibiotic use (sepsis patients in ICU)	No	No	No	Yes	Yes

Data from Schuetz P, Christ-Crain M, Thomann R, et al; ProHOSP Study Group. Effect of procalcitonin-based guidelines vs standard guidelines on antibiotic use in lower respiratory tract infections: the ProHOSP randomized controlled trial. JAMA 2009;302(10):1059–66; and Bouadma L, Luyt CE, Tubach F, et al; PRORATA trial group. Use of procalcitonin to reduce patients' exposure to antibiotics in intensive care units (PRORATA trial): a multicentre randomised controlled trial. Lancet 2010;375(9713):463–74.

Although the literature on PCT-guided antibiotic therapy is encouraging, at this time emergency providers should not be using PCT to direct antibiotic therapy for patients with severe sepsis and septic shock. Currently, standard care in treating severe sepsis and septic shock in the ED requires timely antibiotic administration. In the near future, PCT may have a role in sepsis evaluation in the ED; however, that role is still being defined.

Troponin

Troponin has been most commonly used to diagnose myocardial infarction, with an elevation greater than the 99th percentile in a healthy population meeting criteria for acute coronary syndrome.[50,51] In patients with concern for acute coronary syndrome, troponin has been used to risk stratify patients as well, as seen in the HEART pathway.[52] Troponin testing has also now changed with the introduction of higher-sensitivity assays.[53,54] Cardiac troponin consists of troponin I and T, which are cardiac regulatory proteins that control the calcium-mediated interaction of actin and myosin. This interaction allows for myocardial contraction. Injury of the myocardium causes release of these proteins into the bloodstream.[55–59] Troponin elevation has many etiologies that can be divided into cardiac and noncardiac, shown in **Table 4**.[55–59]

Risk Stratification

In septic patients, elevated troponin level is associated with increased length of stay, increased adverse outcomes, and, most importantly, increased mortality. Rates of

Table 4	
Causes of elevated troponin	
Noncardiac Causes	**Cardiac Causes**
Acute noncardiac critical illness	Acute and chronic heart failure
Acute pulmonary edema	Acute inflammatory myocarditis or endocarditis/
Acute pulmonary embolism	pericarditis
Cardiotoxic drugs	Aortic dissection
Stroke, subarachnoid hemorrhage	Aortic valve disease
Chronic obstructive pulmonary disease	Apical ballooning syndrome
Chronic renal failure	Bradyarrhythmia, heart block
Extensive burns	Cardiac contusion from trauma
Infiltrative disease (amyloidosis)	Cardiac surgery, Postpercutaneous coronary
Rhabdomyolysis with myocyte necrosis	intervention, endomyocardial biopsy
Sepsis	Cardioversion
Severe pulmonary hypertension	Direct myocardial trauma
Strenuous exercise/extreme exertion	Hypertrophic cardiomyopathy
	Tachycardia/tachyarrhythmia

Data from Refs.[55–59]

troponin elevation in patients with sepsis range from 36% to 85%.[58–66] Numerous studies found an association with elevated troponin and increased rates of septic shock and mortality.[58–64]

High-sensitivity troponin assays, now commonly used in Europe, are also correlated with increased mortality.[67] Irrespective of the presence of shock, patients with elevated troponin in the setting of sepsis have 2-fold risk of mortality.[68] Proposed mechanisms of these elevations include demand ischemia from the SIRS response, direct endotoxin damage to the myocardium, cytokine and oxygen free radical damage, and poor cardiac oxygen supply caused by microcirculatory dysfunction.[57,60,61,63,65,68] Left ventricular diastolic dysfunction and right ventricular systolic dysfunction are associated with positive troponin and increased mortality rates.[64]

Early identification of patients with elevated troponin with sepsis can assist providers in focusing resuscitation measures, although further studies are required that use troponin and targeted resuscitation measures guiding treatment. The precise role of troponin, the particular assay, and cutoff levels in sepsis are yet to be determined.

If troponin elevation in the setting of sepsis occurs, an electrocardiogram (ECG) should be obtained. Demand ischemia may be seen in the setting of ischemia, resulting in ECG changes.[56–60] Bedside echocardiogram to evaluate for contractility and wall motion abnormalities should be conducted. Sepsis cardiomyopathy may result in diffuse hypokinesis, but focal wall abnormalities with ECG abnormalities warrant cardiology consultation. Anticoagulation should be discussed with the consultant and primary admission team at that time.[56–61]

Novel Biomarkers

Because of the complex pathophysiology of sepsis, many active substances are released with varying purposes. Multiple biomarkers other than lactate and PCT are currently under study for evaluation of their role in sepsis.[5–8] Few of these markers are regularly available, although proadrenomedullin can be used in the ICU setting.

Endothelial Markers

A key part of sepsis is endothelial activation, associated with changes in hemostatic balance, change in microcirculation, leukocyte trafficking, vascular permeability, and inflammation. Markers of endothelial dysfunction have shown promise in showing increased risk of development of sepsis and septic shock. These endothelial markers include vascular cell adhesion molecule, soluble intercellular adhesion molecule, sE-selectin, plasminogen activator inhibitor, and soluble fms-like tyrosine kinase.[5–8,69–73] Elevation in interleukin (IL)-6, E-selectin, and intercellular adhesion molecule are also associated with increased risk of sepsis development.[72] The increase in levels is associated with sepsis severity, organ dysfunction, and mortality, demonstrating endothelium involvement.[5–8,71,72]

Proadrenomedullin

Proadrenomedullin (ProADM) is a precursor for adrenomedullin, a calcitonin peptide similar to PCT. It is thought that ProADM functions similar to PCT in elevating with acute cytokine release, which occurs in bacterial infection. Adrenomedullin functions as a vasodilator, with additional immune modulating and metabolic effects. However, elevation is also observed in renal failure, cardiovascular disorders, and cancer. ProADM has been used for prognostication and risk stratification in patients with sepsis and severe pneumonia.[73–75] Several studies found that elevated ProADM levels are associated with severity in patients with community-acquired pneumonia and prediction of complications.[76–79]

Perhaps the most efficacious use of this biomarker is in combination with a clinical score. A randomized, controlled study evaluated a risk stratification algorithm using CURB-65 and ProADM levels.[79] CURB-65 is a validated prognostic score for community-acquired pneumonia that evaluates for the presence of several criteria, with 1 point given for each of the following: (1) BUN greater than 19 mg/dL (>7 mmol/L), (2) respiratory rate $\geq$30, (3) systolic blood pressure less than 90 mm Hg or diastolic blood pressure $\leq$ 60 mm Hg, (4) confusion, and (5) age $\geq$65 years.[80] This algorithm tended to reduce hospital stay, with no change in actual clinical outcome when the providers used CURB-65 alone.[79] The use of this marker in combination with clinical scores and gestalt may assist with prognostication, risk stratification, and early discharge of patients, although further evaluation in an ED setting is required.

Acute-Phase Reactants

The body's intrinsic immune system increases cytokine production and inflammatory cell signaling and markers. Lipopolysaccharide-binding protein is an acute-phase reactant that binds a cell wall protein of gram-negative bacteria. During acute-phase reactions, this complex increases drastically, but studies have not been promising, as it does not have literature support for prognostication of disease severity or outcome.[8,81] Pentraxins are pattern recognition receptors that are secreted by immune cells and bind to bacteria and viruses, assisting in destruction. These levels are found to be associated with mortality and severity of sepsis, but literature evaluating the use of this marker for differentiating noninfectious SIRS and sepsis are lacking. Proinflammatory and anti-inflammatory cytokines and chemokines such as IL-6, IL-8, and IL-10 are associated with worse outcome, but further study is required. Macrophage migration inhibitory factor is elevated in sepsis but has failed to distinguish noninfectious SIRS and sepsis. Cell surface markers, including soluble triggering receptor expressed on myeloid cells-1 (sTREM-1), soluble urokinase-type plasminogen activator receptor (suPAR), and CD-64 index, are associated with severity, but further study is required.[8,81]

Cardiac Biomarkers

Although classically used for heart failure and coronary disease, N-terminal pro b-type natriuretic peptide (NT-proBNP) and B-type natriuretic peptide (BNP) have been evaluated for use in septic patients. BNP levels may predict outcome in sepsis, with higher levels associated with prolonged ICU stay and worse outcomes including higher rates of death. Monitoring of BNP in early sepsis can also predict occult cardiac systolic dysfunction, prompting earlier use of inotropic agents.[82–87] Thus, the use of these cardiac biomarkers may assist in prognostication and resuscitation requirements, although further validation of this marker is required. However, these markers lack specificity because of age (causing a false-positive elevation) and other conditions. For example, conditions such as valvular heart disease, atrial fibrillation, pulmonary embolism, chronic obstructive disease, and hyperthyroidism can elevate these markers, whereas obesity may decrease levels.[83–87]

PREDICTING RENAL FAILURE

Predicting acute kidney injury in sepsis provides another avenue for biomarker use. Sepsis often results in acute kidney injury, with rates approaching 25%, and it may predict a higher mortality. Unfortunately, serum creatinine may not be elevated in the acute phase of renal injury. Neutrophil gelatinase–associated lipocalin is a urine marker that is often excreted before elevation in serum creatinine occurs, although its use is controversial.[8,81,87,88]

Multiple biomarkers are under evaluation for use in sepsis diagnosis, prognostication, and resuscitation monitoring. All require further validation in an ED population for further refinement.

SUMMARY

Sepsis is a deadly disease and a common ED condition, but diagnosis and prognostication are not always straightforward. Biomarkers have been advocated and studied in the use of sepsis diagnosis, prognostication, and resuscitation measurement. Lactate has shown great utility in predicting severity of illness and as a marker of resuscitation. Pitfalls exist in lactate use, as many different factors can increase this biomarker. PCT is a new marker that shows promise in antibiotic de-escalation and differentiating between noninfectious SIRS and sepsis, but further refinement is required. Troponin is often elevated in sepsis because of cardiac involvement. Currently, lactate has the best literature support. When used in conjunction with clinical gestalt, biomarkers in sepsis have a bright future to assist providers in prognostication, diagnosis, and resuscitation.

REFERENCES

1. Dellinger RP, Levy MM, Rhodes A, et al. Surviving sepsis campaign: international guidelines for management of severe sepsis and septic shock, 2012. Intensive Care Med 2013;39:165–228.
2. Winters BD, Eberlein M, Leung J, et al. Long-term mortality and quality of life in sepsis: a systematic review. Crit Care Med 2010;38:1276–83.
3. Strehlow MC, Emond SD, Shapiro NI, et al. National study of emergency department visits for sepsis, 1992 to 2001. Ann Emerg Med 2006;48:326–31.
4. Rivers E, Nguyen B, Havstad S, et al. Early goal-directed therapy in the treatment of severe sepsis and septic shock. N Engl J Med 2001;345:1368.
5. Clerico A, Plebani M. Biomarkers for sepsis: an unfinished journey. Clin Chem Lab Med 2013;51(6):1135–8.

6. Rivers EP, Jaehne AK, Nguyen HB, et al. Early biomarker activity in severe sepsis and septic shock and a contemporary review of immunotherapy trials: not a time to give up, but to give it earlier. Shock 2013;39(2):127–37.

7. Schuetz P, Aujesky D, Mueller C, et al. Biomarker-guided personalised emergency medicine for all – hope for another hype? Swiss Med Wkly 2015;145: w14079.

8. Di Somma S, Magrini L, Travaglino F, et al. Opinion paper on innovative approach of biomarkers for infectious diseases and sepsis management in the emergency department. Clin Chem Lab Med 2013;51:1167–75.

9. Jones AE. Lactate clearance for assessing response to resuscitation in severe sepsis. Acad Emerg Med 2013;20(8):844–7.

10. Marik PE, Bellomo R. Lactate clearance as a target of therapy in sepsis: a flawed paradigm. OA Crit Care 2013;1(1):3. Available at: http://www.oapublishinglondon.com/abstract/431.

11. Puskarich MA. Emergency management of severe sepsis and septic shock. Curr Opin Crit Care 2012;18(4):295–300.

12. Gibot S. On the origins of lactate during sepsis. Crit Care 2012;16(5):151.

13. Anderson LW, Mackenhauer J, Roberts JC, et al. Etiology and therapeutic approach to elevated lactate. Mayo Clin Proc 2013;88(10):1127–40.

14. Shapiro NI, Howell MD, Talmor D, et al. Serum lactate as a predictor of mortality in emergency department patients with infection. Ann Emerg Med 2005;45:524–8.

15. Trzeciak S, Dellinger R, Chansky ME, et al. Serum lactate as a predictor of mortality in patients with infection. Intensive Care Med 2007;33:970–7.

16. Singer AJ, Taylor M, Domingo A, et al. Diagnostic characteristics of a clinical screening tool in combination with measuring bedside lactate level in emergency department patients with suspected sepsis. Acad Emerg Med 2014;21(8):853–7.

17. Jones AE, Leonard MM, Hernandez-Nino J, et al. Determination of the effect of in vitro time, temperature, and tourniquet use on whole blood venous point-of-care lactate concentrations. Acad Emerg Med 2007;14:587–91.

18. Adams BD, Bonzani TA, Hunter CJ. The anion gap does not accurately screen for lactic acidosis in emergency department patients. Emerg Med J 2006;23:179–82.

19. Iberti TJ, Leibowitz AB, Papadakos PJ, et al. Low sensitivity of the anion gap as a screen to detect hyperlactatemia in critically ill patients. Crit Care Med 1990;18: 275–7.

20. Puskarich MA, Trzeciak S, Shapiro NI, et al. Whole blood lactate kinetics in patients undergoing quantitative resuscitation for severe sepsis and septic shock. Chest 2013;143(6):1548–53.

21. Mikkelsen ME, Miltiades AN, Gaieski DF, et al. Serum lactate is associated with mortality in severe sepsis independent of organ failure and shock. Crit Care Med 2009;37(5):1670–7.

22. Puskarich MA, Illich BM, Jones AE. Prognosis of emergency department patients with suspected infection and intermediate lactate levels: a systematic review. J Crit Care 2014;29:334–9.

23. Nichol AD, Egi M, Pettila V, et al. Relative hyperlactatemia and hospital mortality in critically ill patients: a retrospective multi-centre study. Crit Care 2010;14:R25.

24. Cady LD Jr, Weil MH, Afifi AA, et al. Quantitation of severity of critical illness with special reference to blood lactate. Crit Care Med 1973;1:75–80.

25. Mizock BA, Falk JL. Lactic acidosis in critical illness. Crit Care Med 1992;20: 80–93.

26. Bakker J, Gris P, Coffernils M, et al. Serial blood lactate levels can predict the development of multiple organ failure following septic shock. Am J Surg 1996; 171:221–6.
27. Nguyen H, Rivers E, Knoblich B, et al. Early lactate clearance is associated with improved outcome in severe sepsis and septic shock. Crit Care Med 2004;32: 1637–42.
28. Arnold RC, Shapiro NI, Jones AE, et al. Multi-center study of early lactate clearance as a determinant of survival in patients with presumed sepsis. Shock 2009; 32:36–9.
29. Jansen TC, van Bommel J, Schoonderbeek FJ, et al. Early lactate-guided therapy in intensive care unit patients a multicenter, open-label, randomized controlled trial. Am J Respir Crit Care Med 2010;182:752–61.
30. Jones AE, Kline JA. Use of goal-directed therapy for severe sepsis and septic shock in academic emergency departments. Crit Care Med 2005;33:1888–9.
31. Jones AE, Shapiro NI, Trzeciak S, et al. Lactate clearance vs central venous oxygen saturation as goals of early sepsis therapy: a randomized clinical trial. JAMA 2010;303:739–46.
32. Dugas AF, Mackenhauer J, Salciccioli JD, et al. Prevalence and characteristics of nonlactate and lactate expressors in septic shock. J Crit Care 2012;27(4):344–50.
33. Hernandez G, Castro R, Romero C, et al. Persistent sepsis-induced hypotension without hyperlactatemia: is it really septic shock? J Crit Care 2011;26(4): 435.e9-14.
34. Jin M, Khan AI. Procalcitonin: uses in the clinical laboratory for the diagnosis of sepsis. Lab Med 2010;41(3):173–7.
35. Pieralli F, Vannucchi V, Mancini A, et al. Procalcitonin kinetics in the first 72 hours predicts 30- day mortality in severely Ill septic patients admitted to an intermediate care unit. J Clin Med Res 2015;7(9):706–13.
36. Assicot M, Gendrel D, Garsin H, et al. High serum procalcitonin concentrations in patients with sepsis and infection. Lancet 1993;341:515–8.
37. Meisner M. Pathobiochemistry and clinical use of procalcitonin. Clin Chim Acta 2002;323:17–29.
38. Muller F, Christ-Crain M, Bregenzer T, et al. Procalcitonin levels predict bacteremia in patients with community-acquired pneumonia: a prospective cohort trial. Chest 2010;138(1):121–9.
39. Schuetz P, Suter-Widmer I, Chaudri A, et al. Prognostic value of procalcitonin in community-acquired pneumonia. Eur Respir J 2011;37(2):384–92.
40. Christ-Crain M, Muller B. Biomarkers in respiratory tract infections: diagnostic guides to antibiotic prescription, prognostic markers and mediators. Eur Respir J 2007;30:556–73.
41. Schuetz P, Christ-Crain M, Thomann R, et al. Effect of procalcitonin-based guidelines vs standard guidelines on antibiotic use in lower respiratory tract infections: the ProHOSP randomized controlled trial. JAMA 2009;302(10):1059–66.
42. Schuetz P, Muller B, Christ-Crain M, et al. Procalcitonin to initiate or discontinue antibiotics in acute respiratory tract infections. Cochrane Database Syst Rev 2012;(9):CD007498.
43. Jensen J, Heslet L, Jensen TH, et al. Procalcitonin as a marker of infection, sepsis, and response to antibiotic therapy. Crit Care Med 2006;34:2596–602.
44. Anand D, Das S, Bhargava S, et al. Procalcitonin as a rapid diagnostic biomarker to differentiate between culture-negative bacterial sepsis and systemic inflammatory response syndrome: a prospective, observational, cohort study. J Crit Care 2015;30(1):218.e7-12.

45. Wacker C, Prkno A, Brunkhorst FM, et al. Procalcitonin as a diagnostic marker for sepsis: a systematic review and meta-analysis. Lancet Infect Dis 2013;13: 426–35.
46. Schuetz P, Briel M, Mueller B. Clinical outcomes associated with procalcitonin algorithms to guide antibiotic therapy in respiratory tract infections. JAMA 2013; 309(7):717–8.
47. Freund Y, Delerme S, Goulet H, et al. Serum lactate and procalcitonin measurements in emergency room for the diagnosis and risk-stratification of patients with suspected infection. Biomarkers 2012;17:590–6.
48. Bouadma L, Luyt CE, Tubach F, et al. Use of procalcitonin to reduce patients' exposure to antibiotics in intensive care units (PRORATA trial): a multicentre randomised controlled trial. Lancet 2010;375(9713):463–74.
49. Hoeboer SH, Van der Geest PJ, Nieboer D, et al. The diagnostic accuracy of procalcitonin for bacteraemia: a systematic review and meta-analysis. Clin Microbiol Infect 2015;21:474–81.
50. Thygesen K, Alpert JS, Jaffe AS, et al. Joint ESC/ACCF/AHA/WHF task force for universal definition of myocardial infarction. Third universal definition of myocardial infarction. J Am Coll Cardiol 2012;60(16):1581–98.
51. Newby LK, Jesse RL, Babb JD, et al. ACCF 2012 expert consensus document on practical clinical considerations in the interpretation of troponin elevations: a report of the American College of Cardiology Foundation task force on Clinical Expert Consensus Documents. J Am Coll Cardiol 2012;60:2427–63.
52. Mahler SA, Riley RF, Hiestand BC, et al. The HEART pathway randomized trial identifying emergency department patients with acute chest pain for early discharge. Circ Cardiovasc Qual Outcomes 2015;8(2):195–203.
53. Thygesen K, Mair J, Giannitsis E, et al. How to use high-sensitivity cardiac troponins in acute cardiac care. Eur Heart J 2012;33:2252–7.
54. Reichlin T, Hochholzer W, Bassetti S, et al. Early diagnosis of myocardial infarction with sensitive cardiac troponin assays. N Engl J Med 2009;361:858–67.
55. Kelley WE, Januzzi JL, Christenson RH. Increases of cardiac troponin in conditions other than acute coronary syndrome and heart failure. Clin Chem 2009; 55(12):2098–112.
56. Korff S. Differential diagnosis of elevated troponins. Heart 2006;92(7):987–93.
57. Court O, Kumar A, Parrillo JE, et al. Clinical review: myocardial depression in sepsis and septic shock. Crit Care 2002;6:500–8.
58. Hamilton MA, Toner A, Cecconi M. Troponin in critically ill patients. Minerva Anestesiol 2012;78(9):1039–45.
59. Patil H, Vaidya O, Bogart D. A review of causes and systemic approach to cardiac troponin elevation. Clin Cardiol 2011;34(12):723–8.
60. Bouhemad B, Nicolas-Robin A, Arbelot C, et al. Acute left ventricular dilatation and shock-induced myocardial dysfunction. Crit Care Med 2009;37:441–7.
61. Wilhelm J, Hettwer S, Schuermann M, et al. Elevated troponin in septic patients in the emergency department: frequency, causes, and prognostic implications. Clin Res Cardiol 2014;103(7):561–7.
62. Bessière F, Khenifer S, Dubourg J, et al. Prognostic value of troponins in sepsis: a meta-analysis. Intensive Care Med 2013;39(7):1181–9.
63. Sheyin O, Davies O, Duan W, et al. The prognostic significance of troponin elevation in patients with sepsis: a meta-analysis. Heart Lung 2015;44(1):75–81.
64. Landesberg G, Jaffe AS, Gilon D, et al. Troponin elevation in severe sepsis and septic shock: the role of left ventricular diastolic dysfunction and right ventricular dilatation. Crit Care Med 2014;42(4):790–800.

65. Clemente G, Tuttolomondo A, Colomba D, et al. When sepsis affects the heart: a case report and literature review. World J Clin Cases 2015;3(8):743–50.

66. Klouche K, Pommet S, Amigues L, et al. Plasma brain natriuretic peptide and troponin levels in severe sepsis and septic shock: relationships with systolic myocardial dysfunction and intensive care unit mortality. J Intensive Care Med 2014;29(4):229–37.

67. Courtney D, Conway R, Kavanagh J, et al. High-sensitivity troponin as an outcome predictor in acute medical admissions. Postgrad Med J 2014; 90(1064):311–6.

68. de Groot B, Verdoorn RC, Lameijer J, et al. High-sensitivity cardiac troponin T is an independent predictor of inhospital mortality in emergency department patients with suspected infection: a prospective observational derivation study. Emerg Med J 2014;31(11):882–8.

69. Skibsted S, Jones AE, Puksarich MA, et al. Biomarkers of endothelial cell activation in early sepsis. Shock 2013;39(5):427–32.

70. Hack CE, Zeerleder S. The endothelium in sepsis: source of and a target for inflammation. Crit Care Med 2001;29:S21–7.

71. Shapiro NI, Schuetz P, Yano K, et al. The association of endothelial cell signaling, severity of illness, and organ dysfunction in sepsis. Crit Care 2010;14:R182.

72. Wang HE, Shapiro NI, Griffin R, et al. Inflammatory and endothelial activation biomarkers and risk of sepsis: a nested case-control study. J Crit Care 2013;28(5): 549–55.

73. Becker KL, Nylen ES, White JC, et al. Procalcitonin and the calcitonin gene family of peptides in inflammation, infection, and sepsis: a journey from calcitonin back to its precursors. J Clin Endocrinol Metab 2004;89(4):1512–25.

74. Elsasser TH, Kahl S. Adrenomedullin has multiple roles in disease stress: development and remission of the inflammatory response. Microsc Res Tech 2002; 57(2):120–9.

75. Struck J, Tao C, Morgenthaler NG, et al. Identification of an Adrenomedullin precursor fragment in plasma of sepsis patients. Peptides 2004;25(8):1369–72.

76. Christ-Crain M, Morgenthaler NG, Struck J, et al. Mid-regional pro-adrenomedullin as a prognostic marker in sepsis: an observational study. Crit Care 2005;9(6):R816–24.

77. Christ-Crain M, Morgenthaler NG, Stolz D, et al. Pro-adrenomedullin to predict severity and outcome in community-acquired pneumonia [ISRCTN04176397]. Crit Care 2006;10(3):R96.

78. Schuetz P, Wolbers M, Christ-Crain M, et al. Prohormones for prediction of adverse medical outcome in community-acquired pneumonia and lower respiratory tract infections. Crit Care 2010;14(3):R106.

79. Albrich WC, Dusemund F, Ruegger K, et al. Enhancement of CURB65 score with proadrenomedullin (CURB65–A) for outcome prediction in lower respiratory tract infections: derivation of a clinical algorithm. BMC Infect Dis 2011;11:112.

80. Lim WS, van der Eerden MM, Laing R, et al. Defining community acquired pneumonia severity on presentation to hospital: an international derivation and validation study. Thorax 2003;58(5):377–82.

81. Reinhart K, Bauer M, Riedemann NC, et al. New approaches to sepsis: molecular diagnostics and biomarkers. Clin Microbiol Rev 2012;25(4):609–34.

82. Cheng H, Fan WZ, Wang SC, et al. N-terminal pro-brain natriuretic peptide and cardiac troponin I for the prognostic utility in elderly patients with severe sepsis or septic shock in intensive care unit: a retrospective study. J Crit Care 2015; 30(3):654.e9-14.

83. Castillo JR, Zagler A, Carrillo-Jimenez R, et al. Brain natriuretic peptide: a potential marker for mortality in septic shock. Int J Infect Dis 2004;8:271–4.
84. Turner KL, Moore LJ, Todd SR, et al. Identification of cardiac dysfunction in sepsis with B-type natriuretic peptide. J Am Coll Surg 2011;213:139–46.
85. Varpula M, Pulkki K, Karlsson S, et al. Predictive value of N-terminal pro-brain natriuretic peptide in severe sepsis and septic shock. Crit Care Med 2007;35: 1277–83.
86. Post F, Weilemann LS, Messow CM, et al. B-type natriuretic peptide as a marker for sepsis-induced myocardial depression in intensive care patients. Crit Care Med Lab Med 2008;46:748–63.
87. Hur M, Kim H, Lee S, et al. Diagnostic and prognostic utilities of multimarkers approach using procalcitonin, B-type natriuretic peptide, and neutrophil gelatinase-associated lipocalin in critically ill patients with suspected sepsis. BMC Infect Dis 2014;14:224.
88. Kim H, Hur M, Cruz DN, et al. Plasma neutrophil gelatinase- associated lipocalin as a biomarker for acute kidney injury in critically ill patients with suspected sepsis. Clin Biochem 2013;46:1414–8.

Pediatric Sepsis

Melanie K. Prusakowski, MD[a],*, Audrey P. Chen, PNP[b]

KEYWORDS

- Pediatric sepsis • Neonatal sepsis • Goal-directed therapy
- Multi-system organ failure

KEY POINTS

- Age-specific vital signs and development-specific clinical parameters complicate the early recognition of pediatric sepsis.
- Early goal-directed therapy in pediatric sepsis differs from adult guidelines in the selection of inotropes and the recommendation to start vasoactive medications peripherally while securing central access.
- Intraosseous needles and umbilical catheters are pediatric-specific modalities for providing sepsis treatment.

INTRODUCTION

Pediatric sepsis is life-threatening organ dysfunction caused by a deleterious host response to infection,[1] and it continues to be a leading cause of death for children in the United States.[2] Neonates, infants, and children with chronic medical conditions comprise a large percentage of those with morbidity and mortality from sepsis or septic shock.[3–5] Pediatric critical care medicine has led epidemiology research efforts over the past 2 decades in an attempt to understand the burden of sepsis in children. The national incidence of pediatric sepsis was 0.56 cases per 1000 (42,364 cases per year nationally) in 1995, with an in-hospital mortality of 10.3%. From 1995 to 2005, there has been an increase in incidence from 0.56 to 0.89 cases per 1000 (with a doubled prevalence of severe sepsis in newborns) and declining mortality rate from 10.3% to 8.9%.[5] The estimated annual health care expenditures for the treatment of pediatric severe sepsis is just under $5 billion in the United States.[5] Although there has been a lack of research looking into rates of pediatric sepsis recognized in the emergency department (ED), a more recent study estimated that close to 100,000 children present to the ED with severe sepsis every year.[6] EDs are at the frontline of recognizing severe sepsis and septic shock and have the resources to initiate

The authors have nothing to disclose.
[a] Departments of Emergency Medicine and Pediatrics, Virginia Tech Carilion School of Medicine, 1 Riverside Circle, Roanoke, VA 24016, USA; [b] Department of Emergency Medicine, Carilion Clinic, 1 Riverside Circle, Roanoke, VA 24016, USA
* Correseponding author.
E-mail address: mkprusakowski@carilionclinic.org

Emerg Med Clin N Am 35 (2017) 123–138
http://dx.doi.org/10.1016/j.emc.2016.08.008
0733-8627/17/© 2016 Elsevier Inc. All rights reserved.

life-saving resuscitation measures. In a landmark study, Han and colleagues[7] demonstrated that, when community hospital EDs recognize pediatric septic shock early and initiate aggressive treatment to reverse the clinical signs of shock (eg, tachycardia, delayed capillary refill, hypotension), morbidity and mortality decrease by 50%. Patients with septic shock have significantly decreased duration of hospital and intensive care unit stays when they received 60 mL/kg of IV fluids and when complete Pediatric Advanced Life Support–directed shock protocol bundles were provided within the first hour of treatment.[8] This article discusses the recognition and management of pediatric severe sepsis and septic shock in the ED.

DEFINITIONS

The definition of pediatric sepsis has evolved from the efforts of the Society of Critical Care Medicine and the American College of Critical Care Medicine (ACCM), who authored the first sepsis guidelines for adults. In 2002, the ACCM in collaboration with the Society of Critical Care Medicine developed the first pediatric sepsis guidelines, highlighting the differences in management of pediatric and neonatal sepsis from adult sepsis.[9] International definitions for pediatric systemic inflammatory response syndrome (SIRS), sepsis, septic shock, and organ dysfunction were agreed on in 2002 by the members of the International Consensus Conference on Pediatric Sepsis. Revised ACCM septic shock guidelines were written in 2007 and are based on the best current literature and expert opinion for the management of neonatal and pediatric septic shock.

The definition of pediatric SIRS differs from the adult definition in its requirement that at least 1 of the diagnostic criteria must be high or low core body temperature or a leukocyte count abnormality (Box 1).[10] Throughout pediatric development, vital signs and laboratory values change requiring, thoughtful attention to age-related norms (Table 1)[11,12] for accurate and early SIRS and sepsis recognition. Tachycardia and pyrexia commonly are seen together, but are often hard to isolate from other variables such as pain, anemia, fluid volume status, respiratory distress, and fear. Unfortunately, there is no established criterion to calculate an age-appropriate heart rate (HR) in the presence of fever.

Pediatric sepsis necessitates that the patient meet the SIRS criteria in the presence of a known or suspected infection (eg, bacterial, viral).[10] Clinical findings that suggest an existing nidus of infection are located in Box 2.[13] Severe sepsis in pediatrics is

---

Box 1
Pediatric systemic inflammatory response syndrome criteria

- Core body temperature (rectal or oral) of greater than 38.5°C or less than 36°C (tympanic, toe, axillary temperature measurements are not recommended)

- Tachycardia

- Tachypnea

- Abnormal high or low leukocyte count for age or bandemia (>10% immature neutrophils)

Systemic inflammatory response syndrome = 2 out of these 4 criteria with at least 1 being abnormality in temperature or leukocyte count.

Data from Goldstein B, Giroir B, Randolph A, et al. International pediatric sepsis consensus conference: definitions for sepsis and organ dysfunction in pediatrics. Pediatric Critical Care Medicine 2005;6(1):2–8.

Table 1
Age-specific vital signs and laboratory values

Age Group	Tachycardia	Bradycardia	Respiratory Rate	Leukocyte Count	Hypotension (SBP)
Birth to 1 wk	>180	<100	>50	>34	<59
1 wk to 1 mo	>180	<100	>40	>19.5 or <5	<79
1 mo to 1 y	>180	<90	>34	>17.5 or <5	<75
2–5 y	>140	—	>22	>15.5 or <6	<74
6–12 y	>130	—	>18	>13.5 or <4.5	<83
13 to <18 y	>110	—	>14	>11 or <4.5	<90

Abbreviation: SBP, systolic blood pressure.
Data from Refs.[10–12]

recognized as sepsis with the development of cardiovascular dysfunction or acute respiratory distress syndrome, or organ dysfunction in at least 2 systems (including renal, hematologic, neurologic, hepatic, or respiratory systems). Septic shock is defined as sepsis with cardiovascular dysfunction manifesting as alterations in HR (tachycardia or bradycardia) and signs of impaired perfusion (**Box 3**). The International Pediatric Sepsis Consensus developed organ dysfunction definitions for cardiac, respiratory, hematologic, neurologic, renal, and hepatic systems (**Box 4**) that can guide the clinician's diagnosis and trajectory of sepsis, severe sepsis, and septic shock. At this time, adult organ system dysfunction guidelines have not been validated in children.[10]

SIMILARITIES BETWEEN PEDIATRIC AND ADULT SEPSIS

Sepsis in the pediatric and neonatal populations is a serious illness associated with considerable mortality(**Box 5**).[14–16] Much like in adults, foundations of care include early recognition of sepsis, aggressive fluid resuscitation, timely administration of

Box 2
Clinical findings suggesting infection in pediatric patients

- Petechiae or purpura + hemodynamic derangement/instability
- Purpura fulminans
- Fever + cough + hypoxemia + pulmonary infiltrates + leukocytosis
- Fever or hypothermia + bulging fontanelle or nuchal rigidity + irritability
- Temperature instability + poor glucose control + irritability (in neonates and premature infants)
- Temperature instability + seizure (in neonate)
- Rash with rapid migration + fever + pain + leukocytosis
- Distended tympanic abdomen + fever + leukocytosis
- Or recognizable infectious mediated clinical syndrome (ie, toxic shock syndrome and staphylococcal scalded skin syndrome, or Rocky Mountain spotted fever) or infectious cutaneous lesion

Data from Refs.[9,10,13]

Box 3
Clinical signs of poor perfusion in pediatric patients

- Cool extremities
- Pale or mottled skin
- Diminished peripheral pulses
- Significant difference between central and peripheral pulses
- Flash capillary refill time or prolonged capillary refill time greater than 2 seconds
- Change in level of consciousness from baseline or irritability
- Decreased urine output (<0.5 mL/kg/h)

Data from Refs.[9,10,13]

---

antibiotics, and source control.[9] Just as comorbid conditions drive the mortality of sepsis in adult patients, medical conditions such as prematurity, congenital heart disease, solid and hematopoietic cancers, and immune deficiencies significantly increase the mortality of pediatric sepsis. The early investigation of sepsis in an infant or child includes source identification (eg, cultures and antigen testing) and inflammatory and biomarker marker evaluation (eg, white blood cell count, erythrocyte sedimentation rate, C-reactive protein analysis, lactate level).[17] Ultrasound imaging and invasive monitoring are used to evaluate resuscitation endpoints. In all populations, disseminated intravascular coagulation (DIC) impacts the likelihood of developing multisystem organ failure.[18]

DIFFERENCES BETWEEN PEDIATRIC AND ADULT SEPSIS

Sepsis in infants and children differs in its pathophysiology, etiology, diagnosis, and management from that of adults. Most of these differences become less pronounced as children get older. The comorbid conditions most often observed in infants with sepsis are congenital heart disease and chronic lung disease, whereas cancer and neuromuscular disease emerge more often in childhood sepsis.[19] The site of infection is also age dependent; infants tend to present with primary bacteremia, whereas older children present most often with respiratory infection and secondary bacteremia.

The pathology of illness in infants and young children is affected by their proportionally higher ratio of extracellular to intracellular fluid. The larger the percentage of extracellular fluid, the more likely decreased intake or increased losses will predispose them to rapid fluid losses. Additionally, the younger the myocardium, the more likely it is functioning at a baseline high contractile state.[20] For this reason, pediatric patients with sepsis depend on increases in HR to generate increased cardiac output (CO) during stress. This concept plays a focal role in the interpretation of vital signs and recognition of sepsis in pediatric patients. Tachycardia is an important mechanism in maintaining CO in pediatric sepsis, but the younger the child, the higher the basal HR and the more unlikely it becomes that CO can be maintained solely by further HR increases.[13] Children with lower CO have the highest risk of mortality.[16] This pathophysiology explains the efficacy of inotropes as first-line therapy in fluid-refractory shock.[16,21] When increasing HR is no longer able to sustain adequate CO, vasoconstriction occurs in response to decreasing stroke volume and contractility. Young infants and neonates are particularly vulnerable to the effects of afterload on left ventricular function.[22] Thus, an abrupt decrease in left ventricular function occurs

Box 4
Organ dysfunction criteria

Cardiovascular (despite ≥40 mL/kg fluid bolus in 1 hour)

Hypotension
   or

Requiring inotrope support
   or

Two of the following:
   Metabolic acidosis: base deficit greater than 5.0 mEq/L
   Increased arterial lactate greater than 2 times the upper limit of normal
   Oliguria: UOP less than 0.5 mL/kg/h
   Delayed capillary refill time: greater than 5 seconds
   Difference between core and peripheral temperature greater than 3°C

Hematologic

INR greater than 2
   or

Platelet count less than 80,000/mm^3 (50% decrease from highest value within 3 days for hematology/oncology patients)

Hepatic

ALT greater than or equal to the upper limit of normal for age ×2
   or

Total bilirubin 4 mg/dL or greater (newborns excluded)

Respiratory

Requiring intubation and mechanical ventilation or noninvasive ventilation measures to maintain adequate oxygenation and ventilation
   or

Oxygen greater than 50% Fio_2 to maintain oxygen saturations 92% or greater
   or

Pao_2/Fio_2 less than 300 with no known cyanotic cardiac defect or previously established lung disease
   or

$Paco_2$ greater than 65 torr or 20 mm Hg over baseline $Paco_2$

Neurologic

GCS of 11 or less
   or

Decline in mental status + change in GCS of 3 or more points from baseline

Renal

Serum creatinine greater than or equal to the upper limit of normal for age ×2 (or baseline creatinine ×2 in patients with chronic kidney disease)

Abbreviations: ALT, alanine aminotransferase; GCS, Glasgow Coma Score; INR, international normalized ratio; UOP, urine output.

Data from Goldstein B, Giroir B, Randolph A, et al. International pediatric sepsis consensus conference: definitions for sepsis and organ dysfunction in pediatrics. Pediatric Critical Care Medicine 2005;6(1):2–8.

Box 5
Key similarities between pediatric and adult sepsis

Comorbid conditions contribute significantly to mortality.

Acute kidney injury is an independent risk factor for mortality in critically ill children and adults.

Disseminated intravascular coagulation impacts the likelihood of developing multisystem organ failure as a complication of sepsis.[14]

Metabolic acidosis is a common and can be monitored with serum lactate.

Ultrasound imaging can guide central line placement, measure contractility or evaluate ventricular filling.

Aggressive fluid resuscitation and prompt administration of antibiotics are goals of therapy.

Low tidal volume strategies are recommended during ventilatory support of sepsis.[15]

---

owing to the increased afterload in the setting of shock and vasoconstriction. This mechanism makes cold shock more likely in the pediatric population (**Table 2**).[23] Pediatric patients demonstrate greater abnormalities in vasoregulation and myocardial dysfunction when compared with adults. The end result is a different role and emphasis on inotropic support in pediatric septic shock.[16] These physiologic differences and other differences between pediatric and adult sepsis are summarized in **Box 6**.[24]

Developmental differences are also present in the physiologic responses of pediatric sepsis patients. Infants and children with sepsis are at greater risk for respiratory collapse than adults owing to a combination of proportionally lower alveolar surface area, lower functional residual capacity, more compliant chest wall dynamics, and relatively greater expenditure of energy to maintain respiratory drive when in distress.[16] Further, ventilation/perfusion mismatch plays a relatively greater role in generating hypoxia as a result of sepsis. In conjunction with a tendency to generate relatively higher systemic vascular resistance, a reduction in oxygen delivery, rather than a defect in oxygen extraction, can be the major determinant of oxygen consumption in pediatric sepsis.[13]

Neonates and young infants may be at increased risk for bleeding complications owing to lower circulating levels of vitamin K–dependent procoagulant factors, decreased thrombin production, lower circulating levels of coagulation inhibitors, and relatively hyporesponsive platelets.[16] Hypocalcemia is a more frequent contributor to cardiac dysfunction in pediatric (especially neonatal) sepsis owing to a variety of developmental factors. Hypoglycemia is relatively common in neonates owing to

---

Table 2
Manifestations of cold and warm shock in pediatrics

Cold Shock: High SVR	Warm Shock: Low SVR
Cool/cold clammy, mottled, or cyanotic extremities	Warm, dry extremities ± flushed skin
Capillary refill >2 seconds	Capillary refill <2 seconds, "flash cap refill"
Diminished or thready peripheral pulses or significant differential in central and peripheral pulses	
	Tachycardia (age specific)
Tachycardia or bradycardia (age specific)	Bounding peripheral pulses
Narrow pulse pressure	Wide pulse pressure

Box 6
Key differences between pediatric and adult sepsis

Epidemiology

- Mortality lower in pediatric (8.9%–10%) than adult (20%–30%) sepsis.[24]
- Some pathogens are relatively restricted to the neonatal population (*Group B Streptococcus*, *Escherichia coli*, *Listeria*, disseminated herpes simplex virus).

Pathophysiology

- Myocardial dysfunction plays a greater role in the clinical picture of pediatric sepsis.
- Younger infants and children more likely to require inotropic support for similar perturbations in clinical status.
- Mortality more often related to diminished cardiac output, rather than low systemic vascular resistance in pediatric sepsis.

Presentation

- Children have greater percentage of body fluids in extracellular compartment, which increases risk of hypovolemia or shock as a component of critical illness.[16]
- Children have limited heart rate reserve compared with adults because they have higher starting heart rates.[13]
- Cold shock is relatively common in pediatric sepsis, where catecholamine-refractory low cardiac output and high vascular resistance septic shock is rare in adults.
- Infants and children are at greater risk of respiratory collapse in critical illness.
- Infants are at particularly high risk of disseminated intravascular coagulation as a result of sepsis.
- Hypocalcemia and hypoglycemia are more likely to complicate pediatric sepsis.

Differential

- Includes etiologies unique to the pediatric population: inborn errors of metabolism, congenital heart disease, perinatally acquired infections, and child abuse.

Initial Recognition and Management

- Recognition of sepsis before the development of hypotension plays critical role in pediatric mortality
- Hypothermia is a more common presenting sign in neonates and infants.
- Relatively large body surface area and immature mechanisms of thermogenesis makes need for external warming more likely in infants.[13]
- Central lines available include umbilical artery and umbilical venous catheters and intraosseous needles in pediatrics.

---

smaller glycogen stores, lower muscle mass, and relatively immature metabolic processes. Finally, genetic, congenital, and acquired factors contribute to the fact that children are more likely to have absolute adrenal insufficiency complicate management of septic shock.[13]

RECOGNIZING PEDIATRIC SEPSIS IN THE EMERGENCY DEPARTMENT

The presentation of a child with sepsis varies with the pathogenesis of the organism as well as characteristics of the host. Illness can be indolent and progressive or sudden and dramatic.

Fever is a common presenting sign of sepsis in the pediatric populations, but is not specific to sepsis as a source of infection. Younger children and infants (much like the elderly) can also present with hypothermia as a manifestation of sepsis. Hypoxia and carbon dioxide retention are frequent findings in sepsis, and can be used to document disease progression. Because children rely greatly on elevation of HR to enhance CO, tachycardia is a frequent finding in pediatric sepsis. Signs of cold shock are more common in children because they use vasoconstriction to maintain blood pressure when stroke volume decreases. This phenomenon manifests as weak or absent distal pulses, prolonged capillary refill, cool extremities, and mottling of the skin. Hypotension is a relatively late and ominous sign in sepsis, signifying the inadequacy of compensatory mechanisms to bolster CO and enhance systemic vascular resistance.[25] Recognizing sepsis and initiating definitive treatment before the development of hypotension is paramount in decreasing mortality associated with pediatric sepsis (2007 Update of the 2002 ACCM Clinical Guidelines for Hemodynamic Support of Neonates and Children with Septic Shock).

Infants and children who present with sepsis may be described as fussy, sleepy, lethargic, irritable, not feeding well, or "just not looking right." Skin can be pale, cyanotic, mottled, exanthematous, or show signs of DIC, such as petechiae or purpura (see **Boxes 2** and **3**). Associated symptoms may include vomiting, diarrhea, chills, respiratory distress, apnea, poor tone, evidence of skin or tissue infection, jaundice, oliguria, altered mental status, anxiety, apnea, shock, or almost any sign of organ injury (see **Box 4**). Given the relative paucity of developmental abilities in neonates, this population is most likely to present with nonspecific, subtle signs of infection and are at greatest risk of having recognition delayed until more ominous mental status or vital sign changes occur.

When caring for the septic-appearing infant or child, the differential diagnosis includes consideration of cardiopulmonary disease (eg, pneumonia, heart failure, pericarditis, myocarditis, pulmonary embolus), metabolic disorders (eg, adrenal insufficiency, diabetes mellitus, diabetes insipidus, inborn errors of metabolism), gastrointestinal pathology (eg, gastroenteritis, peritonitis, hemorrhage, intussusception, volvulus), hematologic disease (eg, anemia, splenic sequestration, proliferative malignancies), neurologic disorders (eg, spontaneous and traumatic bleeds, intoxication, infant botulism), toxic ingestion (eg, clonidine, beta-blocker), anaphylaxis, hemolytic–uremic syndrome,[17] and consideration of child abuse or neglect. The differential in neonatal patients can be further broadened to include pneumonia from aspiration of amniotic fluid, congenital heart lesions causing hypoperfusion and cardiac dysfunction, hypoglycemia related to inborn errors of metabolism, congenital adrenal hyperplasia, and the classic TORCH (toxoplasma, rubella, cytomegalovirus, and herpes simplex) or other perinatally acquired infections.

Metabolic acidosis results when tissues and organ systems are hypoperfused with respect to their oxygen and substrate demands. Infants and children often become tachypneic in the setting of metabolic acidosis, even when the lungs are not the primary source of infection. This situation can result in persistent fetal circulation and severe pulmonary hypertension in neonates and can contribute to cardiac manifestations such as increased right ventricular workload and patent ductus arteriosus. Complete blood cell counts may demonstrate leukocytosis, but leukopenia is a not an uncommon finding in young infants and neonates with sepsis. Hemoglobin and hematocrit values are typically normal unless there is hemolysis from DIC, which is relatively more common in pediatric than adult sepsis. Oliguria and anuria can manifest as elevated creatinine, whereas hepatocellular disease can result in hyperbilirubinemia, transaminitis, and coagulopathy. Finally, hypoglycemia can complicate the presentation and diagnosis of sepsis and contributes to the morbidity.

Similar to adults, the evaluation of sepsis focuses on source identification through cultures, laboratory studies, and imaging as appropriate. Inflammatory markers are less well-studied and supported than in adult sepsis.[25]

MANAGEMENT

Even the most seasoned pediatrician could agree that one of the hardest parts of managing pediatric severe sepsis and septic shock is early recognition. Febrile illness throughout childhood is common and may be a benign viral syndrome or the beginning of sepsis. Classic presentations of pyrexia, vasodilatation, and tachycardia are often seen with benign viral syndromes; however, when combined with signs of poor perfusion (see **Box 3**), sepsis should be suspected.[13] The next sections focus on the acute management of pediatric severe sepsis and septic shock in the ED.

Initial Stabilization

In the setting of pediatric sepsis, the first hour of resuscitation begins with initiating high-flow oxygen delivery by nasal cannula (nasopharyngeal continuous positive airway pressure is also acceptable) or 100% oxygen supplement by nonrebreather mask. Simultaneously, intravenous or intraosseous access should be established within 5 minutes.[13,26,27] Continuous cardiorespiratory and pulse oximetry monitoring should be applied and are useful tools for assessing resuscitation progress. It is recommended to monitor temperature (eg, rectal, oral, bladder catheter), cycle a blood pressure at least every 15 minutes, and track urine output. More invasive monitoring options such as central venous pressure, arterial blood pressure, and superior vena cava oxygen saturation (treatment goal >70%) are helpful in guiding treatment but are limited options in most ED settings, and therefore are not covered in this article. The goals within the first hour are to establish or maintain an airway, optimize oxygenation and ventilation, support circulation and restore adequate perfusion, and administer antibiotics early.[13]

Intravenous fluid resuscitation should begin with a 20 mL/kg rapid bolus of crystalloid.[13] Initial laboratory studies should include peripheral blood culture, culture from indwelling central line or port if applicable, a complete blood count (with automated differential), coagulation studies, DIC studies, complete metabolic panel, ionized calcium, lactic acid, arterial blood gases or venous blood gases, urinalysis with culture, cerebrospinal fluid studies if meningitis is suspected, and other appropriate cultures (eg, wound, sputum).[13] Viral sources are common in pediatrics and targeted testing may be of significant value such as influenza, respiratory syncytial virus, herpes simplex virus, cytomegalovirus, or enterovirus. Inflammatory markers such as C-reactive protein and procalcitonin should be drawn as baseline laboratory values to guide inpatient management. Procalcitonin has shown some promise as a biomarker for distinguishing bacterial from viral illness, delineating SIRS from sepsis, and even helping to guide inpatient antibiotic therapy.[28,29] However, procalcitonin is not ready in the ED for adult or pediatric sepsis to be used in isolation as a determining factor when considering initiation of antibiotics for sepsis.

Ideally, 2 intravenous lines should be established if possible to augment fluid administration and to ensure safe and timely administration of inotropes and antibiotics, because some of these medications must be given in separate intravenous lines (eg, epinephrine is not compatible with vancomycin). Fluid administration by gravity does not deliver resuscitation volume in a timely manner; therefore, it is recommended to give a 20 mL/kg (maximum 1000 mL per bolus) bolus over 5 minutes by syringe push or pressure bag.[30] Repeat fluid boluses over the first 15 minutes while reassessing after each fluid bolus for response to treatment and signs of fluid overload. Often, resuscitation requires 40 to 60 mL/kg of crystalloids, with some children requiring upwards of 200 mL/kg.[13] When sepsis resuscitation efforts in the ED fail to give more than 40 mL/kg within the first hour, the risk for mortality significantly increases.[31]

During fluid resuscitation, the emergency physician should evaluate for signs of improved perfusion such as normalization of vital signs for age. However, attention should also be given to signs of heart failure and fluid overload.[13] Signs of heart failure or fluid overload include the development of rales, cardiomegaly on chest radiograph, increased work of breathing, hypoxemia owing to pulmonary edema, and hepatomegaly. Development of fluid-overload warrants cessation of fluid resuscitation and initiating diuretic therapy and inotropic support.[27] Resuscitation endpoints in the first hour include goals to (1) normalize vital signs for age, (2) normalize mental status, (3) achieve capillary refill of 2 seconds or less, and (4) produce urine output of greater than 1 mL/kg/h. Admission for pediatric sepsis should be to the pediatric intensive care unit.

The ACCM guidelines suggest optimizing oxygen-carrying capacity by transfusing packed red blood cells (10 mL/kg) for hemoglobin levels of less than 10 g/dL. If the patient is actively bleeding during resuscitation, thrombocytopenia of less than or equal to 50,000 should be corrected with platelet transfusions (10 mL/kg in infants and children will increase platelet count by roughly 50,000 μL).[32] Consider prophylactic platelet transfusions for those without active bleeding, but with platelet counts of less than 20,000/mm^3.[27] Fresh frozen plasma infusion (10–15 mL/kg) will increase clotting factors percentage by 20%[32] and is appropriate for those with a prolonged international normalized ratio. This substance should be infused slowly to limit hypotensive side effects.[13]

Roughly 40% of CO is required to sustain respiratory efforts for a child during septic shock.[13] Intubation and mechanical ventilation can help to reverse shock by maximizing CO through reduction in cardiac effort required to maintain work of breathing. Children with declining mentation or those with poor ventilatory effort may benefit from intubation. The 2007 ACCM guidelines do not make specific endorsements for induction medications; however, they do recommend against the use of etomidate and dexmedetomidine in septic shock because there is evidence for worsening outcomes with depression of the adrenal axis and sympathetic nervous system. Prolonged propofol use in children less than 3 years of age is associated with metabolic acidosis and is not recommended.[13] Ketamine is a useful potential alternative induction and sedation agent owing to its favorable hemodynamic profile.

Fluid-Refractory Shock and Vasoactive Support

The ACCM guidelines recommend that fluid-refractory shock should be considered if after giving 40 to 60 mL/kg of isotonic fluids, hypotension or signs of poor perfusion are present. Once fluid refractory shock is recognized, the next step is to consider whether cold shock or warm shock (see **Table 2**) is present. Then, start vasoactive support by peripheral intravenous or intraosseous infusion while attempting to gain central venous access. Dopamine (started at 5 μg/kg/min and titrated up to 10 μg/kg/min) is first line for treating fluid-refractory shock.[13,33] Those who remain in shock despite greater than 10 μg/kg/min of dopamine usually respond to continuous infusions of norepinephrine (0.05–1.5 μg/kg/min)[34] for warm shock, or epinephrine (0.05–0.3 μg/kg/min, maximum of 1 μg/kg/min) for cold shock. There is limited evidence to guide inotrope management in those who are normotensive but persist with signs of shock. Finally, patients with refractory shock should be evaluated for potentially reversible underlying causes of shock (**Table 3**). Extracorporeal membrane oxygenation remains the definitive treatment for patients with refractory septic shock. This treatment should be taken into account when considering transfer options to a tertiary hospital.

Catecholamine-Resistant Shock

Steroid use in pediatric sepsis remains a controversial topic because there are very limited randomized controlled trials to guide recommendations. Children with underlying diseases requiring chronic steroid use, hypothalamic–pituitary–adrenal axis disorders, or those with purpura fulminans or Waterhouse–Friderichen syndrome are at risk of having insufficient cortisol/aldosterone production during shock.[13] The ACCM guidelines reserve recommendation for steroid use only in children who do not respond to epinephrine or norepinephrine infusions (eg, catecholamine-resistant shock) and are suspected to be at risk for adrenal insufficiency or hypothalamic–pituitary–adrenal axis failure. For these patients, a baseline cortisol level should be drawn before administering hydrocortisone stress dose.[13,32,33]

Antibiotic Administration

Antibiotics should be given within the first hour of sepsis and septic shock.[13,27,35] Common choices include ceftriaxone, cefipime, and vancomycin. Factors such as local antibiotic resistance patterns, recent antibiotic use, existing immunosuppression, and drug allergies may factor importantly when choosing antibiotic therapy. **Table 4** outlines some special considerations in treating pediatric sepsis.[36]

Table 3	
Potential causes of refractory shock and associated treatments	
Etiology	**Intervention**
Pericardial effusion	Pericardiocentesis
Pneumothorax	Thoracentesis
Hypoadrenalism	Adrenal hormone replacement
Hypothyroidism	Thyroid hormone replacement
Ongoing blood loss	Replace blood loss, correct coagulopathy
Abdominal compartment syndrome	Peritoneal catheter or surgical abdominal release
Necrotic tissue	Source infection removal and tissue debridement
Inappropriate source control of infection	Nidus removal, intravenous immunoglobulin for toxic shock, appropriate antibiotic use
Excessive immunosuppression	Wean immunosuppressive agents
Immune compromised states	Enhance immune function, white cell growth factors, transfusions

Refractory shock: Shock that persists despite goal-directed use of inotropic agents, vasopressors, vasodilators, and maintenance of metabolic (glucose and calcium) and hormonal (thyroid, hydrocortisone, insulin) homeostasis.
Data from Brierley J, Carcillo JA, Choong K, et al. Clinical practice parameters for hemodynamic support of pediatric and neonatal septic shock: 2007 update from the American College of Critical Care Medicine. Critical Care Medicine 2009;37(2):666–8.

Table 4
Pediatric populations with special considerations in sepsis

Population At-Risk for Sepsis	Typical Pathogens	Antibiotic Recommendations[36]
Surgical and medical splenectomy/asplenia	Encapsulated organisms (*Streptococcus pneumonia, Haemophilus influenza, Neisseria meningitides*)	(Extended-spectrum penicillin or third- or fourth-generation cephalosporin) ± aminoglycoside ± vancomycin
Immune deficiencies/ neutropenia	All pathogens, including opportunistic infections	(Extended-spectrum penicillin or third- or fourth-generation cephalosporin or carbapenem) ± aminoglycoside ± vancomycin, consider antifungals
Medical catheters and hardware	Skin flora (>50% coagulase-negative staphylococci), 20%–30% Gram-negative enteric bacteria, 5%–10% fungi[39]	(Extended-spectrum penicillin or third- or fourth-generation cephalosporin) ± aminoglycoside ± vancomycin
Organ/bone marrow transplantation	All pathogens, including opportunistic infections	(Extended-spectrum penicillin or third- or fourth-generation cephalosporin or carbapenem) ± aminoglycoside ± vancomycin, consider antifungals
Burn victims	*Pseudomonas aeruginosa, Streptococcus aureus,* coagulase-negative staphylococci	Broad-spectrum antibiotics including coverage for *P aeruginosa*
Neonates	*Escherichia coli, group B Streptococcus, Listeria,* herpes simplex virus, pathogens acquired transplacentally	Ampicillin and gentamicin ± vancomycin

Glucose and Calcium Abnormalities

Glucose derangements are common in critically ill children and infants and require prompt recognition and correction by the emergency physician. If unrecognized or treated inappropriately, mortality and the risk for long-term sequelae increase.[13,27] Hypoglycemia is seen more frequently in neonates owing to their limited glycogen stores, increased peripheral glucose use, and inadequate gluconeogenesis. Hypoglycemia can occur in older children as well and could be a sign of severe disease progression (or adrenal insufficiency). Acute hypoglycemia is treated by correcting deficit to normal glucose levels by giving appropriate dextrose-containing solutions for age. It is important to avoid repeated hypoglycemia by initiating infusion of dextrose-containing fluids (D10 isotonic fluid) at age-specific maintenance rates.[13] Hyperglycemia, after initial stress response, can be complicated by impaired insulin production and insulin resistance in sepsis. Also, patients requiring epinephrine infusions are at increased risk for developing hyperglycemia because epinephrine promotes gluconeogenesis and glycogenolysis in addition to inhibiting insulin production. It is recommended to treat hyperglycemia with insulin therapy targeting blood glucose ranges of 80 to 150 mg/dL.[13,27]

Similarly, the ACCM guidelines recommend correcting hypocalcemia (defined as ionized calcium <1.1 mmol/L), because it may contribute to cardiac dysfunction. Intravenous calcium gluconate (50–100 mg/kg) given over 3 to 5 minutes is the treatment for hypocalcemia with cardiac manifestations and a dose of 100 to 200 mg/kg/dose over 20 minutes is recommended for patients with tetany.[32]

PEDIATRIC POPULATIONS WITH ADDITIONAL CONSIDERATIONS IN SEPSIS

Streptococcus pneumonia and *Neisseria meningitidis* emerge as the primary pathogens in sepsis of older infants and children. There are, however, some pediatric patient groups with characteristics that put them at risk of sepsis from other unique pathogens (see **Table 4**).

The risk of sepsis after splenectomy is especially high in children younger than 5 years of age at the time of surgery. *Pneumococcus* accounts for 50% of sepsis after splenectomy, but patients are at risk of invasive infection from all encapsulated microorganisms. Children with sickle cell disease develop a functional asplenia associated with autoinfarction of splenic microvasculature putting this population at several hundredfold higher risk of sepsis from encapsulated organisms such as *S pneumonia*, *Haemophilus influenza*, and *N meningitides*.[37]

Compromised innate or adaptive immunity places patients at greater risk of bacterial sepsis than the average population. Patients with altered ability to mount tissue, inflammatory, or antibody responses are also at risk for sepsis related to organisms of low virulence or even components of normal skin and mucous membrane flora (eg, *Candida albicans*), viruses (including viral pathogens to which they may have been previously immunized) and protozoa (eg, *Pneumocystis carinii*). Neutropenia places infants and children at increased risk of invasive infections, such as sepsis. The reduced white blood cell count and diminished ability to mount an effective host response results in fewer manifestations of inflammation. Neutropenic patients require empiric broad-spectrum antibiotic coverage when febrile,[38] because fever may be the only presenting sign of sepsis. Children and infants can be immunocompromised as a result of long-term steroid use, congenital deficiency syndromes, or acquired illnesses, such as human immunodeficiency virus infection. Children with cancer represent a special population because they can be immunocompromised from their malignancy or chemotherapy. In addition, they often have central lines or ports that increase their exposure to pathogens.

Foreign body reaction can contribute to adherence and proliferation of microorganisms in and on medical hardware and in-dwelling catheters or central lines. Pathogenesis can be related to local contamination and colonization of skin flora at the insertion site, from infection of the lumen of the catheter from contaminated infusate, or from improper handling of infusion site.[39]

Pediatric patients who have undergone organ transplantation are susceptible to sepsis based on their underlying comorbidities and the use of immune modulators to prevent organ rejection. Most notably, bone marrow transplantation results in neutropenia from immune modulators, but also other impaired cell-mediated and humoral immunity, changes in host microbial flora, and compromised skin and mucous membrane integrity.[40] Fever in these patients warrants broad antimicrobial coverage to prevent fulminant sepsis.

Burns compromise the innate immunity of the skin and result in neutrophil dysfunction and abnormal antibody response. Necrotic tissue can be a nidus of infection. Burn victims are at increased risk of sepsis, particularly from *P aeruginosa*, *S aureus*, and *coagulase-negative staphylococci*. Sepsis may also be complicated by inadequate cortisol or aldosterone production in patients with meningococcemia, Waterhouse–Friderichsen syndrome, those on chronic steroid therapy, or those with pituitary or adrenal abnormalities.

The neonate is a special pediatric patient in whom deficits in innate and adaptive immune responses are particularly pronounced.[16] Additionally, this population is not immunized against many common organisms that cause significant morbidity and mortality in infants. Newborns are at risk for infection from *Escherichia coli, Group B streptococcus*, and *Listeria*. Additionally, the source of sepsis may be unique in this age group and can include complications from chorioamnionitis, omphalitis (umbilical stump infection), stage III necrotizing enterocolitis or congenital transmission of pathogens (eg, toxoplasmosis, cytomegalovirus, herpes simplex virus, parvovirus, rubella, and syphilis).

Neonatal sepsis is more often associated with hypothermia than fever.[41] Apnea is a common presenting sign. Severe neonatal sepsis is more likely to be associated with neutropenia than leukocytosis.[41] These features are particularly pronounced in the premature neonate, who is also at particularly high risk for complicated sepsis related to deficiencies in the thyroid and parathyroid axes.[13]

Newborn sepsis can be complicated by cardiac and circulatory factors that are unique to the neonatal period. Sepsis-induced hypoxia and acidosis have direct effects on pulmonary vascular resistance and arterial pressure, and can result in persistent fetal circulation, continued patency of the ductus arteriosus, or persistent pulmonary hypertension of the newborn. For this reason, sepsis can be accompanied by right ventricular failure and excessive pulmonary artery pressures.[13]

SUMMARY

Sepsis continues to be a leading cause of death in the pediatric and neonatal populations. Congenital heart disease and chronic lung disease are the comorbidities most associated with sepsis in infants, who tend to present with primary bacteremia. Cancer and neuromuscular disease emerge more often in secondary bacteremia and childhood sepsis. Age-specific vital signs and development-specific clinical parameters complicate the early recognition of pediatric sepsis, which is crucial if the provider is going to engage in effective treatment. Early goal-directed therapy in pediatric sepsis focuses on source control and support of organ perfusion and function, but differs from management of adult septic shock in the selection of inotropes and the recommendation to start vasoactive medications peripherally while securing central access.

REFERENCES

1. Singer M, Deutschman CS, Seymour CW, et al. The third international consensus definitions for sepsis and septic shock (Sepsis-3). JAMA 2016;315(8):801–10.
2. Osterman MJ, Kochanek KD, MacDorman MF, et al. Annual summary of vital statistics: 2012-2013. Pediatrics 2015;135(6):1115–25.
3. Balamuth F, Weiss SL, Neuman MI, et al. Pediatric severe sepsis in US children's hospitals. Pediatr Crit Care Med 2014;15(9):798–805.
4. Watson RS, Carcillo JA, Linde-Zwirble WT, et al. The epidemiology of severe sepsis in children in the United States. Am J Respir Crit Care Med 2003;167:695–701.
5. Hartman ME, Linde-Zwirble WT, Angus DC, et al. Trends in the epidemiology of pediatric severe sepsis. Pediatr Crit Care Med 2013;14(7):686–93.
6. Singhal S, Allen MW, McAnnally JR, et al. National estimates of emergency department visits for pediatric severe sepsis in the United States. Peer J 2013;1:e79.

7. Han YY, Carcillo JA, Dragotta MA, et al. Early reversal of pediatric-neonatal septic shock by community physicians is associated with improved outcome. Pediatrics 2003;112(4):793–9.

8. Paul R, Neuman MI, Monuteaux MC, et al. Adherence to PALS sepsis guidelines and hospital length of stay. Pediatrics 2012;130(2):e273–80.

9. Carcillo JA, Fields AI, Task Force Committee Members. Clinical practice variables for hemodynamic support of pediatric and neonatal patients in septic shock. Crit Care Med 2002;30(6):1365–78.

10. Goldstein B, Giroir B, Randolph A, et al. International pediatric sepsis consensus conference: Definitions for sepsis and organ dysfunction in pediatrics. Pediatr Crit Care Med 2005;6(1):2–8.

11. Gebara BM. Letters to the editor: values for systolic blood pressure. Pediatr Crit Care Med 2005;6(4):500 (Table 3 – Modified Age-specific systolic blood pressure values; Goldstein B, Giroir B, Randolph A).

12. Haque IU, Zaritsky AL. Analysis of the evidence for the lower limit of systolic and mean arterial pressure in children. Pediatr Crit Care Med 2007;8:138–44.

13. Brierley J, Carcillo JA, Choong K, et al. Clinical practice parameters for hemodynamic support of pediatric and neonatal septic shock: 2007 update from the American College of Critical Care Medicine. Crit Care Med 2009;37(2):666–88.

14. Khemani R, Bart R, Alonzo T, et al. Disseminated intravascular coagulation score is associated with mortality for children with shock. Intensive Care Med 2009;35: 327–33.

15. Hanson J, Flori H. Application of the acute respiratory distress syndrome network low-tidal volume strategy to pediatric acute lung injury. Respir Clin North America 2006;12:349–57.

16. Wheeler DS, Wong HR, Zingarelli B. Pediatric sepsis – part I: "children are not small adults!". Open Inflamm J 2011;4:4–15.

17. Powell K. Sepsis and shock. In: Behrman RE, Kliegman RM, Jenson HB, editors. Nelson textbook of pediatrics. 16th edition. Philadelphia: W.B. Saunders Company; 2000. p. 747–51.

18. Proulx F, Sebastien J, Mariscalco M, et al. The pediatric multiple organ dysfunction syndrome. Pediatr Crit Care Med 2009;10:12–22.

19. Watson R, Carcillo J. Scope and epidemiology of pediatric sepsis. Pediatr Crit Care Med 2005;6(3 Suppl):S3–5.

20. Luce W, Hoffman T, Bauer J. Bench-to-bedside review: developmental influences on the mechanisms, treatment and outcomes of cardiovascular dysfunction in neonatal versus adult sepsis. Crit Care 2007;11:228.

21. Reynolds E, Ryan D, Sheridan R, et al. Left ventricular failure complicating severe pediatric burn injuries. J Pediatr Surg 1995;30:264–70.

22. Crepaz R, Pitscheider W, Radetti G, et al. Age-related variation in left ventricular myocardial contractile state expressed by the stress velocity relation. Pediatr Cardiol 1998;19:463–7.

23. Ceneviva G, Paschall J, Maffei F, et al. Hemodynamic support in fluid refractory pediatric septic shock. Pediatrics 1998;102:e19.

24. Angus DC, Linde-Zwirble WT, Lidicker J, et al. Epidemiology of severe sepsis in the United States: analysis of incidence, outcome, and associated costs of care. Crit Care Med 2001;39:1303–10.

25. Giuliano JS. Septic Shock. Open Pediatr Med J 2013;7(Suppl 1: M6):28–34.

26. Hazinkski MF, Zaritsky A, Nadkarni VM, et al. Pediatric advance life support provider manual. Dallas (TX): American Heart Association; 2002.

27. Dellinger RP, Levy MM, Rhodes A, et al, Surviving Sepsis Campaign Guidelines Committee including the Pediatric Subgroup. Surviving sepsis campaign: international guidelines for management of severe sepsis and septic shock: 2012. Crit Care Med 2013;41(2):580–637.

28. Andreola B, Bressan S, Callegaro S, et al. Procalcitonin and C-reactive protein as diagnostic markers of severe bacterial infections in febrile infants and children in the emergency department. Pediatr Infect Dis J 2007;26(8):672–7.

29. Arkader R, Troster EJ, Lopes MR, et al. Procalcitonin does discriminate between sepsis and systemic inflammatory response syndrome. Arch Dis Child 2006; 91(2):117–20.

30. Stoner MJ, Goodman DG, Cohen DM, et al. Rapid fluid resuscitation in pediatrics: testing the American College of Critical Care Medicine guideline. Ann Emerg Med 2007;50(5):601–7.

31. Carcillo JA, Davis AL, Zaritsky A. Role of early fluid resuscitation in pediatric septic shock. JAMA 1991;266(9):1242–5.

32. Arcara KM, Tschudy MM, editors. The Harriet Lane handbook. 19th edition. Philadelphia: Elsevier; 2012.

33. Irazuzta J, Sullivan KJ, Garcia PC, et al. Pharmacologic support of infants and children in septic shock. J Pediatr (Rio J) 2007;83(2):S36–45.

34. Turner DA, Cheifetz IM. Shock. In: Kliegman RM, Stanton BF, St Geme JW, et al, editors. Nelson's textbook of pediatrics. 20th edition. Philadelphia: Elsevier; 2016. p. 516–27.

35. Kumar A. An alternate pathophysiologic paradigm of sepsis and septic shock: Implications for optimizing antimicrobial therapy. Virulence 2014;5(1):80–97.

36. Simmons ML, Durham SH, Carter CW. Pharmacological management of pediatric patients with sepsis. Adv Crit Care 2012;23(4):437–48.

37. Cohen A. Hematologic emergencies. In: Behrman R, Kliegman R, Jenson H, editors. Nelson textbook of pediatrics. 16th edition. Philadelphia: W.B. Saunders; 2000. p. 865–6.

38. Cohen AR. Hematologic emergencies. In: Fleisher G, Ludwig S, Henretig F, editors. Textbook of pediatric emergency medicine. 4th edition. Philadelphia: Lippincott Williams & Wilkins; 2000. p. 873–4.

39. Flynn P, Barrett F. Infection associated with medical devices. In: Behrman R, Kliegman R, Jenson H, editors. Nelson's textbook of pediatrics. Philadelphia: W.B. Saunders; 2000. p. 788.

40. Hughes W, Pizzo P. Infections in immunocompromised hosts. In: Behrman R, K. RM, J. HB, editors. Nelson's textbook of pediatrics. 16 edition. Philadelphia: W.B. Saunders; 2000. p. 780–8.

41. Selbst S. The septic-appearing infant. In: Fleisher G, Ludwig S, Henretig F, editors. The textbook of pediatric emergency medicine. 16th edition. Philadelphia: Lippincott Williams & Wilkins; 2000. p. 565–72.

Sepsis in Special Populations

Matthew P. Borloz, MD*, Khalief E. Hamden, MD, MS

KEYWORDS

- Sepsis • Pregnancy • Cirrhosis • End-stage renal disease • Obesity

KEY POINTS

- Comorbid conditions and altered physiology lead to delayed recognition of sepsis and complicate its management.
- Medications used to treat sepsis during pregnancy and the puerperium are largely the same as those used in nonpregnant patients.
- Broad-spectrum antibiotic coverage among septic patients with cirrhosis is increasingly important as multidrug-resistant strains are rising in prevalence.
- Patients on hemodialysis have a high incidence of bacteremia; empirical antibiotics should cover methicillin-resistant *Staphylococcus aureus* and gram-negative organisms.
- Obesity limits the sensitivity of physical examination findings as well as clinical assessments of volume status.

INTRODUCTION

The diagnosis and management of sepsis are often complicated by the presence of comorbid conditions or altered physiology (**Box 1**). Although a discussion of every one of these would be outside the scope of this article, the authors have chosen to focus on 4 that are encountered in every emergency department (ED) with some frequency: pregnancy and the puerperium, cirrhosis, end-stage renal disease (ESRD), and obesity.

PREGNANCY AND THE PUERPERIUM
Background

The physiologic adjustments that result from pregnancy and the puerperium (ie, the 6 weeks immediately following delivery) introduce numerous challenges to the prompt recognition and appropriate management of sepsis in this population. Specific

The authors have nothing to disclose.
Department of Emergency Medicine, Virginia Tech Carilion School of Medicine, One Riverside Circle, Roanoke, VA 24016, USA
* Corresponding author.
E-mail address: mpborloz@carilionclinic.org

Emerg Med Clin N Am 35 (2017) 139–158
http://dx.doi.org/10.1016/j.emc.2016.08.006
0733-8627/17/

Box 1
Pitfalls in the diagnosis and treatment of sepsis in special populations

Pregnancy and the puerperium

Pitfall: Falsely attributing the following abnormalities to normal pregnancy instead of sepsis:
- ↑ Heart rate
- ↓ Blood pressure
- ↑ White blood cell count
- ↑ Respiratory rate (tachypnea is *not normal* in pregnancy)
- ↓ Platelet count

Cirrhosis

Pitfall: Falsely attributing the following abnormalities to cirrhosis instead of sepsis:
- ↑ Heart rate
- ↓ Blood pressure
- ↑ Lactate
- ↓ Platelet count

Pitfall: Common modalities to measure volume status are unreliable:
- Inferior vena cava measurements on ultrasound are not validated in this population.
- Passive leg raise is unreliable in the setting of tense ascites with intra-abdominal hypertension.
- Intravascular depletion may be present despite massive extravascular fluid (eg, pleural effusion, ascites, peripheral edema).

Pitfall: Beta-blocker therapy (common in cirrhosis) blunts the tachycardic response often seen in sepsis.

End-stage renal disease

Pitfall: Not recognizing unique sources of infection and difficulty in volume status assessment
- Bacteremia is a common source of infection and lacks specific examination clues.
- Indwelling lines may be the source; providers are often reluctant to remove hemodialysis access.
- Markers of organ failure (ie, creatinine, urine output) are not available as indicators.
- Large swings in volume status at baseline may blunt the physiologic response in acute illness.
- Multiple comorbid conditions and associated chronic medications impair recognition of acute illness (eg, beta-blockers blunt tachycardia).

Obesity

Pitfall: Efforts to identify source of infection limited by body habitus
- Cellulitis may be hidden in skin folds.
- Abdominal, lung, and female pelvic examinations are less reliable.
- Abdominal ultrasound assessment (eg, for acute cholecystitis) is difficult.

Pitfall: Markers of volume status and cardiac function limited
- Jugular venous distention is difficult to see.
- Bedside echo and inferior vena cava ultrasound windows are limited.

---

infectious conditions to which obstetric patients are uniquely susceptible, as well as others to which all patients may be exposed, are mentioned; but a detailed discussion of each of these could fill a volume, and the goal of this section is to highlight patient factors that alter sepsis care compared with the baseline population.

The most recent large, population-based study of pregnancy-associated sepsis cited a rate of 26 hospitalizations per 100,000 pregnancies due to this condition, up from 11 per 100,000 8 years prior. Other differences over that same period included a higher rate of intensive care unit (ICU) admission (78% vs 90%), a higher rate of organ failure (9% vs 35% with ≥3 organ failures), and higher hospital charges (~$25,000 more). Despite what seems to be a sicker population, the mortality rate did not change significantly (**Table 1**).[1] Whether this is due to more effective management, variations in recognition, or other factors is not clear. From 2006 to 2008, sepsis was cited as the leading cause of direct maternal death in the United Kingdom; however, as of 2009 to 2012, it had been supplanted by thromboembolic disease.[2,3]

Diagnosis

Although reports are mixed, most published data suggest that approximately half of pregnancy-related sepsis diagnoses are made in the puerperium.[1,4–8] The most common site of infection among septic pregnant patients reported in the literature is uterine (eg, chorioamnionitis, endometritis), though urinary tract infections (UTIs) exceed these in some reports (**Box 2**).[1,6,8–10] *Escherichia coli* is the most frequently isolated microbe in both antepartum and puerperal sepsis, though group B streptococcus (*strep*) has been implicated most often among patients with intrapartum sepsis.[6,7] Pregnant patients diagnosed with sepsis due to group A *strep* often have rapid progression of illness with high morbidity and mortality according to several reports.[2,4,6] Unfortunately, culture data are often not available or not universally reported in relevant studies of maternal sepsis.[1,6]

Several factors contribute to the potential for delayed recognition of sepsis in obstetric patients. Increased progesterone levels during pregnancy result in a decrease

Table 1 Risk factors for pregnancy-associated sepsis	
	Adjusted Odds Ratio
Chronic liver disease[a]	41.4
Congestive heart failure[a]	20.5
Myocardial infarction[a]	11.0
Cerebrovascular disease[a]	8.6
Peptic ulcer disease[a]	6.5
Chronic kidney disease[a]	5.6
Malignancy[a]	4.7
HIV infection[a]	4.2
Drug abuse	3.4
Peripheral vascular disease[a]	2.8
Connective tissue disease[a]	2.3
Chronic pulmonary disease[a]	1.8
Nongestational diabetes[a]	1.8
Obesity	1.4
Black race	1.4
Preeclampsia/eclampsia	1.3
Poverty	1.3
Absence of health insurance	1.3
Gestational diabetes	0.5

Abbreviation: HIV, human immunodeficiency virus.

[a] Chronic comorbidity.

Data from Oud L, Watkins P. Evolving trends in the epidemiology, resource utilization, and outcomes of pregnancy-associated severe sepsis: a population-based cohort study. J Clin Med Res 2015;7(6):400–16.

Box 2
Infections during pregnancy and the puerperium

Direct (pregnancy related)

Chorioamnionitis

Endometritis/myometritis

Septic abortion

Septic pelvic thrombophlebitis

Wound infection (eg, episiotomy, perineal laceration, cesarean incision)

Indirect (pregnancy increases risk)

Community-acquired pneumonia (bacterial, viral, fungal)

UTI

Listeriosis

Of note, pregnant patients are also susceptible to the same infections as the nonpregnant population, including nosocomial infections. Those listed are merely the sites of infection posing a particularly increased risk.
Data from Morgan J, Roberts S. Maternal sepsis. Obstet Gynecol Clin North Am 2013;40(1):69–87; and Clark SL, Cotton DB, Lee W, et al. Central hemodynamic assessment of normal term pregnancy. Am J Obstet Gynecol 1989;161(6 Pt 1):1439–42.

---

in systemic vascular resistance of approximately 20% and an increase in mean heart rate from 71 beats per minute to 83 to 88 beats per minute.[11–13] As vasodilation and tachycardia are among the classic findings of nonpregnant patients with sepsis, this effectively removes several of the diagnostic features on which clinicians rely. Pregnant patients also typically have an increased minute ventilation due to a larger tidal volume rather than a higher respiratory rate. Consequently, tachypnea should never be ignored in this population.[14,15]

Leukocytosis in the third trimester is not unusual when patients may have white blood cell (WBC) counts approaching 17,000/μL. Normal values are expected by 4 weeks post partum.[16–18]

Elevated lactic acid levels in septic pregnant patients have been associated with an increased risk of positive blood cultures and transfer to a higher level of care.[19] Although the relevant study was small, retrospective, and did not focus on patient-oriented outcomes, the use of lactic acid measurements for prognostication and assessment of response to interventions in the obstetric population is likely similar to that in the nonpregnant population.[20]

The systemic inflammatory response syndrome (SIRS) criteria have been a cornerstone in defining and screening for sepsis. One of the SIRS criteria is heart rate greater than 90 beats per minute, whereas another is WBC greater than 12,000/μL.[21] Pregnant patients without infection may approach or exceed these thresholds even without true sepsis. Indeed, the standard SIRS criteria were found to have such poor specificity in an obstetric population with chorioamnionitis (<20%) that their use has been discouraged.[22] Obstetric SIRS criteria and a Sepsis in Obstetrics Score have been proposed to account for the physiologic changes of pregnancy; they have been used to define cases of maternal sepsis, though they have not been satisfactorily validated to recommend their widespread use.[6,23,24]

Creatinine is depressed (ie, lower than normal) during normal pregnancy, meaning that the emergency provider (EP) may be not be alarmed by a creatinine approaching 1.2 mg/dL.[25] Proposed reference values in previously healthy pregnant women include an upper limit of normal of 0.63 to 0.70 mg/dL.[26] Values between this threshold and 1.2 mg/dL are of uncertain significance in the setting of presumed sepsis.

Management

Pregnant patients have been excluded from each of the major sepsis trials; as a result, guidelines for the care of septic obstetric patients are largely based on inferred data or are simply not included in published recommendations.[27–32]

As with any patient, attention to airway, breathing, and circulation are paramount. Once the first two are secured, attention to hemodynamics follows. Antenatal patients in shock, particularly those in the latter half of pregnancy, should be placed in the left lateral decubitus position to minimize compression of the inferior vena cava by the gravid uterus. Patients exhibiting clinical signs of shock, including but not limited to those who are hypotensive, should be given intravenous crystalloid as the initial resuscitative fluid.[11,33,34] There are no evidence-based guidelines to suggest a particular volume, but the recommendation of 30 mL/kg for nonpregnant patients is likely appropriate in most otherwise healthy obstetric patients.[32] Special attention should be paid to the fact that the colloid osmotic pressure is lower in obstetric patients, so there is a higher risk for pulmonary edema with aggressive fluid loading.[2,11] There is no evidence that colloid solutions (eg, albumin, hydroxyethyl starch) should be used any differently in this population compared with nonpregnant septic patients.[11,33] Recent literature suggesting lower mortality with the use of balanced crystalloid solutions (eg, lactated Ringer) compared with unbalanced solutions (eg, normal saline) do not specifically address this population.[35,36]

Although there has been previous debate about the most appropriate vasopressor to be used in patients with sepsis-induced hypotension refractory to fluid therapy, the most recent guidelines for nonpregnant patients unequivocally recommend norepinephrine as the first-line agent.[32] Several reviews centered on maternal sepsis indicate that, although there is a risk of decreased uteroplacental blood flow with this drug, there is not evidence to suggest that the fetal risk is sufficiently high to recommend an alternative vasopressor.[33,34,37–39]

Table 2 lists commonly used antibacterial agents and a brief summary of their role in pregnancy. In summary, most antibiotic agents used in the care of septic patients who are not pregnant are acceptable for use in those who are. As in nonpregnant patients, source control is of utmost importance. Among pregnant patients with nonobstetric infections as the cause for their sepsis (eg, pneumonia), delivery has not been shown to uniformly improve outcomes for the mother or fetus.[40]

Generally speaking, optimal care for maternal sepsis focuses primarily on early recognition and consideration of infectious conditions unique to pregnancy and the puerperium. Once sepsis is identified, the medical management is actually quite similar to that in the nonobstetric population. Certain conditions that are traditionally managed surgically and coincidentally present during pregnancy (eg, acute appendicitis) are complicated by balancing maternal (and, thus, fetal) well-being in the setting of medically managed disease (eg, intravenous antibiotics) versus fetal viability in the setting of operative intervention.

CIRRHOSIS
Background

Cirrhosis refers to the diffuse fibrotic changes of the liver that may result from any number of causes (eg, chronic alcohol abuse, nonalcoholic steatohepatitis, viral hepatitis). A recent population-based study in the United States estimates a disease prevalence of 0.27%.[41]

Table 2	
Commonly used antibiotic agents and their role during pregnancy	
Penicillins	Preferred class, includes combinations with beta-lactamase inhibitors
Cephalosporins	Preferred class
Aminoglycosides	Acceptable if preferred agents fail Case reports of fetal ototoxicity/nephrotoxicity not supported by larger studies
Carbapenems	No clear risk, imipenem and meropenem preferred
Clindamycin	Recommended only in treatment failures after preferred agents
Fluoroquinolones	No clear risk, norfloxacin and ciprofloxacin preferred
Macrolides	Erythromycin, azithromycin, clarithromycin acceptable when necessary (eg, true penicillin allergy) Erythromycin estolate should not be given during 2nd or 3rd trimester
Metronidazole	Oral preferred over vaginal application for pelvic infection No clear risk with intravenous use
Monobactams	No clear risk with aztreonam
Nitrofurantoin	Acceptable if preferred agents fail or allergy exists Avoid in third trimester
Sulfonamides & trimethoprim	Conflicting data; avoid unless maternal benefit clearly outweighs risk & no alternative
Tetracyclines	Contraindicated after 15 weeks' gestational age Doxycycline preferred in first trimester for relevant infections
Vancomycin	No clear risk

Acceptable indicates that preferred agents should be used if at all possible, but these classes may be employed if life-threatening infection persists or preferred agents are prohibited by severe allergy.
Data from Jenne CN, Kubes P. Immune surveillance by the liver. Nat Immunol 2013;14(10):996–1006.

More than half of patients with cirrhosis admitted to the ICU die in the hospital, and the mean hospital length of stay is nearly 2 weeks.[42] Cirrhosis confers an enormous burden of disease, and these patients exhibit a 4- to 5-fold increase in the rate of infection at the time of, or during, hospitalization compared with the general population.[43] Cirrhosis leads to increased risk of infection due to the following: fibrotic changes in the liver's structure result in a diminished ability to filter bacteria; increased intestinal permeability leads to chronic exposure to translocated bacteria and consequent persistent immune system activation; reduced hepatic synthetic function causes diminished levels of complement and acute phase proteins; circulating immune cells exhibit impaired phagocytic ability; the response to vaccination is blunted.[44]

Spontaneous bacterial peritonitis (SBP) and UTIs are the most common sources of sepsis in this population. Traditionally, Enterobacteriaceae and nonenterococcal strep species have been implicated as the offending agents; however, multidrug-resistant organisms are increasingly being identified. Extended-spectrum beta-lactamase–producing *Enterobacteriaceae*, *Pseudomonas aeruginosa*, and methicillin-resistant *Staphylococcus aureus* (MRSA) were the most frequently isolated in one recent study. Risk factors included hospital-acquired infection, prophylactic or recent antibiotic therapy (especially fluoroquinolones or beta-lactams), and recent history of multidrug-resistant infection.[45]

Diagnosis

Several of the features that suggest sepsis in noncirrhotic patients are already present among nonseptic patients with cirrhosis. Indeed, as many as 30% of noninfected patients with decompensated cirrhosis will exhibit SIRS.[46] Additionally, patients with end-stage liver disease will exhibit tachycardia and hypotension due to arterial vaso-dilation, rendering the presence of these findings difficult to interpret in the setting of infection.[47] Clinical and laboratory findings are less reliable in this patient population, and trends of serial measurements are emphasized over single results. Although the latter is true of many conditions, its importance is particularly highlighted in this population.

Because of decreased clearance of lactate among nonseptic patients with cirrhosis, a single elevated lactate result is of limited value in the evaluation of a patient in whom there exists concern for sepsis. A normal or down-trending lactate, however, is reassuring. There is no specific lactate threshold that is recommended in this population.[48,49]

Assessments of volume status and fluid responsiveness are fraught with problems among patients with cirrhosis. Those with large-volume ascites may develop intra-abdominal hypertension, rendering bedside tests, such as passive leg raise, unreliable.[48,50] Debate remains about the utility of inferior vena cava measurements for assessment of intravascular volume, but there are certainly no studies to date that validate its use in this group of patients.[51–56]

Patients who have developed esophageal varices due to portal hypertension from cirrhosis may be prescribed a nonselective beta-blocker, such as propranolol.[57] These agents may blunt the tachycardia that often cues providers to a significant inflammatory response to infection. Additionally, they may reduce a patient's ability to compensate for the vasodilation characteristic of septic shock.

Acute kidney injury (AKI) is the most common organ failure identified among cirrhotic patients with sepsis, and the degree of injury is associated with prognosis. The 30-day mortality of infected cirrhotic patients with AKI that progressed to a persistent need for renal replacement therapy was 10-fold greater than for those patients without AKI.[58]

Management

Multiple factors complicate the management of patients with concomitant cirrhosis and sepsis. Among these are the impaired ability to trend response to therapy and low plasma oncotic pressure that leads to extravascular fluid shifts and the potential for secondary respiratory and cardiovascular compromise. Furthermore, baseline adrenal insufficiency and coagulopathy make operative source control and other procedural interventions more treacherous.

As a result of increased hydrostatic pressure in the mesenteric vessels (due to portal hypertension) and the decreased plasma oncotic pressure that results from hypoalbuminemia, cirrhotic patients may develop ascites.[59] Aggressive fluid resuscitation with crystalloid exacerbates both of these factors and may lead to intra-abdominal hypertension or abdominal compartment syndrome at the extreme end of the spectrum.[60] The principal consequences of this situation in the setting of sepsis are impaired venous return and decreased diaphragmatic excursion. Should this occur in the setting of tense ascites, therapeutic paracentesis is recommended. Decisions to pursue this intervention should be based on clinical assessment; routine measurement of intra-abdominal pressures is not encouraged.

Intravascularly depleted patients should initially receive crystalloid at a lower-than-standard volume of 10 to 20 mL/kg. There may be a benefit to balanced crystalloid solutions, particularly among those cirrhotic patients with relative hyperchloremia (hyponatremia with normal chloride) or in those already exhibiting a hyperchloremic acidosis.[35,36,48]

Albumin has proven value in 2 particular situations in the management of cirrhotic patients with sepsis: (1) patients undergoing large-volume (ie, ≥5 L) paracentesis in the setting of tense ascites and (2) patients with sepsis due to SBP.[48,61–63] Although no mortality benefit was evident, 2 studies of cirrhotic patients with non-SBP infections showed reduced rates of AKI when they were given albumin.[64,65] As in noncirrhotic patients, those receiving large volumes of crystalloid with a persistent need for volume expansion may benefit from albumin infusion.

Synthetic colloids, such as hydroxyethyl starch, have been shown to increase rates of acute renal failure and the need for renal replacement therapy; one study showed an independent contribution to 90-day mortality with these agents compared with crystalloid.[66–68] Consequently, synthetic colloids are discouraged in cirrhotic patients.

Norepinephrine is the first-line vasopressor agent in this population, as in noncirrhotic patients with septic shock. Central venous catheter (CVC) insertion for administration of these drugs may be complicated by coagulopathy resulting from reduced hepatic synthesis of coagulation factors. A compressible site is recommended in this setting in case of arterial puncture or hematoma formation.

Adrenal insufficiency is common in cirrhotic patients with severe sepsis.[69,70] In fact, it is common in patients with decompensated cirrhosis and may predispose these patients to severe sepsis.[71] The use of corticosteroids is recommended in noncirrhotic patients with septic shock that is refractory to intravenous fluids and vasopressors.[32] Findings have been mixed in patients with cirrhosis, but similar practice is reasonable in this population.[48,70,72]

As in all patients with sepsis, early antibiotic therapy is encouraged. Because of the aforementioned increases in multidrug-resistant bacteria causing infection in this population, initial broad-spectrum coverage is encouraged until cultures allow more tailored therapy. In addition to standard cultures (eg, blood, urine), it is especially important to obtain peritoneal fluid (if ascites is present) in cirrhotic patients with sepsis, as this is a common source.

END-STAGE RENAL DISEASE
Background

In the United States, nearly 14% of adults are estimated to have chronic kidney disease (CKD) and more than 660,000 patients have ESRD.[73] Patients with CKD, and especially those with ESRD, are at increased risk for infection and sepsis and have increased mortality when compared with the general population.[74,75] Infection is the second leading cause of death in dialysis patients and is even more deadly among patients with ESRD not yet on dialysis.[74,76,77] Patients with ESRD are several hundred times more likely to die of sepsis than the general public.[78] The reasons for this increased risk are multifactorial.

Patients with CKD and ESRD are likely to be of older age and[76,79,80] older adults are an increasingly large segment of the population. Adults older than 65 years have a greater incidence of sepsis and higher mortality rates compared with other patients.[81] Older age has been identified as an independent risk factor for sepsis in patients on dialysis.[82]

Patients with ESRD are likely to have other comorbid conditions, such as diabetes and cardiovascular disease.[76,79,82] Comorbidities have been associated with higher rates of infection and sepsis in patients with ESRD.

Poor nutritional status is another risk. Patients on dialysis frequently have anorexia, nausea, and vomiting likely as a consequence of uremic toxicity.[83,84] Low serum albumin is an independent risk factor for sepsis among patients on hemodialysis.[76,82]

Studies have demonstrated an increased risk of infection associated with vascular access catheters, particularly temporary dialysis catheters.[76] The type of vascular access used is an important risk determinant for infection (**Fig. 1**). The highest risk for

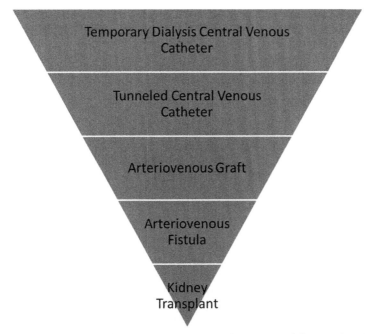

Fig. 1. Decreasing risk of infection based on type of access used for renal replacement therapy.

infection is found in patients who have a nontunneled CVC.[79] For these reasons, it has been recommended that nontunneled dialysis catheters should be avoided and replaced as soon as possible with arteriovenous grafts or fistulas.[83] There is some risk related to repeated disruption of the skin in patients with an arteriovenous graft or native arteriovenous fistula, but it does not exceed the risk inherent in a long-term indwelling catheter.[78] These observations may help to explain the decreased rates of infection observed in patients with a renal transplant, an unexpected finding given the necessity for immunosuppressive medication.[85]

If a temporary CVC must be placed in the ED, the right internal jugular vein is the preferred site for insertion.[86] Despite the fact that jugular venous catheterization is more prone to blood stream infections than subclavian catheterization, the explicit purpose of this recommendation is to decrease the likelihood of stenosis in the subclavian vein, which would preclude later placement of an arteriovenous graft or fistula in the affected extremity.[86,87]

Possibly the most important factor related to the increased incidence of infection and sepsis in patients with CKD and ESRD is increased inflammation and immune compromise related to uremia.[78,88] Renal impairment leads to systemic inflammation.[84] This inflammation, in turn, causes atherosclerosis and cardiovascular disease, which predisposes to circulatory dysfunction and increased risk of infection.[89] Renal impairment also causes immune cell dysfunction and further impairs immunity.[90]

Diagnosis

Patients with ESRD are frequently seen in the ED. The most common presenting complaints in this patient population involve weakness, dyspnea, chest pain, and nausea and vomiting.[91,92] Classic markers used to screen for or identify sepsis, such as temperature, heart rate, respiratory rate, WBC count, and lactic acidosis, are insensitive, especially so in patients with ESRD.[93,94] Reasons for this include large fluctuations in intravascular and extracellular volume, concomitant use of multiple prescription medications, immune dysfunction, comorbidities, and overall poor state of health. Therefore, EPs should be cognizant that the SIRS criteria will be poorly sensitive in this population; vigilance for sepsis in this population is essential because atypical is more commonplace at initial presentation.

Management

ED management of patients with ESRD with severe sepsis or septic shock should begin as it would for any patient with an acute illness. Special attention should be given to the examination of the dialysis access site. Please see **Box 3** for additional clinical considerations.

There is little evidence-based guidance specific to dialysis patients regarding fluid resuscitation, and many providers are reluctant to be aggressive with fluid resuscitation for fear of volume overload.[95,96] Unfortunately, this sometimes leads to a high proportion of septic patients with ESRD who do not receive adequate early fluid resuscitation and antibiotics and have subsequent increased mortality.[93,94] A subgroup analysis of patients with ESRD on hemodialysis was performed on data from the Early Goal Directed Therapy (EGDT) study by Otero and colleagues.[96] This analysis demonstrated that both intubation and mortality rates were higher in the standard care treatment arm compared with the EGDT group. Current recommendations of a 30-mL/kg bolus are reasonable in dialysis patients if intravascular hypovolemia is suspected. Hypovolemia should be suspected in hypotensive patients, and evidence seems to support erring on the side of providing fluid resuscitation.[93,94] If necessary, patients can be intubated and placed on mechanical ventilation for pulmonary edema.

Indirect means by which to assess volume status in patients with ESRD include comparing patients' dry weight with actual weight and asking when patients were last dialyzed. Dry weight is a clinically determined value defined as the postdialysis weight at which a patient has a normal blood pressure without the use of antihypertensive medication.[97] Some dialysis patients may know what their dry weight should be; in other cases you may have to review notes from dialysis sessions or talk with

---

Box 3
Clinical considerations in the treatment of sepsis in patients with end-stage renal disease

Avoid peripheral venous catheterization and application of blood pressure cuffs to an extremity with dialysis access.

Right internal jugular vein is the preferred site for CVC placement followed by the left internal jugular vein.

Give adequate crystalloids to resuscitate septic patients with ESRD.

Avoid succinylcholine during rapid sequence intubation.

Obtain urine, if possible, for analysis and culture.

Remove and culture the tip of any central venous catheter if there is suspicion of a catheter related infection

Provide early empirical antibiotics covering MRSA and gram-negative organisms.

Avoid nephrotoxic medications.

Make dosage adjustments of medications based on renal function

patients' nephrologist. Clues to volume overload on examination include rales, hypertension, jugular venous distention, and peripheral edema. If available, bedside ultrasound imaging of the inferior vena cava may provide more reliable information about intravascular volume and help to direct fluid resuscitation.[98]

Gram-positive bacteria are the predominant organisms isolated in blood cultures from septic patients with ESRD.[79,93] S aureus is the most frequent pathogen cultured from the blood of patients with ESRD.[79,99–101] Given the prevalence of resistant organisms found in dialysis patients, broad-spectrum antibiotics should be selected that cover MRSA and gram-negative organisms. Antibiotic choice should be further guided by local antibiotic susceptibility testing.[86] There is a high incidence of bacteremia in patients with ESRD on dialysis; a high level of suspicion should be maintained for metastatic infections in this patient population, primarily osteoarticular infections and endocarditis.[102]

In summary, septic patients with ESRD are at high risk for mortality and are likely to be the sickest patients in your ED on any given shift. Because of the prevalence of atypical presentations, a high index of suspicion should be maintained for the possibility of sepsis in any patients with CKD or ESRD; early administration of antibiotics and appropriate fluid resuscitation are the interventions most likely to affect survival in this patient population. The SIRS criteria are poorly sensitive in this patient population, and assessment of intravascular volume status can be challenging.

OBESITY
Background

Obesity is an important public health issue that has gained attention as rates of obesity have soared around the world. Nearly 70% of adults in the United States are overweight and more than one-third of all US adults are considered obese by current estimates.[103,104] According to the Centers for Disease Control and Prevention, obesity is defined as a body mass index (BMI) greater than 30 kg/m^2.[105]

Obesity is linked to increased risk for the development of several chronic health conditions, including diabetes, cardiovascular disease, stroke, and certain cancers.[106] It has also been suggested that obesity may increase the risk for infection and sepsis.[107–111] Studies have shown that obese patients have worse outcomes due to infection compared with patients with normal body weight.[107,108,112] Interestingly, some recent studies have demonstrated a decreased risk of mortality in obese septic patients.[113–115]

The so-called "obesity paradox" describes a phenomenon in which obese patients have experienced lower-than-expected mortality compared with lean patients with otherwise similar prognoses.[113–120] This phenomenon is poorly understood, but illness severity scores used to compare study groups have not been validated in obese individuals and they do not typically account for obesity. This point suggests that there may be a bias toward overestimating illness severity in obese patients, which may explain the observed protective effect regarding mortality.[119,121] Some investigators have suggested that because obesity is a chronic inflammatory condition, immunity may be suppressed resulting in a less robust response to sepsis, which may be protective. This position is less convincing as other chronic inflammatory conditions do not share the same survival benefit in sepsis. Although debate continues as to whether obesity increases the risks of sepsis or provides a protective effect against mortality, there is little doubt that obese patients are at higher risk to develop infections.[110,122–127] It is clear from a variety of studies that despite decreased mortality, obese patients with sepsis have significantly more morbidity compared with lean patients.[108,112]

The relationship between obesity and sepsis is not well defined. Similar to other special conditions discussed in this article, obesity is thought to be a chronic inflammatory state.[126] Chronic inflammation in obese patients is likely secondary to several factors, including (1) increased secretion of multiple inflammatory cytokines, (2) activation of inflammatory cells, (3) impairment of innate and adaptive immune function, and (4) insulin resistance.[127]

Diagnosis and Management

There are no obesity-specific guidelines pertaining to the management of septic patients in the ED. Some considerations that may arise include body habitus, lung function, adequacy of fluid replacement, and appropriate choice and dosing of antibiotics and vasopressors.

Obesity has been linked to several disorders of the skin, and skin infections are a common cause of sepsis in obese patients.[121] A careful examination of the skin of obese patients with sepsis, with special attention to skin folds, is an important part of the initial evaluation in this patient population.

Early and aggressive fluid resuscitation is one of the most critical interventions in the ED for septic patients.[122] Current Surviving Sepsis Campaign (SSC) guidelines recommend an initial fluid bolus of at least 30 mL/kg for patients with severe sepsis and septic shock.[123] Guidance has not been provided regarding whether actual body weight should be used for these calculations versus a corrected value (ie, ideal body weight). Studies have demonstrated that obese patients typically receive resuscitative fluid volumes comparable with that given to patients with a normal BMI with no measurable worsening of outcome.[120,121] Some studies have concluded that over-resuscitation may be harmful in septic patients.[124,125] In obese patients with severe sepsis or septic shock, the authors recommend following the SSC guidelines and, thus, providing an initial 30-mL/kg crystalloid bolus and then guiding further fluid resuscitation by objective findings and not solely based on weight.

Similarly, several studies have looked at the dosing of vasopressors for septic shock in obese patients. In these studies, similar mortality was observed in obese patients despite lower doses per kilogram of body weight.[120,121] According to the most recent guidelines from the SSC, norepinephrine is the initial drug of choice when considering vasopressors for refractory hypotension.[123] In the absence of obesity-specific guidelines, norepinephrine should be first line for obese patients. A recent study by Radosevich and colleagues[128] investigating the use of vasopressors in obese patients with septic shock showed a lower weight-based infusion requirement for norepinephrine in obese patients. This finding is fortunate, as norepinephrine is often titrated to effect rather than to a weight-based dose.

Another goal of current guidelines is the early administration of broad-spectrum antibiotics.[123] The efficacy of many antibiotics is altered by volumes of distribution, which are understandably different in obese patients. Many commonly used antibiotics are likely inadequately dosed in obese patients, and there are no generally accepted guidelines regarding appropriate adjustments.[111,129] Antibiotics that likely should be used at higher dosages in obese patients include vancomycin, several of the beta-lactams, macrolides, and fluoroquinolones, among others.[111,129] If available in a timely fashion, the use of a clinical pharmacist may be invaluable when considering appropriate initial dosing of antibiotics in obese patients.

Obese patients present unique respiratory concerns that should be considered in septic patients. Obesity hypoventilation syndrome (Pickwickian syndrome) is defined by acute-on-chronic hypercapneic respiratory failure. This phenomenon can be a significant source of baseline pulmonary dysfunction in some obese patients who may predispose to pulmonary hypertension, cor pulmonale, and pulmonary edema.[130] Therefore, appropriate fluid resuscitation may exacerbate underlying ventilatory insufficiency in these patients and require intervention. Noninvasive ventilatory strategies are considered first line in most instances of acute respiratory failure regardless of body habitus but are more likely to be contraindicated in patients with obesity hypoventilation syndrome due to frequent underlying acidosis and obtundation.[131] If noninvasive support is ineffective or contraindicated, intubation and mechanical ventilation is required. Technical difficulties encountered in obese patients include problems with patient positioning; anatomic differences, such as limited neck mobility and decreased mouth opening; and rapid oxygen desaturation.[132] The provider must presume that these high-risk patients will have a difficult airway, and appropriate preparation should be undertaken.

Obesity is another example of a disease of chronic inflammation that increases susceptibility to infection and likely increases the risk for developing sepsis. There are conflicting data regarding the risk of mortality in obese patients compared with lean patients, and further study is needed on this topic. There is an increasing body of evidence that suggests that antibiotics are underdosed in obese patients. Likewise, further study of appropriate fluid resuscitation in obese patients is warranted. A paradigm shift in medicine toward individually tailored treatment is rapidly approaching; the inclusion of body weight, with particular attention to the treatment of obese patients, will be a significant factor.

SUMMARY

In summary, the EP must remain vigilant to the possibility that the physiologic abnormalities on which they frequently rely in order to identify patients with sepsis may be absent or blunted by comorbid conditions, altered physiology, or chronic medications. Maintaining a high index of suspicion for sepsis in these patients is key to avoid overlooking patients on the verge of acute decompensation. Special considerations regarding diagnostic limitations and the evaluation of response to therapy in each of these patient populations guide subsequent management.

REFERENCES

1. Oud L, Watkins P. Evolving trends in the epidemiology, resource utilization, and outcomes of pregnancy-associated severe sepsis: a population-based cohort study. J Clin Med Res 2015;7(6):400–16.
2. Cantwell R, Clutton-Brock T, Cooper G, et al. Saving mothers' lives: reviewing maternal deaths to make motherhood safer: 2006-2008. The eighth report of the confidential enquiries into maternal deaths in the United Kingdom. BJOG 2011;118(Suppl 1):1–203.
3. Knight M, Kenyon S, Brocklehurst P, et al. Saving lives, improving mothers' care-lessons learned to inform future maternity care from the UK and Ireland confidential enquiries into maternal deaths and morbidity 2009–12. Oxford (MS): National Perinatal Epidemiology Unit, University of Oxford; 2014.
4. Kramer HMC, Schutte JM, Zwart JJ, et al. Maternal mortality and severe morbidity from sepsis in the Netherlands. Acta Obstet Gynecol Scand 2009; 88(6):647–53.
5. Timezguid N, Das V, Hamdi A, et al. Maternal sepsis during pregnancy or the postpartum period requiring intensive care admission. Int J Obstet Anesth 2012;21(1):51–5.

6. Acosta CD, Kurinczuk JJ, Lucas DN, et al. Severe maternal sepsis in the UK, 2011–2012: a national case-control study. PLoS Med 2014;11(7):e1001672.

7. Knowles S, O'Sullivan N, Meenan A, et al. Maternal sepsis incidence, aetiology and outcome for mother and fetus: a prospective study. BJOG 2015;122(5): 663–71.

8. Snyder CC, Barton JR, Habli M, et al. Severe sepsis and septic shock in pregnancy: indications for delivery and maternal and perinatal outcomes. J Matern Fetal Neonatal Med 2013;26(5):503–6.

9. Mabie WC, Barton JR, Sibai B. Septic shock in pregnancy. Obstet Gynecol 1997;90(4 Pt 1):553–61.

10. Mahutte NG, Murphy-Kaulbeck L, Le Q, et al. Obstetric admissions to the intensive care unit. Obstet Gynecol 1999;94:263–6.

11. Morgan J, Roberts S. Maternal sepsis. Obstet Gynecol Clin North Am 2013; 40(1):69–87.

12. Clark SL, Cotton DB, Lee W, et al. Central hemodynamic assessment of normal term pregnancy. Am J Obstet Gynecol 1989;161(6 Pt 1):1439–42.

13. Moertl MG, Ulrich D, Pickel KI, et al. Changes in haemodynamic and autonomous nervous system parameters measured non-invasively throughout normal pregnancy. Eur J Obstet Gynecol Reprod Biol 2009;144:S179–83.

14. Jensen D, Webb KA, O'Donnell DE. Chemical and mechanical adaptations of the respiratory system at rest and during exercise in human pregnancy. Appl Physiol Nutr Metab 2007;32(6):1239–50.

15. Sheffield JS, Cunningham FG. Community-acquired pneumonia in pregnancy. Obstet Gynecol 2009;114(4):915–22.

16. Cunningham FG. Laboratory values in normal pregnancy. In: Queenan JT, Hobbins JC, Spong CY, editors. Protocols for high-risk pregnancies: an evidence-based approach. 5th edition. Chichester (United Kingdom): Wiley-Blackwell; 2010. p. 588.

17. Chandra S, Tripathi AK, Mishra S, et al. Physiological changes in hematological parameters during pregnancy. Indian J Hematol Blood Transfus 2012;28(3): 144–6.

18. Edelstam G, Lowbeer C, Kral G, et al. New reference values for routine blood samples and human neutrophilic lipocalin during third-trimester pregnancy. Scand J Clin Lab Invest 2001;61(8):583–91.

19. Albright C, Ali T, Lopes V, et al. Lactic acid measurement to identify risk of morbidity from sepsis in pregnancy. Am J Perinatol 2014;32(5):481–6.

20. Jones AE, Shapiro NI, Trzeciak S, et al. Lactate clearance vs central venous oxygen saturation as goals of early sepsis therapy: a randomized clinical trial. JAMA 2010;303(8):739–46.

21. Bone RC, Balk RA, Cerra FB, et al. Definitions for sepsis and organ failure and guidelines for the use of innovative therapies in sepsis. The ACCP/SCCM Consensus Conference Committee. American College of Chest Physicians/Society of Critical Care Medicine. Chest 1992;101(6):1644–55.

22. Lappen JR, Keene M, Lore M, et al. Existing models fail to predict sepsis in an obstetric population with intrauterine infection. Am J Obstet Gynecol 2010; 203(6):573.e1-5.

23. Waterstone M, Murphy JD, Bewley S, et al. Incidence and predictors of severe obstetric morbidity: case-control study. BMJ 2001;322(7294):1089–94.

24. Albright CM, Ali TN, Lopes V, et al. The sepsis in obstetrics score: a model to identify risk of morbidity from sepsis in pregnancy. Am J Obstet Gynecol 2014;211(1):39.e1-8.

25. Singer M, Deutschman CS, Seymour CW, et al. The Third International Consensus Definitions for Sepsis and Septic Shock (Sepsis-3). JAMA 2016; 315(8):801–10.
26. Larsson A, Palm M, Hansson L-O, et al. Reference values for clinical chemistry tests during normal pregnancy. BJOG 2008;115(7):874–81.
27. Rivers E, Nguyen B, Havstad S, et al. Early goal-directed therapy in the treatment of severe sepsis and septic shock. N Engl J Med 2001;345(19):1368–77.
28. The ProCESS Investigators. A randomized trial of protocol-based care for early septic shock. N Engl J Med 2014;370(18):1683–93.
29. The ARISE Investigators and the ANZICS Clinical Trials Group. Goal-directed resuscitation for patients with early septic shock. N Engl J Med 2014;371(16): 1496–506.
30. Mouncey PR, Osborn TM, Power GS, et al. Trial of early, goal-directed resuscitation for septic shock. N Engl J Med 2015;372(14):1301–11.
31. Sprung CL, Annane D, Keh D, et al. Hydrocortisone therapy for patients with septic shock. N Engl J Med 2008;358(2):111–24.
32. Dellinger RP, Levy MM, Rhodes A, et al. Surviving Sepsis Campaign: international guidelines for management of severe sepsis and septic shock, 2012. Intensive Care Med 2013;39(2):165–228.
33. Cordioli RL, Cordioli E, Negrini R, et al. Sepsis and pregnancy: do we know how to treat this situation? Rev Bras Ter Intensiva 2013;25(4):334–44.
34. Barton JR, Sibai BM. Severe sepsis and septic shock in pregnancy. Obstet Gynecol 2012;120(3):689–706.
35. Raghunathan K, Shaw A, Nathanson B, et al. Association between the choice of iv crystalloid and in-hospital mortality among critically ill adults with sepsis. Crit Care Med 2014;42(7):1585–91.
36. Rochwerg B, Alhazzani W, Sindi A, et al. Fluid resuscitation in sepsis: a systematic review and network meta-analysis. Ann Intern Med 2014;161(5):347.
37. Neligan PJ, Laffey JG. Clinical review: special populations-critical illness and pregnancy. Crit Care 2011;15(4):227.
38. Pacheco LD, Zwart JJ. Sepsis. In: van de VM, Scholefield H, Plante LA, editors. Maternal critical care: a multidisciplinary approach. New York: Cambridge University Press; 2013. p. 346–55.
39. Oud L. Pregnancy-associated severe sepsis: contemporary state and future challenges. Infect Dis Ther 2014;3(2):175–89.
40. Paruk F. Infection in obstetric critical care. Best Pract Res Clin Obstet Gynaecol 2008;22(5):865–83.
41. Scaglione S, Kliethermes S, Cao G, et al. The epidemiology of cirrhosis in the United States: a population-based study. J Clin Gastroenterol 2015;49(8):690–6.
42. Olson JC, Wendon JA, Kramer DJ, et al. Intensive care of the patient with cirrhosis. Hepatology 2011;54(5):1864–72.
43. Jalan R, Fernandez J, Wiest R, et al. Bacterial infections in cirrhosis: a position statement based on the EASL Special Conference 2013. J Hepatol 2014;60(6): 1310–24.
44. Jenne CN, Kubes P. Immune surveillance by the liver. Nat Immunol 2013;14(10): 996–1006.
45. Fernández J, Acevedo J, Castro M, et al. Prevalence and risk factors of infections by multiresistant bacteria in cirrhosis: a prospective study. Hepatology 2012;55(5):1551–61.
46. Fernández J, Gustot T. Management of bacterial infections in cirrhosis. J Hepatol 2012;56(Suppl 1):S1–12.

47. Al-hamoudi W. Cardiovascular changes in cirrhosis: pathogenesis and clinical implications. Saudi J Gastroenterol 2010;16(3):145.
48. Nadim MK, Durand F, Kellum JA, et al. Management of the critically ill patient with cirrhosis: a multidisciplinary perspective. J Hepatol 2016;64(3):717–35.
49. Funk GC, Doberer D, Kneidinger N, et al. Acid-base disturbances in critically ill patients with cirrhosis. Liver Int 2007;27(7):901–9.
50. Mahjoub Y, Touzeau J, Airapetian N, et al. The passive leg-raising maneuver cannot accurately predict fluid responsiveness in patients with intra-abdominal hypertension. Crit Care Med 2010;38(9):1824–9.
51. Barbier C, Loubières Y, Schmit C, et al. Respiratory changes in inferior vena cava diameter are helpful in predicting fluid responsiveness in ventilated septic patients. Intensive Care Med 2004;30(9):1740–6.
52. Corl K, Napoli AM, Gardiner F. Bedside sonographic measurement of the inferior vena cava caval index is a poor predictor of fluid responsiveness in emergency department patients. Emerg Med Australas 2012;24(5):534–9.
53. Feissel M, Michard F, Faller J-P, et al. The respiratory variation in inferior vena cava diameter as a guide to fluid therapy. Intensive Care Med 2004;30(9):1834–7.
54. Ferrada P, Anand RJ, Whelan J, et al. Qualitative assessment of the inferior vena cava: useful tool for the evaluation of fluid status in critically ill patients. Am Surg 2012;78(4):468–70.
55. Muller L, Bobbia X, Toumi M, et al. Respiratory variations of inferior vena cava diameter to predict fluid responsiveness in spontaneously breathing patients with acute circulatory failure: need for a cautious use. Crit Care 2012;16(5):1–7.
56. Nagdev AD, Merchant RC, Tirado-Gonzalez A, et al. Emergency department bedside ultrasonographic measurement of the caval index for noninvasive determination of low central venous pressure. Ann Emerg Med 2010;55(3):290–5.
57. Aguilar-Olivos N, Motola-Kuba M, Candia R, et al. Hemodynamic effect of carvedilol vs. propranolol in cirrhotic patients: systematic review and meta-analysis. Ann Hepatol 2014;13(4):420–8.
58. Wong F, O'Leary JG, Reddy KR, et al. New consensus definition of acute kidney injury accurately predicts 30-day mortality in patients with cirrhosis and infection. Gastroenterology 2013;145(6):1280–8.e1.
59. Moore CM. Cirrhotic ascites review: pathophysiology, diagnosis and management. World J Hepatol 2013;5(5):251.
60. Aspesi M, Gamberoni C, Severgnini P, et al. The abdominal compartment syndrome. Clinical relevance. Minerva Anestesiol 2002;68(4):138–46.
61. Bernardi M, Caraceni P, Navickis RJ, et al. Albumin infusion in patients undergoing large-volume paracentesis: a meta-analysis of randomized trials. Hepatology 2012;55(4):1172–81.
62. Kwok CS, Krupa L, Mahtani A, et al. Albumin reduces paracentesis-induced circulatory dysfunction and reduces death and renal impairment among patients with cirrhosis and infection: a systematic review and meta-analysis. Biomed Res Int 2013;2013:295153.
63. Sort P, Navasa M, Arroyo V, et al. Effect of intravenous albumin on renal impairment and mortality in patients with cirrhosis and spontaneous bacterial peritonitis. N Engl J Med 1999;341(6):403–9.
64. Guevara M, Terra C, Nazar A, et al. Albumin for bacterial infections other than spontaneous bacterial peritonitis in cirrhosis. A randomized, controlled study. J Hepatol 2012;57(4):759–65.

65. Thévenot T, Bureau C, Oberti F, et al. Effect of albumin in cirrhotic patients with infection other than spontaneous bacterial peritonitis. A randomized trial. J Hepatol 2015;62(4):822–30.

66. Schortgen F, Lacherade J-C, Bruneel F, et al. Effects of hydroxyethylstarch and gelatin on renal function in severe sepsis: a multicentre randomised study. Lancet 2001;357(9260):911–6.

67. Perner A, Haase N, Guttormsen AB, et al. Hydroxyethyl starch 130/0.42 versus Ringer's acetate in severe sepsis. N Engl J Med 2012;367(2):124–34.

68. Müller RB, Haase N, Lange T, et al. Acute kidney injury with hydroxyethyl starch 130/0.42 in severe sepsis: acute kidney injury with starch. Acta Anaesthesiol Scand 2015;59(3):329–36.

69. Tsai M-H, Peng Y-S, Chen Y-C, et al. Adrenal insufficiency in patients with cirrhosis, severe sepsis and septic shock. Hepatology 2006;43(4):673–81.

70. Fernández J, Escorsell A, Zabalza M, et al. Adrenal insufficiency in patients with cirrhosis and septic shock: effect of treatment with hydrocortisone on survival. Hepatology 2006;44(5):1288–95.

71. Acevedo J, Fernández J, Prado V, et al. Relative adrenal insufficiency in decompensated cirrhosis: relationship to short-term risk of severe sepsis, hepatorenal syndrome, and death. Hepatology 2013;58(5):1757–65.

72. Arabi YM, Aljumah A, Dabbagh O, et al. Low-dose hydrocortisone in patients with cirrhosis and septic shock: a randomized controlled trial. Can Med Assoc J 2010;182(18):1971–7.

73. United States Renal Data System United States Renal Data System. 2015 USRDS annual data report: epidemiology of kidney disease in the United States. Bethesda (MD): National Institutes of Health, National Institute of Diabetes and Digestive and Kidney Diseases; 2015. Available at: http://www.usrds.org/2015/view/Default.aspx. Accessed April 6, 2016.

74. James MT, Laupland KB, Tonelli M, et al. Risk of bloodstream infection in patients with chronic kidney disease not treated with dialysis. Arch Intern Med 2008;168(21):2333–9.

75. Wang HE, Gamboa C, Warnock DG, et al. Chronic kidney disease and risk of death from infection. Am J Nephrol 2011;34(4):330–6.

76. Powe NR, Jaar B, Furth SL, et al. Septicemia in dialysis patients: incidence, risk factors, and prognosis. Kidney Int 1999;55(3):1081–90.

77. Lukowsky LR, Kheifets L, Arah OA, et al. Patterns and predictors of early mortality in incident hemodialysis patients: new insights. Am J Nephrol 2012;35(6):548–58.

78. Sarnak MJ, Jaber BL. Mortality caused by sepsis in patients with end-stage renal disease compared with the general population. Kidney Int 2000;58(4):1758–64.

79. Gauna TT, Oshiro E, Luzio YC, et al. Bloodstream infection in patients with end-stage renal disease in a teaching hospital in central-western Brazil. Rev Soc Bras Med Trop 2013;46(4):426–32.

80. Prakash S, O'Hare AM. Interaction of aging and CKD. Semin Nephrol 2009;29(5):497–503.

81. Starr ME, Saito H. Sepsis in old age: review of human and animal studies. Aging Dis 2014;5(2):126–36.

82. Jaar BG, Hermann JA, Furth SL, et al. Septicemia in diabetic hemodialysis patients: comparison of incidence, risk factors, and mortality with nondiabetic hemodialysis patients. Am J Kidney Dis 2000;35(2):282–92.

83. The National Kidney Foundation. K/DOQI clinical practice guidelines for chronic kidney disease: evaluation, classification and stratification. Am J Kidney Dis 2002;39:S1–266.

84. Carrero JJ, Stenvinkel P. Inflammation in end-stage renal disease–what have we learned in 10 years? Semin Dial 2010;23(5):498–509.

85. Shen T-C, Wang I-K, Wei C-C, et al. The risk of septicemia in end-stage renal disease with and without renal transplantation: a propensity-matched cohort study. Medicine (Baltimore) 2015;94(34):e1437.

86. Vanholder R, Canaud B, Fluck R, et al. Catheter-related blood stream infections (CRBSI): a European view. Nephrol Dial Transplant 2010;25(6):1753–6.

87. CDC -Terminology and Estimates of Risk - 2011 BSI Guidelines - HICPAC. Available at: http://www.cdc.gov/hicpac/BSI/02-bsi-summary-of-recommendations-2011.html. Accessed April 17, 2016.

88. Vaziri ND, Pahl MV, Crum A, et al. Effect of uremia on structure and function of immune system. J Ren Nutr 2012;22(1):149–56.

89. Ishani A, Collins AJ, Herzog CA, et al. Septicemia, access and cardiovascular disease in dialysis patients: The USRDS Wave 2 Study1. Kidney Int 2005; 68(1):311–8.

90. Girndt M, Sester U, Sester M, et al. Impaired cellular immune function in patients with end-stage renal failure. Nephrol Dial Transplant 1999;14(12):2807–10.

91. Sacchetti A, Harris R, Patel K, et al. Emergency department presentation of renal dialysis patients: indications for EMS transport directly to dialysis centers. J Emerg Med 1991;9(3):141–4.

92. Sacchetti A, Stuccio N, Panebianco P, et al. ED hemodialysis for treatment of renal failure emergencies. Am J Emerg Med 1999;17(3):305–7.

93. Rojas L, Muñoz P, Kestler M, et al. Bloodstream infections in patients with kidney disease: risk factors for poor outcome and mortality. J Hosp Infect 2013;85(3): 196–205.

94. de Carvalho MA, Freitas FGR, Silva Junior HT, et al. Mortality predictors in renal transplant recipients with severe sepsis and septic shock. PLoS One 2014; 9(11):e111610.

95. Abou Dagher G, Harmouche E, Jabbour E, et al. Sepsis in hemodialysis patients. BMC Emerg Med 2015;15:30.

96. Otero RM, Nguyen HB, Huang DT, et al. Early goal-directed therapy in severe sepsis and septic shock revisited: concepts, controversies, and contemporary findings. Chest 2006;130(5):1579–95.

97. Gunal AI. How to determine "dry weight"? Kidney Int Suppl 2013;3(4):377–9.

98. Dipti A, Soucy Z, Surana A, et al. Role of inferior vena cava diameter in assessment of volume status: a meta-analysis. Am J Emerg Med 2012;30(8): 1414–9.e1.

99. Engemann JJ, Friedman JY, Reed SD, et al. Clinical outcomes and costs due to Staphylococcus aureus bacteremia among patients receiving long-term hemodialysis. Infect Control Hosp Epidemiol 2005;26(6):534–9.

100. Steinberg JP, Clark CC, Hackman BO. Nosocomial and community-acquired staphylococcus aureus bacteremias from 1980 to 1993: impact of intravascular devices and methicillin resistance. Clin Infect Dis 1996;23(2):255–9.

101. Thomson PC, Stirling CM, Geddes CC, et al. Vascular access in haemodialysis patients: a modifiable risk factor for bacteraemia and death. QJM 2007;100(7): 415–22.

102. Vandecasteele SJ, Boelaert JR, Vriese ASD. Staphylococcus aureus infections in hemodialysis: what a nephrologist should know. Clin J Am Soc Nephrol 2009;4(8):1388–400.
103. Ogden CL, Carroll MD, Kit BK, et al. Prevalence of childhood and adult obesity in the United States, 2011-2012. JAMA 2014;311(8):806–14.
104. FastStats. Available at: http://www.cdc.gov/nchs/fastats/obesity-overweight. htm. Accessed April 3, 2016.
105. Defining Adult Overweight and Obesity | Overweight & Obesity | CDC. Available at: http://www.cdc.gov/obesity/adult/defining.html. Accessed April 27, 2016.
106. Adult Obesity Facts | Data | Adult | Obesity | DNPAO | CDC. Available at: http:// www.cdc.gov/obesity/data/adult.html. Accessed March 4, 2016.
107. Louie JK, Acosta M, Samuel MC, et al. A novel risk factor for a novel virus: obesity and 2009 pandemic influenza A (H1N1). Clin Infect Dis 2011;52(3): 301–12.
108. Orr K, Chien P. Sepsis in obese pregnant women. Best Pract Res Clin Obstet Gynaecol 2015;29(3):377–93.
109. Wang HE, Gamboa C, Warnock DG, et al. Chronic Kidney Disease and Risk of Death from Infection. Am J Nephrol 2011;34(4):330–6.
110. Falagas ME, Kompoti M. Obesity and infection. Lancet Infect Dis 2006;6(7): 438–46.
111. Huttunen R, Syrjänen J. Obesity and the risk and outcome of infection. Int J Obes 2013;37(3):333–40.
112. Maley N, Gebremariam A, Odetola F, et al. Influence of obesity diagnosis with organ dysfunction, mortality, and resource use among children hospitalized with infection in the United States. J Intensive Care Med 2016. [Epub ahead of print].
113. King P, Mortensen EM, Bollinger M, et al. Impact of obesity on outcomes for patients hospitalised with pneumonia. Eur Respir J 2013;41(4):929–34.
114. Kuperman EF, Showalter JW, Lehman EB, et al. The impact of obesity on sepsis mortality: a retrospective review. BMC Infect Dis 2013;13:377.
115. Wurzinger B, Dünser MW, Wohlmuth C, et al. The association between body-mass index and patient outcome in septic shock: a retrospective cohort study. Wien Klin Wochenschr 2010;122(1–2):31–6.
116. Dixon JB, Lambert GW. The obesity paradox–a reality that requires explanation and clinical interpretation. Atherosclerosis 2013;226(1):47–8.
117. Badheka AO, Rathod A, Kizilbash MA, et al. Influence of obesity on outcomes in atrial fibrillation: yet another obesity paradox. Am J Med 2010;123(7):646–51.
118. Diong C, Jones PP, Tsuchimochi H, et al. Sympathetic hyper-excitation in obesity and pulmonary hypertension: physiological relevance to the "obesity paradox". Int J Obes (Lond) 2016;40(6):938–46.
119. Wardell S, Wall A, Bryce R, et al. The association between obesity and outcomes in critically ill patients. Can Respir J 2015;22(1):23–30.
120. Wacharasint P, Boyd JH, Russell JA, et al. One size does not fit all in severe infection: obesity alters outcome, susceptibility, treatment, and inflammatory response. Crit Care 2013;17(3):R122.
121. Arabi YM, Dara SI, Tamim HM, et al. Clinical characteristics, sepsis interventions and outcomes in the obese patients with septic shock: an international multi-center cohort study. Crit Care 2013;17(2):R72.
122. Pike F, Yealy DM, Kellum JA, et al. Protocolized Care for Early Septic Shock (Pro-CESS) statistical analysis plan. Crit Care Resusc 2013;15(4):301–10.

123. Dellinger RP, Levy MM, Rhodes A, et al. Surviving Sepsis Campaign: international guidelines for management of severe sepsis and septic shock: 2012. Crit Care Med 2013;41(2):580–637.
124. Marik P, Bellomo R. A rational approach to fluid therapy in sepsis. Br J Anaesth 2016;116(3):339–49.
125. Boyd JH, Forbes J, Nakada T, et al. Fluid resuscitation in septic shock: a positive fluid balance and elevated central venous pressure are associated with increased mortality. Crit Care Med 2011;39(2):259–65.
126. Cottam DR, Mattar SG, Barinas-Mitchell E, et al. The chronic inflammatory hypothesis for the morbidity associated with morbid obesity: implications and effects of weight loss. Obes Surg 2004;14(5):589–600.
127. Kolyva AS, Zolota V, Mpatsoulis D, et al. The role of obesity in the immune response during sepsis. Nutr Diabetes 2014;4:e137.
128. Radosevich JJ, Patanwala AE, Erstad BL. Norepinephrine dosing in obese and nonobese patients with septic shock. Am J Crit Care 2016;25(1):27–32.
129. Falagas ME, Karageorgopoulos DE. Adjustment of dosing of antimicrobial agents for bodyweight in adults. Lancet 2010;375(9710):248–51.
130. Piper AJ, Grunstein RR. Obesity hypoventilation syndrome. Am J Respir Crit Care Med 2011;183(3):292–8.
131. Jones SF, Brito V, Ghamande S. Obesity hypoventilation syndrome in the critically ill. Crit Care Clin 2015;31(3):419–34.
132. Vissers RJ, Gibbs MA. The high-risk airway. Emerg Med Clin North Am 2010; 28(1):203–17, ix–x.

Sepsis Resuscitation in Resource-Limited Settings

Brian Meier, MD[a,b],*, Catherine Staton, MD, MScGH[a,b]

KEYWORDS

- Sepsis • Community emergency departments • Low- and middle-income countries

KEY POINTS

- Protocols may aid identification and initial treatment of patients presenting with sepsis to community emergency departments.
- Aggressive fluid resuscitation and early administration of antimicrobials are key to effective care.
- Major differences, including patient characteristics and resource availability, limit the generalizability of current sepsis guidelines to low- and middle-income countries.
- Further research, specific to low-resource settings, is necessary to set priorities for expanding sepsis care globally.

INTRODUCTION

As we have seen throughout this issue, the approach to identifying and treating sepsis can be complicated. Additionally, most research investigating the best practices in identifying and treating sepsis has been done in large academic centers in high-income countries (HICs). Despite the recommendations, studies show that the current sepsis guidelines can be difficult to carry out in both large academic emergency departments (EDs)[1] and low- and middle-income countries (LMICs).[2,3] Limiting factors such as equipment availability and staffing issues can be found not only in low-resource settings[2,3] but also in HICs.[1,4] Additionally, the failure of sepsis protocols in some LMICs leads to questions about how we classify sepsis in these settings.[5,6] How do providers in community EDs (CED) translate the results of these studies into daily practice? Which are the most cost-effective strategies in delivering quality sepsis care with limited resources? This article focuses on sepsis in low-resource settings, ranging from a CED in the United States to hospitals in LMICs. This article

The authors have nothing to disclose.
a Division of Emergency Medicine, Department of Surgery, Duke University Medical Center, DUMC Box 3096, 2301 Erwin Road, Duke North, Suite 2600, Durham, NC 27710, USA; b Duke Global Health Institute, Trent Hall, 310 Trent Drive, Durham, NC 27710, USA
* Corresponding author. Division of Emergency Medicine, Department of Surgery, Duke University Medical Center, DUMC Box 3096, 2301 Erwin Road, Duke North, Suite 2600, Durham, NC 27710.
E-mail address: brian.meier@duke.edu

identifies the most common barriers to providing quality sepsis care, recommendations for maximizing current resources, and priorities for future directions of care.

SURVIVING SEPSIS IN THE COMMUNITY
Guidelines and Sepsis Bundles

The 2012 Surviving Sepsis Campaign (SSC) Guidelines, although generally based on research in large academic centers, are designed to allow initiation of sepsis care in any setting, including CEDs.[7] The current guidelines represent a modified version of the original guidelines released in 2004. In the years after the publication of the original guidelines, several studies looked at complete and component specific compliance with the guidelines. The 2 largest of these, conducted in academic centers around the world, found that compliance with the complete bundle overall was less than 30%.[7,8] The individual components with the highest compliance were measurement of lactate (61%–78%), obtaining blood cultures (64%–84%), fluid/vasopressor initiation (60%–77%), and ventilator plateau-pressure control (80%–85%).[7,8] A study of implementation in a CED had similar results, finding that although patients often received antimicrobials (78%) and vasopressors (79%), few received central venous pressure measurement (27%) or central venous oxygen saturation measurement (15%).[9] Despite the overall low compliance, it was believed that increased compliance led to improved mortality outcomes.[10,11]

It was, therefore, generally accepted that overall, protocol-based care was beneficial, even if there was debate on which components should be included. The revised 2012 SSC guidelines continued to promote protocol-based care, but the individual components were streamlined to include only those that had solid supporting evidence.

The concept of strict protocol-based care, however, has since been called into question, as several large studies found no mortality difference compared with standard care.[12–14] However, a more recent study seems to confirm the benefits of protocol-based care.[15] There are several proposed reasons for the variation in these results largely involving a change in usual care provided in sepsis management and the complex infrastructure and resources required for protocol implementation.[16,17]

Early Recognition of Sepsis

Early recognition of sepsis is critical and yet provides potentially the greatest obstacle in achieving further improvements in decreased mortality. Recognition ideally begins in the prehospital setting and in triage where increased education and improved screening protocols for suspected sepsis reduce time to diagnosis and treatment.[18–20] However, a subjective component remains involved in the diagnosis of sepsis such that the provider has to attribute systemic dysfunction to an underlying infectious process. Early recognition is challenging in first-world large academic EDs let alone in CEDs or LMICS.

Measuring Lactate

Serum lactate is classically thought to result from anaerobic metabolism, either systemic or regional, and it is used as a surrogate marker for tissue hypoperfusion. An elevated serum lactate level is associated with worse outcomes in septic patients.[21–23] In recent sepsis trials, an elevated lactate was found in 30% to 50% of patients without hypotension[24,25] and was found to be associated with increased mortality independent of blood pressure.[26,27] For this reason, early measurement of serum lactate is necessary to avoid the missing patients with so-called "cryptic shock"(ie, lactate $\geq$4 mmol/L and normotension).[26]

Consequently, early lactate testing in patients suspected of having sepsis should be part of standard practice. In most cases, the costs associated with testing can be offset by the costs associated with earlier recognition and treatment.[28,29] Point-of-care lactate correlates well with laboratory lactate[30] and is preferred, as it leads to expedited diagnosis and treatment.[31] The costs of point-of-care compared with laboratory lactates vary depending on institution.

Antimicrobials

Numerous studies have shown that early administration of appropriate antibiotics improves outcomes in septic patients,[32–34] other studies have shown mixed results,[35] and still others have shown no benefit.[36,37] So does time to antibiotics matter? The answer of course is, it depends. Most studies that show mortality benefits for early antibiotics were done in patients with septic shock.[32,35,36] There is some evidence that this also extends to the elevated lactate ($\geq$4 mmol/L) group (regardless of blood pressure).[33] When looking at less-severe septic patients or grouping all sepsis patients together, the results are less impressive.[35,37] What is perhaps most notable is that no study has ever used the 3-hour rule that the guidelines use as a benchmark.

How does this translate to the CED or LMIC? In general, the goal should be to strive for early and appropriate antimicrobial administration. In patients with severe sepsis and septic shock, earlier is better. However, appropriate antibiotic therapy is also important. Inappropriate antibiotics (ie, antibiotic did not cover isolated pathogen) can lead to increased mortality.[38,39] Thus, any ED protocol for septic patients should include triggers for empiric antibiotics for patients with severe sepsis and septic shock. These broad-spectrum antibiotics should be immediately available in the ED and based on the ED antibiogram.[40]

Fluid Resuscitation

The complex physiologic processes of sepsis that lead to tissue hypoperfusion are still being elucidated. As of now, it is thought that this is caused by some combination of decreased circulating volume, increased insensible losses, and vasodilation,[41] which is compounded in certain cases by cardiac, renal, and other end-organ dysfunction.[42] The guidelines recommend a 30-mL/kg crystalloid fluid bolus for patients with hypotension or elevated lactate.[40] The actual practice of fluid resuscitation, however, is much more complex than this and is covered in (See Rob Loflin and Michael E. Winters' article, "Fluid Resuscitation in Severe Sepsis", in this issue).

The choice of which fluids to use for resuscitation in sepsis is an ongoing debate. The current general consensus is that we should choose crystalloids over colloids, and lactated Ringer's is preferable to normal saline.[41,43,44] The amount of fluids required for resuscitation is patient specific. At the time of recognition of severe sepsis or septic shock, a 30-mL/kg bolus is recommended. Then, reassessment of the patient's fluid status is recommended before any additional fluid administration (**Fig. 1**).

Miscellaneous Recommendations

Staff resources

Although emergency physicians are ultimately responsible for identifying and treating septic patients, sepsis is a resource intensive disease, and numerous ED health care personnel are involved. Nurse-driven protocols assist in earlier identification of septic

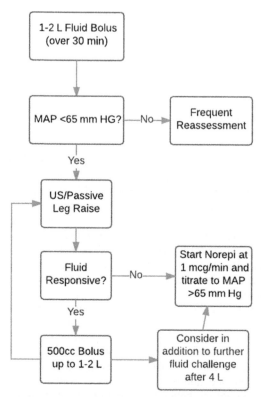

Fig. 1. Flow chart of fluid resuscitation.

patients and decreased time to obtaining blood cultures, lactate, and administering antibiotics.[45–47] Conversely, insufficient nursing resources have been cited as a barrier to implementation of sepsis guidelines.[1] Based on these findings, a nurse-driven protocol, including methods to allow temporary one-to-one nursing care, should be developed to facilitate compliance with sepsis guidelines. These methods can be further enhanced with the development of nurse or physician "champions" who promote sepsis education and provide feedback to foster a team-based culture for treating sepsis.[48]

Transfer decisions
One of the most important decisions to consider for a septic patient presenting to a CED is their ultimate disposition. The decision to admit to the floor versus intensive care unit (ICU) is often simplified in community settings based on the lack of monitoring availability outside of the ICU. However, does the patient require transfer? This decision will vary widely by location based on transport times and resources in the community hospital. Often, patients with severe sepsis and septic shock will be transferred out of a CED. This can, however, delay time to appropriate resuscitation and antibiotic administration.[49] The approach to sepsis transfers should be similar to that of trauma transfers. Consideration for transfer should begin immediately when recognizing that a patient may exceed institutional capabilities. The priority, however, should be initiation of aggressive fluid resuscitation and antibiotic administration while simultaneously arranging early transfer.

Summary of Goals of Sepsis Care in the Community Emergency Department or Low- and Middle-Income Country Emergency Department

---

- Nearly all sepsis management research has been done in large academic centers.
- Lack of benefit in the literature from sepsis protocols is likely a result of overall improvements in care and knowledge of guidelines.
- Protocols may benefit community hospitals by streamlining care and improving adherence to guidelines.
- Protocols should include prehospital or triage screening for sepsis.
- Point-of-care lactate measurement is easy to perform, can identify patients at risk for bad outcomes, and can be followed as a resuscitation endpoint.
- Blood cultures should be drawn early without impeding antibiotic delivery.
- Appropriate broad-spectrum antimicrobials should be given as early as possible and readily available to nurses.
- Septic patients should be aggressively resuscitated with hypotension (mean arterial pressure < 65 mm Hg) or an elevated lactate (>4 mmol/L) with a balanced crystalloid solution.
- Fluid resuscitation after the initial bolus should be guided by assessment of intravascular volume.
- Norepinephrine is the vasopressor of choice in septic shock.
- Septic patients are resource intensive; initial one-to-one nursing care improves adherence to guidelines.
- The ultimate disposition of septic patients in a CED (ICU vs transfer) should be considered early in their care so as not to delay definitive care.

SEPSIS IN LOW- AND MIDDLE-INCOME COUNTRIES

Accurate sepsis incidence and mortality data are still lacking in LMICs. A Brazilian study showed an incidence of sepsis and septic shock of 61.4 and 30 per 1000 patient-days, respectively, with mortality rates from sepsis of 35% and 52% from septic shock.[50] This finding was similar to that of a report from Zambia that showed a sepsis-related mortality rate of approximately 55%.[51] Results can vary widely, however, as a study from Asian ICUs showed rates of sepsis ranging from 10% in Bangladesh to 54% in Nepal.[52] The true incidence of sepsis in LMICs is unknown, as a recent review found no population-level estimates from LMICs.[53]

In the coming sections, the great disparity in the ability to diagnose and treat sepsis between countries and within the borders of a single country is explored. An example of this disparity is the availability of ICU beds. In the United States there are 20 ICU beds per 100,000 population; this number decreases to 8.9 in South Africa, 3.9 in China, and 1.6 in Sri Lanka.[54] Underlying pathologic and comorbid conditions can also vary widely. LMICs face an increased burden of disease from human immunodeficiency virus (HIV), malaria, and tuberculosis that complicate treatment. This variation in underlying conditions and comorbidity is believed to be partly responsible for the conflicting results of studies attempting to bring early, goal-directed therapy protocols to LMICs.[55,56]

Case Studies

A limited amount of research suggests that utilization of sepsis bundles and protocols in LMICs is associated with improved outcomes. This section looks at a few specific studies that have promising results. Similar to related research in HICs, however, these success stories are mostly found in academic settings, limiting the generalizability of their results.

CHINA

Wang and colleagues[57] conducted a study looking at mortality before and after implementation of a protocol designed to identify and treat severe sepsis and septic shock. They included patients based on the more nuanced definitions of severe sepsis (eg, end-organ dysfunction) and septic shock (eg, persistent hypotension or lactate ≥ 4)[40] and had a protocol based on the 2004 version of the SSC guidelines[58] broken down into a resuscitation bundle and management bundle. The results are summarized in **Table 1**. These results show that although full compliance with the protocol was not remarkably high (8.5%), even this modest adherence may have led to significantly better outcomes in mortality and various performance indicators. However, also notable was the large increase in early antibiotic delivery and aggressive fluid administration, which may explain the outcomes.

In addition to these findings, the investigators identified numerous barriers to completing the protocol. They found that there was often a delay in antibiotic administration, as a representative of the patient's family had to go to the pharmacy to purchase antibiotics and bring them back to the patient. In addition, nurses would simply carry out orders in the order in which they were written; thus, if antibiotics were at the bottom of the orders, they would be given last.[57] These types of delays are common in LMICs (and to a lesser extent in US CEDs) but are examples of barriers that could be overcome with increased awareness and education.

BRAZIL

A report in 2003 found that despite spending more than $8 billion on hospital care for patients,[59] mortality from sepsis was 56% in Brazil. This rate was notably higher than the 45% figure for other developing nations surveyed in the study.[60] The implementation of the SSC guidelines in Brazil is under the direction of the Latin American Sepsis Institute. The Latin American Sepsis Institute uses a combination of education campaigns, manuals, and data collection to coordinate care across Latin America and has resulted in widespread use of sepsis protocols at many hospitals in Brazil. Literature coming out of this work has shown that increased awareness toward diagnosing

Table 1 Chinese sepsis protocol study		
	Preprotocol	Postprotocol
Patients	78	117
% Severe sepsis	70.5%	69.2%
% Septic shock	29.5%	30.8%
In-hospital mortality	35 (44.8%)	37 (31.6%)[a]
% ICU	39%	27%
% Boarders	54%	43%
% Compliance with bundle	1.3%	8.5%[a]
% Fluid bolus (20 mL/kg)	27%	82.9%[a]
% Antibiotics <3 h of triage	25.6%	69.2%[a]

[a] P-value less than .05 compared with preprotocol.

sepsis and early administration of fluids and antibiotics can lead to reduction in sepsis-related mortality.[61,62]

A study by Westphal and colleagues[62] looked at the difference in diagnosis of sepsis when applying the SSC guidelines diagnostic criteria to all patients rather than just those already with an infection. The study took place at 2 hospitals in southern Brazil with "average to advanced levels of care."[62] They used the expanded definition of severe sepsis (eg, end-organ dysfunction) and usual definition of septic shock (eg, hypotension, elevated lactate). The protocol consisted of nursing technicians screening patients for criteria that would qualify for either severe sepsis or septic shock. Then, a ward nurse would review the case and consult a physician for treatment if he or she thought the patient met criteria. This protocol took place in EDs, ICUs, and the wards. The initial phase only screened patients with infection, whereas the intervention phase screened all patients.[62] Although overall compliance did not significantly change, the increased screening led to significant improvements in time to diagnosis and mortality. The relevant results are summarized in **Table 2**.

SEPSIS CARE IN AFRICA—QUESTIONING THE GUIDELINES

Despite the promising findings in middle-income countries such as Brazil and China, little research has been carried out in low-income settings. Furthermore, when this research has been carried out, the results have been mixed at best. The following sections examine 3 trials looking at implementing SSC guidelines in sub-Saharan Africa.

FEAST TRIAL

The Fluid Expansion as Supportive Therapy (or FEAST) trial by Maitland and colleagues[63] was the first large study looking at aggressive fluid resuscitation in pediatric shock and severe infection. It took place in 6 clinical centers in 3 African countries (Uganda, Tanzania, and Kenya). The trial included children (age 60 days to 12 years) with severe febrile illness and evidence of impaired perfusion. These patients were then further subdivided into those with (stratum A) and without (stratum B) severe hypotension. Stratum A patients were randomly assigned 1:1:1 into normal saline (20 mL/kg bolus over 1 hour), 5% albumin (20 mL/kg bolus over 1 hour), and maintenance fluid groups (2.5–4 mL/kg/h). Patients in stratum B were randomly assigned to receive either a normal saline bolus (40 mL/kg) or 5% albumin bolus (40 mL/kg).[63]

Surprisingly, the trial was stopped early when an interim analysis found that patients in stratum A had a significantly higher 48-hour mortality rate in both the saline bolus group (10.6%) and the albumin bolus group (10.5%) compared with the maintenance fluid group (7.3%, $P = .01$). The relative risk of mortality when receiving any bolus compared with control was 1.45 (95% CI, 1.13–1.86). There was no significant

Table 2				
Implementation of surviving sepsis guidelines in Brazil				
	Results from Brazilian Sepsis Studies (all Results $P<.05$)			
	Time to Diagnosis	**% In-Hospital Mortality**	**28-d Mortality**	**Bundle Compliance**
Westphal et al,[62] 2011				
Baseline	34 h ± 48 h	61.7%	47%	32.3%*
Postintervention	11 h ± 17 h	36.5%	24.3%	28.7%*

All results $P<.05$, except those with *.

difference between normal saline bolus compared with albumin bolus in either stratum. Further, there were no differences in any other outcome including pulmonary edema, neurologic sequelae, or increased intracranial pressure.[63]

Some critics of the trial argue the inclusion criteria for signs of poor perfusion were too broad, namely, that they only required one of the following: delayed cap refill, cool extremities, weak radial pulses, or severe tachycardia.[63] In contrast to this, the World Health Organization (WHO) recommends fluid resuscitation only for the combination of these findings.[64] Other critics feel that overzealous fluid resuscitation in a population with such high levels of anemia was bound to have negative consequences because of hemodilution.[65] The FEAST authors have since published further subgroup analyses that show increased mortality in all subgroups including the WHO definition of hypoperfusion and when controlling for severe anemia on presentation. They additionally argue that the increase in mortality is more likely a result the loss of sympathetically mediated physiologic compensation (cardiovascular collapse) rather than fluid overload.[56] Although the findings of the FEAST trial have not resulted in drastic policy changes (the WHO continues to recommend fluid boluses in this group),[66] it certainly raises concern when considering the administration of SSC guidelines in low-resource settings.

PROMOTING RESOURCE-LIMITED INTERVENTIONS FOR SEPSIS MANAGEMENT IN UGANDA GROUP

The first sepsis study in sub-Saharan Africa looking at adult patients was published in 2009 by the Promoting Resource-Limited Interventions for Sepsis Management in Uganda (PRISM-U) study group. This observational study showed an in-hospital mortality rate for patients with severe sepsis of 23.7% and a further 22.3% mortality rate within 30 days of discharge. Also notable from this study was the high percentage of advanced HIV found in septic patients (84.9% with HIV, mean CD4 count of 52 cells/mm^3) and the minimal amount of fluids administered (median 500 mL in the first 6 hours).[67]

As a result of these findings, this group carried out a before and after trial looking at the effect of implementing a strategy of early, monitored management in patients with severe sepsis.[5] The authors defined severe sepsis as suspected infection, 2 or more SIRS (Systemic Inflammatory Response Syndrome) criteria (without white blood cell count), hypotension (systolic blood pressure <100 mm Hg), and a lactate greater than 2.5 mmol/L or a Karnofsky Performance Score ≤40. The intervention called for a 1000-mL bolus given over 60 minutes and repeat 500-mL boluses every 30 minutes for continued hypotension. Additionally, enrolled patients received 1:1 monitoring from a study officer to assess vital signs and need for continued fluids. The intervention lasted for the first 6 hours after enrollment, after which the patient received "usual care".[5]

The relevant results are shown in **Table 3**. Overall, the study showed improvements in time to initial fluids, amount of fluids, time to antibiotics, and 30-day mortality. Early

Table 3 PRISM-U study group in Uganda		
	Fluids Given in First 6 h[a]	Received Any Fluids in 1st h
Control group	500 mL (300–1000 mL)	55.1%
Intervention group	3000 mL (2500–4000 mL)	97.1%

All results with P-values less than .05.
[a] Median (interquartile range).

antibiotic administration was independently associated with decreased mortality, but there was not a direct correlation between mortality and incrementally shorter time to antibiotics. One caveat, the large number of "inappropriate antimicrobials," complicates these findings. A factor that may have influenced outcomes was increased monitoring. In addition to the study nurses, the group used a novel design wherein a patient's friend or family member was required to be at the bedside to alert nurses to completion of fluids.[5] Low cost (or no cost) interventions such as these can have remarkable influences on patient care.

ZAMBIA

After the publication of the FEAST and PRISM-U trials, Andrews and colleagues[51] set out to test a fluid-based resuscitation protocol at a large hospital in Lusaka, Zambia. The trial enrolled patients with severe sepsis either at presentation or within 24 hours of arrival, provided the patient was still in the ED and within 6 hours of meeting inclusion criteria. The group used a definition for severe sepsis that included signs of end-organ dysfunction. The fluid intervention was based on measurements of jugular venous pressure. Patients in the control group received usual care, with the addition of a dedicated nurse to ensure completion of orders and notify providers of changes in the patient's condition. The intervention group had a similar study nurse with the addition of an initial 2000-mL bolus (normal saline or lactated Ringer's) within 1 hour, and an additional 2000 mL was given over 4 hours for decreased jugular venous pressure after reassessment. The choice of adjunctive therapies such as antimicrobials was left up to physician discretion.[51]

Similar to the FEAST trial, this trial was stopped early. This decision was due to concerns of increased mortality in a certain subgroup of patients who had an initial respiratory rate greater than 40 breaths per minute and oxygen saturation less than 90%. Fifteen of 18 (83%) patients in this group died including 100% (8 of 8) in the intervention group. Overall, there was no significant difference in in-hospital mortality between the treatment and control groups (64.2% vs 60.7%) nor in 28-day mortality (71.4% vs 66.7%). No significant difference in time to antimicrobials from admission was found between treatment groups. There was, however, a significant difference in the amount of fluids administered in the first 6 hours (treatment group 2.9 L vs control group 1.6 L).[51]

IS SEPSIS DIFFERENT IN SUB-SAHARAN AFRICA?
Different Patients

Why are these findings so different from those that we find in other parts of the world when dealing with septic patients? Several different patient and system factors result in the disparities of outcomes in sepsis. Perhaps the most obvious is the prevalence of HIV/acquired immune deficiency syndrome (AIDs) in sub-Saharan Africa. In the 2 African studies discussed above, the percentage of HIV-positive patients was 80.7% in Zambia[51] and 84.8% in Uganda.[5] Further, the CD-4 counts (per cubic millimeter) on admission in these studies were 55.4[51] and 55.7,[5] respectively, suggesting advanced disease (eg, AIDS). HIV/AIDS was found to be associated with increased mortality in both HICs[68] and LMICs.[69]

The pathogenesis of sepsis is also different in sub-Saharan Africa compared with most other settings. In most HICs, the most common organisms isolated from septic patients are either staphylococcus/streptococcus or gram-negative bacilli, such as Escherichia coli, Klebsiella, and Pseudomonas.[70] In contrast, nontyphoidal Salmonella has been reported in approximately 20% of positive blood cultures in sub-Saharan

Table 4
Availability of resources in African hospitals

SSC Bundle Components	% Always Available
Broad-spectrum antibiotics	25.2
Lactate	21.7
Treatment of hypotension	90.2
Equipment	
Blood pressure measurement	93.8
O_2 Saturation measurement	76.8
Ventilator	71.9
Antibiogram	70.4
Disposable materials	
Intravenous cannula	97.3
Oxygen facemask	96.6
Central venous catheter	48.8

Africa.[67,71] Further complicating matters is the association of *Mycobacterium tuberculosis* and *Cryptococcus neoformans* in HIV patients.[51,67,71] Additionally, the availability and reliability of laboratory facilities in these settings makes diagnostic confirmation a challenge.[72] Because of this, initial diagnosis is often clinical and commonly thought to be related to malaria. A recent study found that 60.7% of patients who presented to Tanzanian EDs with a fever received a diagnosis of malaria; however, this was the actual cause of fever in only 1.6% of these patients.[73] In fact, 26.2% of these patients had evidence of an acute bacterial zoonotic infection,[73] which is particularly concerning to those of us who rarely consider such a diagnosis.

The potential for marked delay in presentation is also a consideration. In the Andrews study, the duration of the chief complaint ranged from 3 to 30 days.[51] Perhaps most astounding is that 74.3% of patients were nonambulatory at the time of admission and they had been so for an average of 5 days.[51] Many have tried home remedies or been treated for malaria before eventual arrival at the hospital.

Different Resources

Consideration must also be given to resource availability when caring for septic patients. A survey of providers at the Fourth All Africa Anesthesia Congress in 2011 found key differences in the resources available in LMICs compared with HICs.[3] This survey showed that only 1.5% of the providers from African countries felt they could consistently implement all of the recommendations of the SSC 2008 guidelines. This was in contrast to 81.8% of providers from HICs present at the conference. Sub-Saharan countries were also analyzed independently from Northern African countries and South Africa. The availability of some specific components is listed in **Table 4**.[3] The authors of this article also mention that this is likely an overestimate of resources, given that their respondents were mostly from university or private hospitals.[3]

SUMMARY AND RECOMMENDATIONS

As can be seen from the above discussion, myriad factors limit the ability to treat sepsis in LMICs. Some limitations are common in all geographic regions such as infrastructure and diagnostic capabilities; whereas others are unique to specific regions. Because of these limitations, general guidelines that apply to all LMICs are challenging. The WHO has devised a set of recommendations that stress early recognition and resuscitation of sepsis, while considering context-specific comorbidities, and are consistent with those developed by other groups.[74,75] Highlights from these recommendations are:

- Early recognition is key especially in patients with abnormal vital signs, alteration in mental status, or a new decrease in functional status.
  - An early warning scoring system may assist sepsis recognition by nurses.
- Resources for correcting abnormal vital signs such as oxygen and fluids must be immediately available and administered early.
- Vital signs need to be repeated at least every hour until consistently normal.
- Antimicrobial treatments should be administered as quickly as possible based on suspected source of infection.
  - If possible, rapid diagnostic testing for HIV, malaria, and influenza should be used to help guide initial treatments.

In addition, recommendations for system-based improvements include:

- Training programs for recognition and early treatment of sepsis designed for nurses, physicians, and other providers
- Quality metrics for measuring adherence to guidelines and identifying common gaps in care
- Facility improvements to strengthen critical care capacity, laboratory services, and emergency department resources
- Coordination of district and regional hospitals to share resources and streamline transfer processes

The broadness of these recommendations, on both a patient and a systems level, reveal the challenge at hand. Additionally, in many LMICs, the specialty of emergency medicine is either nascent or nonexistent. In fact, nearly all of the trials referenced in this section have been led by Internal Medicine or Critical Care providers. As emergency medicine grows in LMICs, there is an opportunity for emergency medicine providers to lead the fight against sepsis on the front lines. This includes partnerships for education and research to take the unique skills of the emergency medicine provider and translate them for use in low-resource settings. The challenges of treating sepsis in LMICs, similar to those found in community EDs, necessitate a unique approach that seeks to both maximize the resources at hand while also identifying key areas for improvement.

REFERENCES

1. Carlbom DJ, Rubenfeld GD. Barriers to implementing protocol-based sepsis resuscitation in the emergency department—Results of a national survey. Crit Care Med 2007;35:2525–32.
2. Mahavanakul W, Nickerson EK, Srisomang P, et al. Feasibility of modified surviving sepsis campaign guidelines in a resource-restricted setting based on a cohort study of severe S. aureus sepsis. PLoS One 2012;7:e29858.
3. Baelani I, Jochberger S, Laimer T, et al. Availability of critical care resources to treat patients with severe sepsis or septic shock in Africa: a self-reported, continent-wide survey of anaesthesia providers. Crit Care 2011;15:R10.
4. Burney M, Underwood J, McEvoy S, et al. Early detection and treatment of severe sepsis in the emergency department: identifying barriers to implementation of a protocol-based approach. J Emerg Nurs 2012;38:512–7.

5. Jacob ST, Banura P, Baeten JM, et al. The impact of early monitored management on survival in hospitalized adult Ugandan patients with severe sepsis: a prospective intervention study. Crit Care Med 2012;40:2050–8.

6. Chimese SM, Andrews B, Lakhi S. The etiology and outcome of adult patients presenting with sepsis to the University Teaching Hospital, Lusaka, Zambia. Med J Zambia 2014;39:19–22.

7. Levy MM, Artigas A, Phillips GS, et al. Outcomes of the Surviving Sepsis Campaign in intensive care units in the USA and Europe: a prospective cohort study. Lancet Infect Dis 2012;12:919–24.

8. Levy MM, Dellinger RP, Townsend SR, et al. The surviving sepsis campaign: results of an international guideline-based performance improvement program targeting severe sepsis. Intensive Care Med 2010;36:222–31.

9. O'Neill R, Morales J, Jule M. Early goal-directed therapy (EGDT) for severe sepsis/septic shock: which components of treatment are more difficult to implement in a community-based emergency department? J Emerg Med 2012;42: 503–10.

10. Levy MM, Rhodes A, Phillips GS, et al. Surviving sepsis campaign: association between performance metrics and outcomes in a 7.5-year study. Intensive Care Med 2014;40:1623–33.

11. Kortgen A, Niederprüm P, Bauer M. Implementation of an evidence-based "standard operating procedure" and outcome in septic shock. Crit Care Med 2006;34: 943–9.

12. Yealy DM, Kellum JA, Huang DT, et al. A randomized trial of protocol-based care for early septic shock. N Engl J Med 2014;370:1683–93.

13. Peake SL, Delaney A, Bailey M, et al. Goal-directed resuscitation for patients with early septic shock. N Engl J Med 2014;371:1496–506.

14. Mouncey PR, Osborn TM, Power GS, et al. Trial of early, goal-directed resuscitation for septic shock. N Engl J Med 2015;372:1301–11.

15. Rhodes A, Phillips G, Beale R, et al. The surviving sepsis campaign bundles and outcome: results from the international multicentre prevalence study on sepsis (the IMPreSS study). Intensive Care Med 2015;41:1620–8.

16. Angus D, Barnato A, Bell D, et al. A systematic review and meta-analysis of early goal-directed therapy for septic shock: the ARISE, ProCESS and ProMISe Investigators. Intensive Care Med 2015;41:1549–60.

17. Campaign SS. Surviving Sepsis Campaign Responds to ProCESS Trial. Available at: http://www.survivingsepsis.org/SiteCollectionDocuments/SSC-Responds-Process-Trial.pdf2014. Accessed February 14, 2016.

18. Seymour CW, Rea TD, Kahn JM, et al. Severe sepsis in pre-hospital emergency care. Am J Respir Crit Care Med 2012;186:1264–71.

19. Guerra WF, Mayfield TR, Meyers MS, et al. Early detection and treatment of patients with severe sepsis by prehospital personnel. J Emerg Med 2013;44: 1116–25.

20. Studnek JR, Artho MR, Garner CL Jr, et al. The impact of emergency medical services on the ED care of severe sepsis. Am J Emerg Med 2012;30:51–6.

21. Arnold RC, Shapiro NI, Jones AE, et al. Multicenter study of early lactate clearance as a determinant of survival in patients with presumed sepsis. Shock 2009;32:35–9.

22. Mikkelsen ME, Miltiades AN, Gaieski DF, et al. Serum lactate is associated with mortality in severe sepsis independent of organ failure and shock. Crit Care Med 2009;37:1670–7.

23. Nguyen HB, Rivers EP, Knoblich BP, et al. Early lactate clearance is associated with improved outcome in severe sepsis and septic shock. Crit Care Med 2004;32:1637–42.

24. Trzeciak S. Lac-time? Crit Care Med 2004;32:1785–6.

25. Rivers E, Nguyen B, Havstad S, et al. Early goal-directed therapy in the treatment of severe sepsis and septic shock. N Engl J Med 2001;345:1368–77.

26. Donnino MW, Nguyen B, Jacobsen G, et al. Cryptic septic shock: a sub-analysis of early, goal-directed therapy. Chest 2003;124(4_MeetingAbstracts):90S-b.

27. Howell MD, Donnino M, Clardy P, et al. Occult hypoperfusion and mortality in patients with suspected infection. Intensive Care Med 2007;33:1892–9.

28. Talmor D, Greenberg D, Howell MD, et al. The costs and cost-effectiveness of an integrated sepsis treatment protocol. Crit Care Med 2008;36:1168–74.

29. van Horssen R, Schuurman TN, de Groot MJM, et al. Lactate point-of-care testing for acidosis: cross-comparison of two devices with routine laboratory results. Pract Lab Med 2016;4:41–9.

30. Boldt J, Kumle B, Suttner S, et al. This article has been retracted: point-of-care (POC) testing of lactate in the intensive care patient. Acta Anaesthesiol Scand 2001;45:194–9.

31. Sean S, Christopher SR, Rahul K, et al. Point-of-care lactate measurement in an emergency department is associated with expedited early goal-directed management of severe sepsis and septic shock. D53 SEPSIS: mechanisms and implications for management. New York: American Thoracic Society; 2010. A6141-A.

32. Kumar A, Roberts D, Wood KE, et al. Duration of hypotension before initiation of effective antimicrobial therapy is the critical determinant of survival in human septic shock. Crit Care Med 2006;34:1589–96.

33. Gaieski DF, Mikkelsen ME, Band RA, et al. Impact of time to antibiotics on survival in patients with severe sepsis or septic shock in whom early goal-directed therapy was initiated in the emergency department. Crit Care Med 2010;38:1045–53.

34. Ferrer R, Martin-Loeches I, Phillips G, et al. Empiric antibiotic treatment reduces mortality in severe sepsis and septic shock from the first hour: results from a guideline-based performance improvement program. Crit Care Med 2014;42:1749–55.

35. Puskarich MA, Trzeciak S, Shapiro NI, et al. Association between timing of antibiotic administration and mortality from septic shock in patients treated with a quantitative resuscitation protocol. Crit Care Med 2011;39:2066–71.

36. de Groot B, Ansems A, Gerling DH, et al. The association between time to antibiotics and relevant clinical outcomes in emergency department patients with various stages of sepsis: a prospective multi-center study. Crit Care 2015;19:194.

37. Sterling SA, Miller WR, Pryor J, et al. The impact of timing of antibiotics on outcomes in severe sepsis and septic shock: a systematic review and meta-analysis. Crit Care Med 2015;43:1907–15.

38. Garnacho-Montero J, Gutiérrez-Pizarraya A, Escoresca-Ortega A, et al. Adequate antibiotic therapy prior to ICU admission in patients with severe sepsis and septic shock reduces hospital mortality. Crit Care 2015;19:302.

39. Kumar A, Ellis P, Arabi Y, et al. Initiation of inappropriate antimicrobial therapy results in a fivefold reduction of survival in human septic shock. Chest 2009;136:1237–48.

40. Dellinger RP, Levy MM, Rhodes A, et al. Surviving Sepsis Campaign: international guidelines for management of severe sepsis and septic shock, 2012. Intensive Care Med 2013;39:165–228.

41. Daniels R. Surviving the first hours in sepsis: getting the basics right (an intensivist's perspective). J Antimicrob Chemother 2011;66:ii11–23.
42. Madhusudan P, Tirupakuzhi Vijayaraghavan BK, Cove ME. Fluid resuscitation in sepsis: reexamining the paradigm. Biomed Res Int 2014;2014:984082.
43. Karakala N, Raghunathan K, Shaw AD. Intravenous fluids in sepsis: what to use and what to avoid. Curr Opin Crit Care 2013;19:537–43.
44. Yunos NM, Bellomo R, Hegarty C, et al. Association between a chloride-liberal vs chloride-restrictive intravenous fluid administration strategy and kidney injury in critically ill adults. JAMA 2012;308:1566–72.
45. Moore LJ, Jones SL, Kreiner LA, et al. Validation of a screening tool for the early identification of sepsis. J Trauma 2009;66:1539–47.
46. Bruce HR, Maiden J, Fedullo PF, et al. Impact of nurse-initiated ED sepsis protocol on compliance with sepsis bundles, time to initial antibiotic administration, and in-hospital mortality. J Emerg Nurs 2015;41:130–7.
47. Coates E, Villarreal A, Gordanier C, et al. Sepsis power hour: a nursing driven protocol improves timeliness of sepsis care. J Hosp Med 2015;10(Suppl 2). Available at: http://www.shmabstracts.com/abstract/sepsis-power-hour-a-nursing-driven-protocol-improves-timeliness-of-sepsis-care/. Accessed February 13, 2016.
48. Campbell J. The effect of nurse champions on compliance with Keystone Intensive Care Unit Sepsis-screening protocol. Crit Care Nurs Q 2008;31:251–69.
49. Faine BA, Noack JM, Wong T, et al. Interhospital transfer delays appropriate treatment for patients with severe sepsis and septic shock: a retrospective cohort study. Crit Care Med 2015;43:2589–96.
50. Silva E, Pedro MA, Sogayar AC, et al. Brazilian sepsis epidemiological study (BASES study). Crit Care 2004;8:R251.
51. Andrews B, Muchemwa L, Kelly P, et al. Simplified severe sepsis protocol: a randomized controlled trial of modified early goal-directed therapy in Zambia. Crit Care Med 2014;42:2315–24.
52. Phua J, Koh Y, Du B, et al. Management of severe sepsis in patients admitted to Asian intensive care units: prospective cohort study. BMJ 2011;342:d3245.
53. Fleischmann C, Scherag A, Adhikari NKJ, et al. Assessment of global incidence and mortality of hospital-treated sepsis. current estimates and limitations. Am J Respir Crit Care Med 2015;193:259–72.
54. Adhikari NK, Fowler RA, Bhagwanjee S, et al. Critical care and the global burden of critical illness in adults. Lancet 2010;376:1339–46.
55. Myburgh J, Finfer S. Causes of death after fluid bolus resuscitation: new insights from FEAST. BMC Med 2013;11:67.
56. Maitland K, George EC, Evans JA, et al. Exploring mechanisms of excess mortality with early fluid resuscitation: insights from the FEAST trial. BMC Med 2013;11:68.
57. Wang Z, Xiong Y, Schorr C, et al. Impact of sepsis bundle strategy on outcomes of patients suffering from severe sepsis and septic shock in China. J Emerg Med 2013;44:735–41.
58. Dellinger RP, Carlet JM, Masur H, et al. Surviving sepsis campaign guidelines for management of severe sepsis and septic shock. Intensive Care Med 2004;30:536–55.
59. Teles JMM, Silva E, Westphal G, et al. Surviving sepsis campaign in Brazil. Shock 2008;30:47–52.

60. Beale R, Reinhart K, Dobb G, et al. Progress (promoting global research excellence in severe sepsis): a preliminary report of an international internet-based sepsis registry. Chest 2003;124(4_MeetingAbstracts):224S-b.
61. Noritomi DT, Ranzani OT, Monteiro MB, et al. Implementation of a multifaceted sepsis education program in an emerging country setting: clinical outcomes and cost-effectiveness in a long-term follow-up study. Intensive Care Med 2013;40:182–91.
62. Westphal GA, Koenig Á, Filho MC, et al. Reduced mortality after the implementation of a protocol for the early detection of severe sepsis. J Crit Care 2011;26: 76–81.
63. Maitland K, Kiguli S, Opoka RO, et al. Mortality after fluid bolus in African children with severe infection. N Engl J Med 2011;364:2483–95.
64. Organization WHO. Pocket book of hospital care for children: guidelines for the management of common illnesses with limited resources. Geneva (Switzerland): World Health Organization; 2005.
65. Southall DP, Samuels MP. Treating the wrong children with fluids will cause harm: response to 'mortality after fluid bolus in African children with severe infection'. Arch Dis Child 2011;96(10):905–6.
66. Kiguli S, Akech SO, Mtove G, et al. WHO guidelines on fluid resuscitation in children: missing the FEAST data. BMJ 2014;348:f7003.
67. Jacob ST, Moore CC, Banura P, et al. Severe sepsis in two ugandan hospitals: a prospective observational study of management and outcomes in a predominantly HIV-1 infected population. PLoS One 2009;4:e7782.
68. Mrus JM, Braun L, Michael SY, et al. Impact of HIV/AIDS on care and outcomes of severe sepsis. Crit Care 2005;9:R623.
69. Japiassú AM, Amâncio RT, Mesquita EC, et al. Sepsis is a major determinant of outcome in critically ill HIV/AIDS patients. Crit Care 2010;14:1–8.
70. Bochud P-Y, Calandra T. Pathogenesis of sepsis: new concepts and implications for future treatment. BMJ 2003;326:262–6.
71. Crump JA, Ramadhani HO, Morrissey AB, et al. Invasive bacterial and fungal infections among hospitalized HIV-infected and HIV-uninfected adults and adolescents in Northern Tanzania. Clin Infect Dis 2011;52:341–8.
72. Petti CA, Polage CR, Quinn TC, et al. Laboratory medicine in Africa: a barrier to effective health care. Clin Infect Dis 2006;42:377–82.
73. Crump JA, Morrissey AB, Nicholson WL, et al. Etiology of severe non-malaria febrile illness in Northern Tanzania: a prospective cohort study. PLoS Negl Trop Dis 2013;7:e2324.
74. Crump JA, Gove S, Parry CM. Management of adolescents and adults with febrile illness in resource limited areas. BMJ 2011;343:d4847.
75. Dünser MW, Festic E, Dondorp A, et al. Recommendations for sepsis management in resource-limited settings. Intensive Care Med 2012;38:557–74.

Prehospital Sepsis Care

Jerrilyn Jones, MD, MPH[a],*, Benjamin J. Lawner, DO, MS, EMT-P[a,b]

KEYWORDS

- Prehospital • Emergency medical services • Sepsis • Advanced life support
- Paramedic

KEY POINTS

- Early recognition of sepsis in the prehospital environment can improve patient outcomes.
- Early recognition and aggressive fluid therapy (when appropriate) are important components of a prehospital sepsis protocol.
- Early notification of the receiving hospital and measurement of serum lactate concentrations may expedite care of the septic patient encountered in the prehospital environment.
- Additional research is needed to determine the necessary components of a prehospital sepsis protocol.

INTRODUCTION

Emergency medical services (EMS) personnel frequently provide care for individuals with time-critical illnesses and injuries. One such condition is sepsis, which represents a broad spectrum of clinical presentations requiring early recognition and rapid intervention. Interventions such as the administration of antibiotics and intravenous (IV) fluids within the first few hours have been linked to lower mortalities.[1,2] In the United States, EMS systems have a long-standing tradition of care coordination. For example, trauma victims are conveyed speedily to designated trauma centers and victims of ST-segment elevation myocardial infarction (STEMI) are delivered to waiting cardiac catheterization laboratories. Because sepsis represents a distinct medical entity that would benefit from timely medical intervention, it logically follows that a systematic approach to prehospital recognition and treatment would benefit this distinct group of patients. That said, the recognition of a sepsis syndrome during the prehospital phase of care is far more complex than teaching EMS providers to recognize varying degrees of hemodynamic instability.

Modern EMS systems incorporate a variety of professionals, and each level of EMS provider has been trained to a different level of understanding with respect to human

Disclosures: None.
[a] Department of Emergency Medicine, University of Maryland School of Medicine, 110 S. Paca Street, 6th floor, Suite 200, Baltimore, MD 21201, USA; [b] Baltimore City Fire Department, Emergency Medical Services, 3500 West Northern Parkway, Baltimore, MD 21215, USA
* Corresponding author.
E-mail address: jjones@em.umaryland.edu

Emerg Med Clin N Am 35 (2017) 175–183
http://dx.doi.org/10.1016/j.emc.2016.08.009
0733-8627/17/© 2016 Elsevier Inc. All rights reserved.

anatomy and physiology. Basic emergency medical technicians (EMTs) can interpret abnormalities in vital signs but might not be familiar with the underlying physiology. Paramedics understand the physiologic implications of a septic state but might not appreciate subtle or occult presentations of sepsis in immunosuppressed or chronically ill individuals. Because early recognition and intervention are associated with a decreased mortality, it is imperative to engage EMS systems in a comprehensive approach to the treatment of sepsis. This article explores current practices and available medical decision-making tools, job aids, and point-of-care (POC) tests in order to articulate an evidence-based approach to the prehospital recognition of sepsis.

EXISTING TRIAGE TOOLS

In 2009 and 2010, researchers from Harborview Medical Center attempted to quantify EMS providers' understanding of sepsis.[3] Providers from 3 EMS agencies, at all levels of EMS education and training, participated in an online 10-question survey focused on sepsis recognition. The study population included firefighter (FF)//EMTs, other EMTs, and paramedics. Seven hundred eighty-six EMS providers completed the survey: 408 FF/EMTs (52%), 276 other EMTs (21%), and 102 paramedics (13%). Almost all (97%) of the participants had "heard of sepsis" and appreciated its association with increased in-hospital mortality.[3] However, knowledge gaps were found when participants were asked about their understanding of sepsis. EMTs were less likely than paramedics to identify the correct definition of sepsis, and this finding persisted following logistic regression analysis. Importantly, 55% of respondents agreed that EMS providers could play a role in the early identification of patients at risk for sepsis. These results lend credence to the idea of a systemic, protocolized approach to sepsis care. Important limitations surfaced in the analysis of the study. Each EMS system has different training programs, and the results may not be readily generalizable. The survey did not incorporate clinical scenarios, and researchers were therefore unable to test a provider's ability to engage in more complex medical decision making. However, paramedics' broad and more refined familiarity with sepsis suggested that these providers could be integrated into more specific and widespread prehospital treatment strategies.

Guerra and colleagues[4] examined the utility of an aggressive, goal-directed, prehospital sepsis protocol. Before this study's results are examined, it is helpful to appreciate aspects of the regional EMS system that made such important research possible. First, physicians from a single group staffed all the emergency departments (EDs) involved in the study. The EMS system used an "all-advanced life support" (all-ALS) model of care, meaning that each ambulance crew included at least one credentialed paramedic.[4] Finally, medical direction was provided by board-certified emergency physicians affiliated with area hospitals and EMS system. Although such a collaborative arrangement might seem logical, the reality of physician oversight in EMS is far less consistent. This study featured a rather fortuitous pairing of engaged medical direction and an all-ALS system. Although basic life support (BLS) providers have a pivotal role to play in terms of recognition, EMTs are not often authorized to insert IV lines or administer medication therapy. The authors used an evidence-based triage screening tool and incorporated POC lactic acid testing into the prehospital sepsis algorithm. Patients who met predefined prehospital triage parameters were directed into a "sepsis alert" protocol. Essentially, patients had to fulfill 4 criteria: (1) age greater than 18 years and not pregnant, (2) presence of 2 systemic inflammatory response criteria, (3) suspected infection, and (4) hypoperfusion manifested by prehospital systolic hypotension or an elevated lactic acid level (>4 mmol/L). The study population comprised 112 patients. Paramedics correctly identified 32 of 67 patients (48%) who were subsequently diagnosed as having severe sepsis. Patients dropped out of the "sepsis alert" protocol for reasons apart from provider familiarity with the sepsis definition. Of the 35 septic patients who were not identified by EMS personnel, 5 had vital signs that did not meet criteria. Thirteen additional septic patients were identified during their ED stay as a result of an elevated white blood cell count. In an unadjusted analysis that examined survival as a primary endpoint, patients classified by EMS personnel as having severe sepsis had an odds ratio of 3.19 in favor of survival (95% confidence interval [CI], 1.14–8.88). The authors also reported a lower mortality for EMS patients identified with the sepsis alert protocol as opposed to those not identified with the sepsis alert protocol. This study affirms that paramedic-level providers can identify severe sepsis and initiate appropriate treatment. Furthermore, the use of an "alert" protocol could have several positive downstream effects. Patients identified as having a time-sensitive condition are more likely to undergo timely interventions. Potentially negative effects of this specific protocol included false-positive sepsis activations and increased costs associated with paramedic education and training. It is logical to infer, however, that additional investment in training costs would be offset by the benefits gleaned from aggressive prehospital resuscitation of septic patients.

A recent retrospective study examined more than 66,000 EMS encounters for the purpose of developing a prehospital sepsis score (PRESS).[5] This score can be used by a broad range of EMS providers to facilitate the early treatment and rapid transport of septic patients to definitive care. The investigators looked at dispatch and patient characteristics associated with adverse outcomes. In an urban, 2-tiered (BLS and ALS) EMS system, a few variables emerged that were persistently linked to the inpatient diagnosis of severe sepsis or septic shock: advanced age, hot tactile temperature, low systolic blood pressure, and low oxygen saturation. Compared with other currently available triage schemes, the PRESS relies mostly on clinical assessment and 9-1-1 triage. Indeed, prehospital POC lactate analysis is not readily available in most EMS agencies, and compliance with rigorous protocols may depend at least in part on the ambulance crew's level of training. The sensitivity of the score was 91% in the derivation group and 78% in the validation group. When the predefined threshold of 2 or more points is met, the sensitivity of the PRESS increases to 86%.

This scoring technique has several important limitations. Patients in the derivation group had already met criteria for the systemic inflammatory response syndrome (SIRS). Patients deemed "at risk" for sepsis had to meet all the criteria in the prehospital setting: elevated heart rate, elevated respiratory rate, and systolic blood pressure less than 100 mm Hg. Therefore, the PRESS's respectable sensitivity would suffer following validation in an external cohort.

EARLY WARNING SCORES

The concept of an early warning score (EWS) was developed in an effort to identify deteriorating hospitalized patients rapidly.[6] These scores, most often a composite of physiologic and/or laboratory values, have become the standard of care in many parts of the world.[6] However, the utility of an EWS in the prehospital environment is less well established. There is precedent for timely prehospital intervention directed at time-sensitive conditions such as stroke, STEMI, and penetrating trauma. It follows that sepsis, which is also a time-critical illness, would benefit from the same treatment strategy. Although early treatment of sepsis shows a greater morbidity and mortality benefit than early thrombolysis and balloon angioplasty for patients with acute coronary syndrome, until recently it received less attention and research funding.[7,8] There is current interest in developing a prehospital EWS to identify patients with critical illness and facilitate their early access to appropriate, definitive care.[6]

Developing an EWS for sepsis presents unique challenges. The first challenge is the lack of a consensus definition for sepsis. Sepsis is a clinical syndrome for which the inclusion and exclusion criteria have been changed over the years. The most recent definition by the International Committee on Sepsis was published in *Journal of the American Medical Association* in 2016.[9] The authors of that article anticipate that, as one becomes more knowledgeable about the biology behind the clinical manifestations of sepsis, the definition of the disease will be refined. For example, the term "severe sepsis" is now considered redundant, so it has been removed from the clinical spectrum.[9] Changing the nomenclature poses a problem when it comes to research and establishing evidence-based practices. Much of the data produced so far used "severe sepsis" criteria in determining whether an intervention was successful. The lack of a clear definition, as well as a lack of consensus on measurable outcomes, makes the existing body of literature heterogeneous and difficult to compare.[6] Establishing a universal EWS under these circumstances becomes complex.

The first prehospital EWS was the Rapid Acute Physiology Score (RAPS), which is an abbreviation of the APACHE-II (Acute Physiology and Chronic Health Evaluation) score.[6] RAPS was developed and tested for the aeromedical transport of critically ill patients. There are several in-hospital EWS currently in use. Attempts have been made to translate in-hospital EWSs into the prehospital environment via scoring systems such as the Modified EWS (MEWS), with varying success.[6,10]

Guerra and colleagues[4] developed a "sepsis alert" protocol that incorporates modified SIRS criteria along with prehospital lactate measurements to identify severe sepsis patients. The Robson screening tool takes into account temperature, heart rate, respiratory rate, mental status, plasma glucose concentrations, and a history suggestive of new infection.[8] The BAS tool is based on the following vital signs: oxygen saturation less than 90%, respiratory rate greater than 30, and systolic blood pressure less than 90 mm Hg (BAS 90–30–90).[1,6,11]

In 2015, German researchers developed the Prehospital Early Sepsis Detection score (PRESEP), which gives weighted values to abnormal vital signs (**Table 1**). The cutoff indicating potential septic disease is greater than or equal to 4.[7] The authors compared their scoring system with MEWS, BAS 90-30-90, and the Robson screening tool. The PRESEP score performed better than MEWS and BAS 90-30-90 in terms of sensitivity, specificity, as well as positive and negative predictive value. The Robson

Table 1
Prehospital early sepsis detection score

Vital Sign	Points
Temperature >38 C	4
Temperature <36 C	1
Heart rate >90 bpm	2
Respiratory rate >22 breaths/min	1
Oxygen saturation <92%	2
Systolic blood pressure <90 mm Hg	2

A score greater than or equal to 4 suggests sepsis.
From Bayer O, Schwarzkopf D, Stumme C, et al. An early warning scoring system to identify septic patients in the prehospital setting: the PRESEP score. Acad Emerg Med 2015;22:868–71.

score, however, had a higher sensitivity and negative predictive value but a lower specificity and positive predictive value.[7] It is important to note that the German model of prehospital care differs significantly from the American model. In Germany, ambulance crews typically include physicians. In addition, in the United States, body temperatures are not always measured by prehospital care providers, which could limit the generalizability of a scoring system that requires it.[12]

As previously mentioned, the PRESS score is 86% sensitive when the threshold of 2 points is met or exceeded.[13] The score incorporates several pieces of data that are collected routinely by both dispatch and EMS providers in the United States in order to identify patients at risk for severe sepsis.[13] Each criterion is weighted (see **Table 1**). The maximum is 24 points, and the threshold of 2 or more points can be met with a single criterion. This scoring system has several limitations, and additional validation studies are required before it can be put into widespread practice.

In a recent article in *Journal of the American Medical Association*, the Sepsis-3 Committee recommended use of the Sequential Organ Failure Assessment (SOFA) score as a marker of organ dysfunction. The SOFA score, which incorporates laboratory values such as bilirubin and creatinine levels, has been used primarily in the intensive care setting. A score greater than or equal to 2 is associated with an in-hospital mortality greater than 10%. The authors propose using a truncated SOFA score in out-of-hospital, ED, and general ward settings to identify patients at increased risk of worse outcomes related to sepsis. The criteria for this quick SOFA score (qSOFA) are respiratory rate greater than or equal to 22 breaths/min, systolic blood pressure less than or equal to 100 mm Hg, and altered mentation. The presence of 2 of these 3 criteria had similar predictive validity to the full SOFA score outside the ICU.[9]

EWSs and the prehospital care provider's ability to act on them could have the greatest impact in areas where transport times are prolonged. The mainstays of sepsis treatment are antimicrobial therapy, source control, and supportive therapy (eg, IV fluids, vasopressors) to maintain tissue perfusion.[14] Seymour and colleagues[15] found that, after multivariable adjustment, placement of a prehospital catheter with or without prehospital fluid administration was associated with a reduced odds of hospital mortality. It must be noted that decisions to administer fluids or insert a catheter were not driven by any sepsis-specific protocol. Instead, patients in whom an IV line was placed were viewed by the medics as having life-threatening or urgent conditions according to the EMS severity index.[15] These patients also had lower blood pressures, lower Glasgow Coma Scale scores, higher heart rates, and higher respiratory rates compared with those who did not have the intervention. Essentially, the patients who had an IV catheter placed with or without fluid administration were perceived by the prehospital providers to be sicker.[15] The average amount of fluid administered was a mere 500 mL, leading some to think that the hospital mortality benefit was due to early hospital notification and reduced time to intervention in the ED.[10] Indeed, some have questioned whether prehospital warnings have any measurable effect on the overall mortality.[12] Even if the actual impact of early prehospital notification remains unproven, an EMS treatment strategy that prioritizes recognition of sepsis syndromes and aggressive fluid administration when appropriate is consistent with sound medical practice.

AN IDEAL PREHOSPITAL SEPSIS PROTOCOL

Prehospital care in the United States is protocol driven. EMS providers are expected to know the protocols in their jurisdiction and to operate within and venture outside of them only in consultation with real-time medical direction. Within a given jurisdiction, the protocols will differ according to provider level. EMTs have the baseline skill set allowed for prehospital transport. Their scope of practice is limited to obtaining vital signs, applying oxygen, and delivering a limited number of medications.[16] These individuals can recognize abnormalities but are limited in the ways they may intervene. Conversely, paramedics provide the highest level of routine prehospital care. They possess all the skills of an EMT plus are able to establish IV lines and administer IV drugs, provide cardiac care such as cardioversion and transcutaneous pacing, as well as provide definitive airway management (ie, intubation).[16] Various models of prehospital care are used—some operate solely with EMTs, some with solely paramedics, and others with a combination of the 2 levels of training and practice.

The ideal prehospital protocol for sepsis would not only provide accurate recognition but also dictate what action should follow the recognition. It should be simple to apply and take into account skills possessed by both EMTs and paramedics so that it could be applied in a wide range of systems. In light of the recommendations by the Sepsis-3 Committee, a prehospital sepsis protocol could incorporate the elements of qSOFA with the addition of a POC lactate measurement. The qSOFA components are readily calculable and easy to recall, because each component is given one point. The addition of POC lactate measurement would add specificity when used in the correct clinical context, as 2 of 3 points with qSOFA alone could be amassed in many clinical scenarios (eg, drug overdose).

POC lactate measurements correlate well with measurements from whole blood. Gaieski and colleagues[17] compared the accuracy of fingertip POC and whole blood POC lactate measurements with the reference method for lactate analysis. They also examined the time differential from fingertip POC lactate results to that obtained from the laboratory. Both fingertip and whole blood POC lactate measurements showed excellent agreement with the reference method, with intraclass correlation coefficients of 0.90 and 0.92, respectively. In addition, the average time between obtaining POC and reference laboratory results was 65 minutes (95% CI, 30–103). Although the sample size was small, the findings suggest that POC fingertip lactate results are accurate, quickly available, and suitable for use in the prehospital setting.

At present, POC lactate monitors are not widely used in the prehospital environment. Body fluid testing for information that may influence patient care decisions is regulated by the Centers for Medicare and Medicaid Services through the Clinical Laboratory Improvement Amendments (CLIA).[18] Several standards must be met before an agency can be authorized to perform the test. CLIA has established 3 categories of laboratory tests based on criteria that involve the equipment and the knowledge required to interpret the results. The categories are high complexity, moderate complexity, and waived testing. Measurement of POC lactate is considered moderate complexity, so an EMS service must be accredited and certified at that level before it can implement POC lactate testing. Whole blood glucose testing, in comparison, has been granted CLIA-waived status.[18] Several POC lactate measurement devices have been approved for clinical use by the US Food and Drug Administration. However, obtaining and maintaining these devices as well as ensuring that prehospital care providers are trained in their proper use can be costly to the system.

When a septic patient is identified, steps should be taken to ensure transport to definitive care as quickly as possible. A "sepsis alert" should be given to the receiving hospital so that the patient can be triaged in a timely manner and appropriate treatment initiated immediately. Hayden and colleagues[19] sought to determine if a triage sepsis alert and sepsis protocol reduced time to fluids and antibiotics in the ED. They found that by identifying certain sepsis criteria at triage and thus triggering a system that automated "sepsis bundle" treatment, the mean time to a fluid bolus was reduced by 31 minutes and the mean time to antibiotics was reduced by 59 minutes.[19] Such a system triggered from the field could reduce times to fluids and antibiotics even further.

In a 2-tiered system, a sepsis protocol should include parameters that dictate when prehospital care should be escalated to ALS. Placing IV catheters and starting IV fluids is outside the scope of practice for an EMT. Any such intervention must be done by a paramedic. En route to the hospital, it might be reasonable for a paramedic to administer a fluid bolus to a hypotensive patient with sepsis. Additional therapy, such as antibiotics, should be administered only after considering transport times and in consultation with medical control. For example, in a rural EMS system for which transport times are routinely 2 hours or longer, there is likely little downside in starting broad-spectrum antibiotics for a patient who presents in septic shock. The ability to do so depends on the availability of the medication and the skill of the prehospital care providers who are present. The transport team should obtain real-time online medical direction before the administration of antibiotics. In most cases, the prehospital use of antibiotics should not be a standing order within a sepsis protocol.

Finally, an ideal sepsis protocol would give guidance regarding where patients should be transported. In systems in which ambulance diversion is used, prehospital identification of a patient in septic shock could allow an ambulance to bypass the nearest hospital for a more appropriate one if the first does not have critical care capability. Authorization for such measures would be coordinated at a regional or state level in the same way that trauma and cardiac systems of care are organized.

PARTNERS IN CARE

Prehospital personnel are often the first health care providers to reach patients with life-threatening illnesses and injuries, including sepsis. EMS units transport more patients with sepsis than with stroke or acute myocardial infarction.[20] Based on a review of 16 published studies, Lane and colleagues[20] calculated that roughly half of all patients admitted to a hospital with severe sepsis arrive by ambulance service. This volume suggests that EMS providers are uniquely positioned to play a role not only in early notification systems to hospitals when transporting a septic patient but also in illness surveillance within the community. Community paramedicine is a new model of community-based health care delivery that uses EMS personnel and systems to address issues of wellness, prevention, postdischarge care, care for the chronically ill, and medical compliance within a local population.[21] Initially designed to expand access to care in underserved rural areas, these providers perform assessments and interventions on an outpatient basis and usually do not transport patients to hospitals. Community paramedicine can be used to monitor for illness trends among high-risk populations such as nursing home residents. Using EMS skills in this way could allow identification of septic patients even earlier in their disease process and prevent adverse outcomes. Early identification and management of sepsis may allow patients to avoid the hospital all together, which could save up to $50,000 per patient, translating to annual nationwide savings of $17 billion.[22]

CHALLENGES AND THE PATH FORWARD

The clinical syndrome of sepsis is not yet completely understood. This incomplete understanding, coupled with the previously undervalued importance of the disease, has led to gaps in prehospital training modules. After all, formal, state-funded EMS systems were established in the 1970s in response to the large numbers of out-of-hospital deaths caused by trauma.[23] Studies have shown that prehospital personnel have low rates of sepsis identification when judgment alone is used.[3] These findings indicate a need for increased education regarding the presentations of occult sepsis and for the development of protocols that incorporate objective data into the process by which septic patients can be identified. Accurate recognition of sepsis in the prehospital environment can prevent delays in definitive care and presumably improve patient outcomes.

In addition to improving the prehospital recognition of sepsis, additional research is needed in terms of delineating which parameters and biomarkers are most important in sepsis classification. Outcomes research is needed to determine whether there is a mortality benefit to prehospital intervention in sepsis and, if so, which EMS treatment conveys that benefit. Elucidating these parameters will help determine education guidelines and can help to justify the cost of additional equipment and training surrounding the out-of-hospital management of sepsis.

SUMMARY

Similar to acute myocardial infarction and stroke, sepsis is a time-sensitive condition that would benefit from early recognition and management. Many patients with sepsis and septic shock are transported to EDs via EMS. Data indicate that prehospital care providers' recognition of sepsis is low when based solely on clinical judgment. At present, there is no universally accepted scoring system that can be used to identify septic patients in the prehospital setting. In addition, there are no guidelines indicating what treatment should be initiated for a septic patient in the prehospital environment. There is suggestion that a "sepsis alert" triggered by EMS personnel might reduce the time to administration of antibiotics and fluids. Giving EMS care providers the education and tools they need to detect sepsis in the field could lead to even earlier detection of this potentially life-threatening condition and thereby improve patient outcomes. Additional research is needed to determine what role EMS should play in the chain of survival when it comes to this serious clinical syndrome.

ACKNOWLEDGMENTS

The article was copyedited by Linda J. Kesselring, MS, ELS, the technical editor/ writer in the Department of Emergency Medicine at the University of Maryland School of Medicine.

REFERENCES

1. Rivers EP, Coba V, Whitmill M. Early goal-directed therapy in severe sepsis and septic shock: a contemporary review of the literature. Curr Opin Anaesthesiol 2008;21:128–40.
2. Rivers E, Nguyen B, Havstad S, et al. Early goal-directed therapy in the treatment of severe sepsis and septic shock. N Engl J Med 2001;345:1368–77.
3. Seymour CW, Carlbom D, Engelberg RA, et al. Understanding of sepsis among emergency medical services: a survey study. J Emerg Med 2012;42:666–77.
4. Guerra WF, Mayfield TR, Meyers MS, et al. Early detection and treatment of patients with severe sepsis by prehospital personnel. J Emerg Med 2013;44:1116–25.
5. Baez AA, Cochon L. Acute Care Diagnostics Collaboration: assessment of a Bayesian clinical decision model integrating the Prehospital Sepsis Score and point-of-care lactate. Am J Emerg Med 2016;34:193–6.

6. Williams TA, Tohira H, Finn J, et al. The ability of early warning scores (EWS) to detect critical illness in the prehospital setting: a systematic review. Resuscitation 2016;102:35–43.

7. Bayer O, Schwarzkopf D, Stumme C, et al. An early warning scoring system to identify septic patients in the prehospital setting: The PRESEP score. Acad Emerg Med 2015;22:868–71.

8. Robson W, Nutbeam T, Daniels R. Sepsis: a need for prehospital intervention? Emerg Med J 2009;26:535–8.

9. Singer M, Deutschman CS, Seymour CW, et al. The third international consensus definitions for sepsis and septic shock (Sepsis-3). JAMA 2016;315:801–10.

10. Sterling SA, Puskarich MA, Jones AE. Prehospital treatment of sepsis: what really makes the "golden hour" golden? Crit Care 2014;18:697.

11. Wallgren U, Castren M, Svennson AEV, et al. Identification of adult septic patients in the prehospital setting: a comparison of two screening tools and clinical judgement. Eur J Emerg Med 2014;21(4):260–5.

12. Cone DC. The Prehospital Sepsis Screen: a test in search of an application? Acad Emerg Med 2015;22:845–6.

13. Polito CC, Isakov A, Yancey AH, et al. Prehospital recognition of severe sepsis: development and validation of a novel EMS screening tool. Am J Emerg Med 2015;33:1119–25.

14. Studnek JR, Artho MR, Garner CL, et al. The impact of emergency medical services on the ED care of severe sepsis. Am J Emerg Med 2012;30:51–6.

15. Seymour CW, Cooke CR, Heckbert SR, et al. Prehospital intravenous access and fluid resuscitation in severe sepsis: an observational cohort study. Crit Care 2014; 18:533.

16. The National Highway Traffic Safety Administration. National EMS Scope of Practice Model, 2007. Available at: www.nhtsa.gov/people/injury/ems/EMSScope.pdf. Accessed May 25, 2016.

17. Gaieski DF, Drumheller BC, Goyal M, et al. Accuracy of handheld point-of-care fingertip lactate measurement in the emergency department. West J Emerg Med 2012;14:58–62.

18. Collopy KT, Kivlehan SM, Snyder S. What's the point of point-of-care testing? EMS World 2014;43:34–42.

19. Hayden GE, Tuuri RE, Scott R, et al. Triage sepsis alert and sepsis protocol lower times to fluids and antibiotics in the ED. Am J Emerg Med 2016;34:1–9.

20. Lane D, Ichelson RI, Drennan IR, et al. Prehospital management and identification of sepsis by emergency medical services: a systematic review. Emerg Med J 2016;33:408–13.

21. Choi BY, Blumberg C, Williams K. Mobile integrated health care and community paramedicine: an emerging emergency medical services concept. Ann Emerg Med 2015;67(3):1–6.

22. Tsertsvadze A, Royle P, McCarthy N. Community-onset sepsis and its public health burden: protocol of a systematic review. Syst Rev 2015;4:119.

23. NHTSA. Emergency medical services education agenda for the future: a systems approach, 2000. Available at: www.nhtsa.gov/people/injury/ems/EdAgenda/final/index.html. Accessed May 25, 2016.

Pitfalls in the Treatment of Sepsis

Lars-Kristofer N. Peterson, MD[a,b],*, Karin Chase, MD[c,d]

KEYWORDS

- Sepsis • SIRS • qSOFA • Medical errors • Emergency medicine • Critical care

KEY POINTS

- There have been recent changes in the diagnostic criteria for sepsis due to criticism of prior definitions.
- The diagnosis of sepsis is challenging in special patient populations (eg, the elderly, children, patients taking medications that alter typical physiologic responses).
- There is significant controversy in "bundled" care for septic patients because it is unclear which aspects are most helpful and which aspects may pose the potential for harm.
- The disposition of a septic patient out of the emergency department may be one of the most consequential decisions the treating clinician can make. It should be approached considering not only the patient's condition in the emergency department but also their likely trajectory following admission.
- Strong consideration for transfer to a higher level of care should be made if it is not clear the resources required for the severity of illness can be met at their present institution.

INTRODUCTION

Emergency departments (ED) and emergency providers (EPs) have a vital role to play in the treatment and management of septic patients. Indeed, presentation and admission via the ED have been associated with more favorable outcomes.[1,2] However, sepsis care in the ED has also been shown to have quality concerns, which include incorrect antimicrobial choice, delay to diagnosis, and failure to implement evidence-based treatments.[3–5] In this article, the authors describe potential pitfalls in ED sepsis diagnosis and treatment and how to avoid or mitigate them. It should be noted that to avoid redundant content, this is not exhaustive.

The authors of this article have nothing to disclose.
[a] Department of Medicine, Cooper Medical School of Rowan University, Camden, NJ, USA;
[b] Department of Emergency Medicine, Cooper Medical School of Rowan University, Camden, NJ, USA; [c] Pulmonary and Critical Care Medicine Division, Department of Medicine, University of Rochester Medical Center, 601 Elmwood Avenue, Rochester, NY 14642, USA; [d] Department of Emergency Medicine, University of Rochester Medical Center, 601 Elmwood Avenue, Rochester, NY 14642, USA
* Corresponding author. Cooper University Hospital, One Cooper Plaza, Camden, NJ 08103.
E-mail address: peterson-lars@cooperhealth.edu

DIFFICULTY IN DIAGNOSIS
Systemic Inflammatory Response Syndrome

The original definition of sepsis relied on the presence of 2 or more criteria outlined in the systemic inflammatory response syndrome (SIRS). In fact, the SIRS criteria acted as the building blocks for identifying and diagnosing sepsis, severe sepsis, and septic shock. SIRS incorporated changes in heart rate, body temperature, respiratory rate, and white blood cell count. If there was a known or suspected infection in a patient with 2 or more SIRS criteria, the patient was diagnosed with sepsis (**Box 1**).

It is known that systemic inflammation can occur in several different noninfectious conditions, decreasing the specificity of SIRS. **Fig. 1** illustrates the presences of SIRS in some of the more common noninfectious conditions, including trauma and pancreatitis.

A diagnostic error may occur when the clinician prematurely excludes the diagnosis of sepsis in a patient where one of these other noninfectious systemic inflammatory states is present. This premature closure may result in delayed identification and treatment of a concurrent infection. The converse is also true; not all patients with systemic inflammation are infected and, in these patients, antibiotics are not indicated. In the ED, the undifferentiated nature of the patient and lack of initial clinical data compound these issues.

In addition, a recent study showed that SIRS criteria also lacked sensitivity for defining sepsis. Diseases like sepsis that are associated with significant morbidity and mortality demand a highly sensitive screening tool for diagnosis. Kaukonen and colleagues[6] showed that 1 in 8 patients in the intensive care unit (ICU) with infection and organ dysfunction did not have 2 or more SIRS criteria. These SIRS-negative patients had a lower, but substantial, mortality associated with severe sepsis. Because of the shortcomings of the SIRS criteria as well as a better understanding of the pathophysiology of sepsis, the Sepsis 3.0 definition was developed.

Quick Sequential Organ Failure Assessment

It remains to be seen if the new sepsis definition will result in a more accurate and rapid diagnosis of sepsis. The authors of the new definition propose stepping away from using the SIRS criteria because they were considered to be unhelpful and confused both the adaptive and the maladaptive physiologic response to infection. They introduced the Quick Sequential Organ Failure Assessment (qSOFA) score

---

Box 1
Systemic inflammatory response syndrome

Two or more of the following:

- Temperature greater than 38°C or less than 36°C
- Heart rate greater than 90 beats per minute
- Respiratory rate greater than 20 breaths per minute or $Paco_2$ less than 32 mm Hg
- White blood cell count greater than 12,000/mm^3 or less than 4000/mm^3 or greater than 10% immature bands

Data from Bone RC, Balk RA, Cerra FB, et al. Definitions for sepsis and organ failure and guidelines for the use of innovative therapies in sepsis. The ACCP/SCCM Consensus Conference Committee. American College of Chest Physicians/Society of Critical Care Medicine. Chest 1992;101:1644–55.

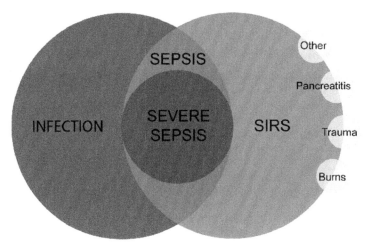

Fig. 1. Spectrum of infection, SIRS, sepsis, and severe sepsis. (*Data from* Bone RC, Balk RA, Cerra FB, et al. Definitions for sepsis and organ failure and guidelines for the use of innovative therapies in sepsis. The ACCP/SCCM Consensus Conference Committee. American College of Chest Physicians/Society of Critical Care Medicine. Chest 1992;101:1644–55.)

to be used as a clinical score in patients outside the ICU with suspected infection that are more likely to have poor outcomes typical of sepsis.[7,8] The qSOFA score consists of 3 variables: respiratory rate, altered mentation, and systolic blood pressure (**Box 2**).

Concerns have been raised about the qSOFA score and its ability to provide useful guidance in patients with infection and suspected sepsis.[9] It should also be noted that the qSOFA score was designed to predict worse outcomes in sepsis and not as a screening tool to be deployed in the ED.

Lack of a Gold-Standard Test

Another reason the diagnosis of sepsis can be difficult to make and may be missed is the lack of a reliable gold-standard test. The gold standard for identifying an infection is positive microbiological data, which is almost never available in the ED. EPs encountering a patient for the first time need to rely on other elements of the clinical picture in conjunction with the sepsis diagnostic criteria. There has been a great deal of investigative work into the role of various biomarkers aiding in the diagnosis of patients presenting with SIRS.[10–12] Despite many

---

Box 2
Quick sequential organ failure assessment

- Respiratory rate greater than or equal to 22 breaths per minute

- Altered mentation

- Systolic blood pressure less than 100 mm Hg

From Singer M, Deutschman CS, Seymour CW, et al. The third international consensus definitions for sepsis and septic shock (sepsis-3). JAMA 2016;315(8):805.

publications, the role of a single biomarker has yet to be incorporated into daily clinical practice.

Special Populations and Effects of Medication

There are particular populations of patients that manifest subtle signs and symptoms of infection. This subtlety can lead to making the diagnosis of infection, and therefore sepsis, challenging. The elderly, the severely malnourished, and the immunosuppressed have abnormal responses to infection. It has been reported that fever will be absent in 20% to 30% of elderly patients with a known infection. They are more likely to present with nonspecific symptoms, such as altered mental status, fatigue, and anorexia.[13–15]

The clinician often faces similar challenges with the immunosuppressed patient. Once again, typical responses to infection may be absent and mislead those caring for the patient. In addition, patients who are taking medications that blunt typical physiologic responses or alter clinical data due to their effect may have a delay to diagnosis. For example, β-blockade can limit tachycardia, whereas leukocytosis in a patient using steroids can be falsely attributed to the medication rather than an underlying infection.

Sepsis Is a Dynamic Process

Patients with an infection may decompensate while undergoing evaluation in the ED. For this reason, constant reassessment is necessary. The young college student with cough who had normal triage vital signs and initial suspicion of a simple upper respiratory infection may develop tachycardia, fever, and tachypnea, raising concern for pneumonia. The patient is now manifesting signs of sepsis and will likely need more care than initially thought. Sepsis is a dynamic process, and for this reason, patients require frequent reassessment by both nurses and EPs. Failure to do so may result in missing the diagnosis of sepsis.

Assuming a Bacterial Cause

Not all sepsis is caused by a bacterial infection. Failing to consider other causes of infection, such as fungal or viral causes, can result in a delay to diagnosis and ultimately a delay in appropriate treatment.[16]

Fig. 2, from Martin and colleagues,[16] demonstrates that the incidence of sepsis is increasing, but also highlights an increase in the frequency of fungal causes of sepsis. The most common fungal infections in humans are species of Candida and Aspergillus.[17] However, depending on the patient's risk factors, other fungal infections may be present such as Cryptococcus, Pneumocystis jirovecii, or regionally prevalent organisms. The EP must review the history of the septic patient (eg, immunosuppression, travel, previous infectious causes), carefully consider if there is risk for either fungal or viral sepsis, and initiate the appropriate empiric treatment. Consultation with an infectious disease specialist may also be prudent in unclear or high risk cases (**Box 3, Table 1**).

End Organ Failure as the Initial Presentation of Sepsis

End organ failure may be the only presenting sign of sepsis.[22] Although EPs are accustomed to searching for end organ failure if sepsis is already suspected, what happens if incidental end organ failure is noted in the absence of suspected sepsis? These patients could easily be overlooked in terms of a concurrent infection if the apparent new abnormality is viewed in isolation. In the ED, this presentation of sepsis is especially challenging because data supporting whether the changes are acute or chronic

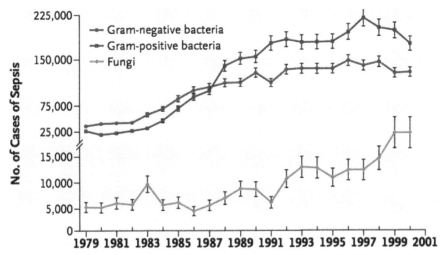

Fig. 2. Number of sepsis cases by cause. (*Data from* Martin GS, Mannino DM, Eaton S, et al. The epidemiology of sepsis in the United States from 1979 through 2000. N Engl J Med 2003;348(16):1546–54.)

processes may not be accessible. In their publication defining the new definition of sepsis and septic shock, Singer and colleagues[7] caution that even in the setting of a negative qSOFA screen, if there is suspicion for sepsis, further examination of end organ function should be performed. The EP should also view this in the opposite direction as well: if unexplained end organ failure is discovered, then underlying sepsis should be considered.

Sepsis can be a difficult diagnosis to make. Both failure to make the diagnosis and overdiagnosing sepsis can have significant consequences. When the diagnosis is missed, there is a delay in early interventions, including intravenous fluids (IVF) and antibiotics, which can lead to worse outcomes.[23] Conversely, overdiagnosing sepsis can result in inappropriate antibiotic administration or IVF, resulting in complications such as the development of resistant organisms, *Clostridium difficile* colitis, or iatrogenic volume overload.[24]

Box 3
Risk factors for invasive fungal infection

- Immunosuppression (see **Table 1**)
- Exposure in endemic regions (Ohio and Mississippi River valleys, the desert Southwest)
- Use of invasive indwelling vascular catheters (peripherally inserted central catheter, hemodialysis catheter, tunneled central lines)
- Use of long-term urinary catheters or presence of nephrostomy/urostomy
- Use of total parenteral nutrition
- Widespread burns
- Intestinal injury or conditions that weaken intestinal mucosal barriers

Data from Refs.[18–21]

Table 1 Examples of immunosuppression	
Pathogenesis	**Condition**
Physiologic	• Extremes of age • Pregnancy
Acquired	• HIV/AIDS • Diabetes • Malnutrition • Malignancy/chemotherapy • Radiation treatment • Medications (steroids)
Congenital	Inherited immunodeficiencies
Other	• Cystic fibrosis • Systemic inflammation

Adapted from Leach R. The immune compromised patient. In: Leach R, Editor. Critical care at a glance. Hoboken: Wiley-Blackwell; 2014. p. 133–4.

PITFALLS IN THE TREATMENT OF SEPSIS
Failure to Communicate to the Treatment Team

The management of sepsis is a team sport. The clinician may order fluids, antibiotics, and diagnostic studies, but unless the whole treatment team is aware of the concerns about the patient and their risk for decline, other patients or tasks may take priority. ED crowding, a proxy measure for how busy the clinical environment is, has been implicated as a factor causing delays to antibiotic treatment.[25] Similarly, ED crowding has been associated with decreased sepsis resuscitation protocol compliance and contamination of bacterial blood cultures.[26,27] Ensuring that each member of the treatment team has a shared mental model of how to manage the seriously ill patient is the responsibility of the treating EP as well as the department.

Invasive Mechanical Ventilation

Introducing the element of invasive mechanical ventilation adds complication to the treatment of sepsis and septic shock. Which patients that are septic or in septic shock require invasive mechanical ventilation? If mechanical ventilation is required, when is the ideal time to do it?

Type IV respiratory failure is found in patients who are in shock. These patients are placed on invasive mechanical ventilation during the resuscitation process with the goal of reducing the effort exerted by respiratory muscles, thereby lowering their oxygen consumption. Animal studies have shown that roughly 20% of cardiac output can be expended on the respiratory muscles.[28] Invasive mechanical ventilation may benefit patients in septic shock by reducing respiratory muscle work and lowering total oxygen consumption, therefore increasing oxygen delivery to other vital organs, such as the heart, brain, and kidneys.[29] The patient with septic shock may also have other types of respiratory failure, which can be supported by mechanical ventilation. These benefits need to be weighed against the potential adverse events that may occur during the process of intubation or while the patient remains intubated. **Fig. 3** illustrates the risks and benefits of mechanical ventilation in septic shock.

If the decision is made to proceed with invasive mechanical ventilation, when is the ideal time to perform it? Unfortunately, the literature is lacking when it comes to this question. If the patient is in respiratory distress or has a depressed neurologic status and cannot protect their airway, early airway intervention is warranted. However, if

| **Risks** | **Benefits** |

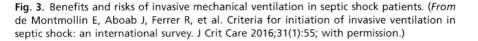

- Hemodynamic deterioration
- Ventilator-induced lung injury
- Ventilator-acquired pneumonia
- Ventilator-induced diaphragmatic dysfunction

- Adequate oxygenation
- Reduced work of breathing and redistribution of cardiac output
- Prevention of inflammatory diaphragmatic dysfunction

Fig. 3. Benefits and risks of invasive mechanical ventilation in septic shock patients. (*From* de Montmollin E, Aboab J, Ferrer R, et al. Criteria for initiation of invasive ventilation in septic shock: an international survey. J Crit Care 2016;31(1):55; with permission.)

other pressing concerns are not present, then intubation may be safely delayed. The answer to this dilemma is best made at the bedside by the treating clinician.

Intubation of the patient in shock of any kind carries significant risk of adverse events. The traditional process of rapid sequence induction applied to the septic patient can cause severe hypotension, prolonged cardiac depression, and even death. Hypotension following intubation has been associated with significantly higher in-hospital mortality as well as longer length of stay in the ICU and hospital.[30] Avoiding complications when controlling the airway of the patient in shock requires advanced planning, aggressive resuscitation, and optimization before beginning intubation. In addition, there needs to be anticipation of rapid physiologic changes and the ability to act quickly when they occur. The authors refer the reader to excellent online resources for further information on avoiding adverse events related to intubation and mechanical ventilation in the patient with shock physiology.[31,32]

Bundled Care

Care bundles and protocols can provide a good framework or even checklist when treating a patient with sepsis. The early-goal directed therapy (EGDT) trial by Rivers and colleagues[33] produced the first prospectively trialed protocol for sepsis care. Since that publication, the Surviving Sepsis Campaign has published guidelines including sepsis care bundles.[34] The most recent Surviving Sepsis Campaign bundle was published in 2013 and is shown in **Box 4**.

The issue with protocols and care bundles arises from the heterogeneity of sepsis. Following protocols without attention to the clinical context can lead to unnecessary, time-consuming, and potentially harmful interventions. Specifically, focusing on bundled care for sepsis, the necessity of placing a central venous catheter (CVC), and following central venous pressure (CVP) and central venous oxygen saturation ($ScvO_2$) has been questioned. Similarly, the practice of providing IVF to a patient who is not intravascularly depleted is controversial, and some assert is harmful. Three recently published trials: ProCESS, ProMISe, and ARISE, showed that "usual care" in sepsis is as good as protocolized care.[35–37] The 3 trials examined differences in mortality in patients treated with the EGDT sepsis protocol versus a "usual care" arm (ie, provider discretion for all interventions) and found no difference in the primary outcome. The patients in the "usual" care arm received fewer CVCs; CVP was rarely monitored, and $ScvO_2$ was not followed as often. However, the physicians in the

---

Box 4
Surviving sepsis campaign bundles

To be completed within 3 hours:

- Measure lactate level

- Obtain blood cultures before administration of antibiotics

- Administer broad spectrum antibiotics

- Administer 30 mL/kg crystalloid for hypotension or lactate greater than or equal to 4 mmol/L

To be completed within 6 hours:

- Apply vasopressors (for hypotension that does not respond to initial fluid resuscitation to maintain a mean arterial pressure) greater than or equal to 65 mm Hg

- In the event of persistent arterial hypotension despite volume resuscitation (septic shock) or initial lactate greater than 4 mmol/L:
  - Measure CVP[a]
  - Measure ScvO$_2$[a]

- Remeasure lactate if initial lactate was elevated[a]

[a] Targets for quantitative resuscitation included in the guidelines area CVP of greater than or equal to 8 mm Hg, ScvO$_2$ of greater than or equal to 70%, and normalization of lactate.
From Dellinger RP, Levy MM, Rhodes A, et al. Surviving sepsis campaign: international guidelines for management of severe sepsis and septic shock: 2012. Crit Care Med 2013;41:580–637.

"usual care" arm were trained in the era of EGDT and bundled care—raising the question of how much these practices influenced the treatment in the "usual care" arm. The take-home point from these studies is that early recognition, aggressive IVF resuscitation, and early broad-spectrum antibiotics are the cornerstones in managing patients with severe sepsis and septic shock. Protocolized care may be beneficial in certain clinical settings (see Brian Meier and Catherine Staton's article, "Sepsis Resuscitation in Resource Limited Settings," in this issue) but certainly does not seem mandatory for ideal patient outcomes in sepsis.

PITFALLS IN THE DISPOSITION OF THE SEPTIC PATIENT
Failure to Ensure Follow-up, Failure to Admit to the Correct Level of Care

"Disposition is destiny" is a maxim in emergency medicine revealing the importance of determining where the patient is to go at the end of their ED encounter. Answering the question, "can this patient be safely discharged?" is sometimes vexing. In addition, if the patient is admitted, what level of care should the patient be assigned?

There is a small subset of patients who are at high risk for severe infection, but after their ED assessment may not clearly require admission. Patients with concern for neutropenic fever but ultimately have a benign workup may fall into this category. In these patients, the choice of disposition will depend on several factors, including the patient's home environment, available caregivers, the long-term health risk related to the feared condition, and availability of follow-up. In the patient who is to be discharged with the potential of a significant infection, follow-up is mandatory. It is incumbent on the EP to ensure this follow-up is adequate and, perhaps most importantly, available. In the busy primary care practice, the "routine ED follow-up" may be triaged as relatively nonacute. One way to bridge this potential gap in care is to reach out to the outpatient treatment team responsible for follow-up. For some patients, their primary care physician may be the best resource, and simply getting in touch with the on-call physician for the practice is the only step required. For more complicated patients, such as the patient receiving chemotherapy, seeing their oncologist in the next 24 hours may be the best course. Furthermore, it may be prudent to order additional outpatient testing ahead of the follow-up encounter. If follow-up care cannot be definitively established, the best course of action for the EP and the patient may be observation or possibly full admission.

Once the decision to admit the patient has been made, it is incumbent on the EP to admit that patient to the appropriate level of care. Patients inappropriately admitted to a general medical floor who require transfer to an ICU within 24 to 48 hours after admission have worse clinical outcomes than patients who are admitted to an ICU at the start of their in-patient stay.[1,38,39] In the surgical quality literature, unplanned admissions to intensive care are considered a meaningful part of quality metrics due to the interplay between antecedent patient safety/quality issues, ICU admission, and worse outcome.[40] It is hypothesized that the causes of the observed worse outcomes include the following: (1) a delay to recognition of the patient's changing status; (2) decreased availability of equipment and personnel adapted to resuscitation; (3) decreased team experience with resuscitation on the floor; (4) possibly more severe disease trajectories with a falsely reassuring indolent initial course.[41–47]

Although patient condition, objective data, clinical experience, and hospital system factors may clearly dictate which patients should be admitted to the floor versus an ICU, there are some patients who do not neatly fit into a specific level of care. Given the poorer outcomes in patients who are admitted to the floor but then transferred to the ICU, it is important to be wary of these patients. In these cases, using a combination of patient demographic factors, laboratory data, and comorbid conditions may serve as "triggers" for closer scrutiny. Some of these factors may be intuitive, but even if they are transient and resolved in the ED, it may point to signs of a rockier clinical course after the time of admission (**Box 5**).

Once the patient is identified as being at increased risk for unplanned ICU transfer following admission, the EP should work with the admitting team (and intensivist if one is available) to identify the best level of care. If the patient's risk is thought to be low enough that a floor admission is safe, then a plan regarding frequent rounding, closer nursing assessment, and other interventions to mitigate the risk of an unanticipated decline should be implemented.

Box 5
Predisposing factors for delayed intensive care unit admission

Depressed bicarbonate

Altered mental status

Significant comorbidities (congestive heart failure, chronic obstructive pulmonary disease, vascular disease, kidney disease)

Tachycardia

Respiratory infection as primary sepsis cause

Age >65

Respiratory dysfunction

Transient hypotension

Anemia, thrombocytopenia, elevated bands

Data from Refs.[42,44,48–50]

Box 6
Triggers to consider transfer of the septic patient

- Inability to manage the severity of illness on presentation
- Lack of experience or expertise in managing septic shock and other aspects of the patient's treatment (ARDS)
- Requirement of procedure or intervention unavailable at the presenting institution
- The patient has pertinent significant history or other complicating factors primarily managed at a higher level of care

---

Failure to Transfer

For some institutions, particularly those in a rural or small community setting, the decision to admit the septic patient may have another level of complexity: the need for transfer to an institution capable of handling the patient's needs (**Box 6**). The surgical literature is replete with studies demonstrating that facilities performing specific procedures more frequently tend to have better outcomes related to that procedure. Robust data paralleling this trend in septic patients are lacking. However, limited studies have shown that hospitals with higher case volumes of both severe sepsis and mechanically ventilated patients tend to have lower mortalities related to these conditions.[51,52] Institutions with smaller volumes of admissions via the ED have a higher unplanned ICU admission rate (with known increased risk of worse outcomes).[50] Although the cause for this trend is unknown and likely multifactorial, it may speak to the relative infrequency of caring for patients who acutely decline or patients with significant comorbidities. As outlined in the preceding articles, the care of the septic patient has a range of intensity: some patients only require appropriate antibiotic agents and IVF, whereas others require specialized intervention through surgical or interventional radiology consultation. It is vital that the EP not only make the appropriate diagnosis but also understand the likely course of the illness and the ability of the local institution to manage it.

One of the primary indications for transfer is the severity of illness at presentation. For example, in a patient with septic shock who is found to be in acute renal failure in the ED, it would be prudent to consider transfer to an institution with the capability of initiating dialysis. Similarly, patients who present with sepsis complicated by acute respiratory distress syndrome (ARDS) will require ventilator management with an experienced respiratory therapist who can guard against ventilator-associated lung injury. In severe ARDS, patients have been shown to benefit from both prone positioning and chemical paralysis.[53,54] The EP may not necessarily be the one to initiate these therapies, but they should ensure the receiving admitting team is comfortable with managing such interventions. Along the same lines, if a septic patient requires a procedure for source control that is unavailable at the local institution, transferring that patient should be considered a core part of the treatment plan.

Outside of the severity or cause of the presenting illness, septic patients may have connection to a medical home secondary to an element of their past medical or surgical history prompting transfer. Patients who are actively receiving chemotherapy, have hematologic malignancies, or have been recipients of bone marrow transplants may benefit from consultation or transfer to the site where they receive their oncologic treatment. Similarly, patients with recent operations or a significant surgical history and are septic from a source related to that history may have a better outcome if treated at the center familiar with their case and relevant anatomy. Another important population to consider transferring to their "home" institution is the patient status post solid organ transplantation because they will also have significant anatomic and immunologic changes that require appropriate management with teams familiar with such complexities.

If the institution does not have the needed personnel, equipment, or experience in caring for the severely ill septic patient, strong consideration for interhospital transfer to a facility that can meet the patient's needs should be made while active treatment is initiated in the ED. Delay to appropriate ICU treatment is detrimental to the patient as well as the health care system in terms of mortality and length of stay.[55] Admitting the patient to a local ICU that cannot meet their needs is analogous to admitting the patient to the incorrect level of care.

Failure to Mitigate Transfer Risks

It is vital for the referring EP to continue treating the septic patient until the transfer is completed. Appropriate sepsis resuscitation should not be delayed while a transfer is arranged. It has been shown that patients who have undergone interhospital transfer from some referring EDs for sepsis have delays to appropriate antibiotic administration. It is hypothesized that in the zero sum environment of the ED, the logistical burden of transferring the patient interferes with appropriate resuscitation.[56] Clinicians should be mindful of this and actively direct their resuscitative efforts to overcome this challenge.

The EP should also make an attempt to predict the patient's course while waiting for transfer resources to arrive and ensure the patient has been appropriately stabilized before leaving the originating facility. Stabilization may include securing the patient's airway when needed, providing adequate access to administer needed antibiotics and vasoactive medications if required, and creating plans for the transfer team to manage changes in the patient's condition. The sending EP should ensure the transferring emergency medical services crew has appropriate medical direction.

SUMMARY

Sepsis is the most challenging disease process faced in the ED environment for myriad reasons. This article has outlined some of the key pitfalls EPs may encounter when caring for patients with suspected sepsis in the ED. Pitfalls begin with the failure to consider sepsis and the numerous ways it can present and carry on through the consideration of various underlying causes, the complex and intensive management, and finally, the consideration of disposition whether that ends up being the original institution or at a facility for appropriate transfer.

ACKNOWLEDGMENTS

Dr. Peterson would like to thank the Division of Pulmonary and Critical Care Medicine and the Department of Emergency Medicine of the University of Rochester Medical School of Medicine & Dentistry for supporting his authorship of this article.

REFERENCES

1. Escarce JJ, Kelley MA. Admission source to the medical intensive care unit predicts hospital death independent of APACHE II score. JAMA 1990;264(18): 2389–94.
2. Powell ES, Khare RK, Courtney DM, et al. Lower mortality in sepsis patients admitted through the ED vs direct admission. Am J Emerg Med 2012;30(3): 432–9.

3. Carlbom DJ, Rubenfeld GD. Barriers to implementing protocol-based sepsis resuscitation in the emergency department—Results of a national survey. Crit Care Med 2007;35(11):2525–32.

4. De Miguel-Yanes JM, Andueza-Lillo JA, González-Ramallo VJ, et al. Failure to implement evidence-based clinical guidelines for sepsis at the ED. Am J Emerg Med 2006;24(5):553–9.

5. Chen HC, Lin WL, Lin CC, et al. Outcome of inadequate empirical antibiotic therapy in emergency department patients with community-onset bloodstream infections. J Antimicrob Chemother 2013;68(4):947–53.

6. Kaukonen KM, Bailey M, Pilcher D, et al. Systemic inflammatory response syndrome criteria in defining severe sepsis. N Engl J Med 2015;372(17):1629–38.

7. Singer M, Deutschman CS, Seymour CW, et al. The third international consensus definitions for sepsis and septic shock (sepsis-3). JAMA 2016;315(8):801–10.

8. Seymour CW, Liu VX, Iwashyna TJ, et al. Assessment of clinical criteria for sepsis. JAMA 2016;315(8):762–813.

9. Simpson SQ. New sepsis criteria: a change we should not make. Chest 2016; 149(5):1117–8.

10. de Montmollin E, Annane D. Year in review 2013: critical care—sepsis. Crit Care 2014;18(5):165–8.

11. Biron BM, Ayala A, Lomas-Neira JL. Biomarkers for sepsis: what is and what might be? Biomark Insights 2015;10(Suppl 4):7–17.

12. Cho SY, Choi JH. Biomarkers of sepsis. Infect Chemother 2014;46(1):1–12.

13. Nasa P, Juneja D, Singh O. Severe sepsis and septic shock in the elderly: an overview. World J Crit Care Med 2012;1(1):23–30.

14. Gavazzi G, Krause KH. Ageing and infection. Lancet Infect Dis 2002;2(11): 659–66.

15. Norman DC, Yoshikawa TT. Fever in the elderly. Infect Dis Clin North Am 1996; 10(1):93–9.

16. Martin GS, Mannino DM, Eaton S, et al. The epidemiology of sepsis in the United States from 1979 through 2000. N Engl J Med 2003;348(16):1546–54.

17. Ellis D, Marriott D, Hajjeh RA, et al. Epidemiology: surveillance of fungal infections. Med Mycol 2000;38(Suppl 1):173–82.

18. Richardson MD. Changing patterns and trends in systemic fungal infections. J Antimicrob Chemother 2005;56(Suppl 1):i5–11.

19. Leach R. Common fungal and protozoal infections. Chapter 67. In: Leach RM, editor. Critical care at a glance. Hoboken: Wiley-Blackwell; 2014. p. 130–2.

20. Blumberg HM, Jarvis WR, Soucie JM, et al. Risk factors for candidal bloodstream infections in surgical intensive care unit patients: the NEMIS prospective multicenter study. The National Epidemiology of Mycosis Survey. Clin Infect Dis 2001;33(2):177–86.

21. Leach R. The immune compromised patient. In: Leach R, editor. Critical care at a glance. Hoboken: Wiley-Blackwell; 2014. p. 133–4.

22. Shankar-Hari M, Deutschman CS, Singer M. Do we need a new definition of sepsis? Intensive Care Med 2015;41(5):909–11.

23. Kumar A, Roberts D, Wood KE, et al. Duration of hypotension before initiation of effective antimicrobial therapy is the critical determinant of survival in human septic shock. Crit Care Med 2006;34(6):1589–96.

24. Nathan C, Cars O. Antibiotic resistance–problems, progress, and prospects. N Engl J Med 2014;371(19):1761–3.

25. Kennebeck SS, Timm NL, Kurowski EM, et al. The association of emergency department crowding and time to antibiotics in febrile neonates. Acad Emerg Med 2011;18(12):1380–5.

26. Lee CC, Lee NY, Chuang MC, et al. The impact of overcrowding on the bacterial contamination of blood cultures in the ED. Am J Emerg Med 2012;30(6):839–45.

27. Shin TG, Jo IJ, Choi DJ, et al. The adverse effect of emergency department crowding on compliance with the resuscitation bundle in the management of severe sepsis and septic shock. Crit Care 2013;17(5):R224.

28. Viires N, Sillye G, Aubier M, et al. Regional blood flow distribution in dog during induced hypotension and low cardiac output. Spontaneous breathing versus artificial ventilation. J Clin Invest 1983;72(3):935–47.

29. Manthous CA, Hall JB, Kushner R, et al. The effect of mechanical ventilation on oxygen consumption in critically ill patients. Am J Respir Crit Care Med 1995; 151(1):210–4.

30. Heffner AC, Swords D, Kline JA, et al. The frequency and significance of postintubation hypotension during emergency airway management. J Crit Care 2012; 27(4):417.e9-13.

31. Weingart SD. Laryngoscope as a Murder Weapon (LAMW) Series—Hemodynamic Kills. EMCrit. 2013. Available at: http://emcrit.org/podcasts/intubation-patient-shock/. Accessed May 27, 2016.

32. Nickson C. Rapid sequence intubation of the shock patient. Life in the Fast Lane. Available at: http://lifeinthefastlane.com/ccc/rapid-sequence-induction-of-the-shock-patient/.

33. Rivers E, Nguyen B, Havstad S, et al. Early goal-directed therapy in the treatment of severe sepsis and septic shock. N Engl J Med 2001;345(19):1368–77.

34. Dellinger RP, Levy MM, Rhodes A, et al. Surviving sepsis campaign: international guidelines for management of severe sepsis and septic shock: 2012. Crit Care Med 2013;41:580–637.

35. ProCESS Investigators, Yealy DM, Kellum JA, et al. A randomized trial of protocol-based care for early septic shock. N Engl J Med 2014;370(18):1683–93.

36. Mouncey PR, Osborn TM, Power GS, et al. Trial of early, goal-directed resuscitation for septic shock. N Engl J Med 2015;372(14):1301–11.

37. The ARISE Investigators, ANZICS Clinical Trials Group, Peake SL, et al. Goal-directed resuscitation for patients with early septic shock. N Engl J Med 2014; 371(16):1496–506.

38. Parkhe M, Myles PS, Leach DS, et al. Outcome of emergency department patients with delayed admission to an intensive care unit. Emerg Med (Fremantle) 2002;14(1):50–7.

39. Renaud B, Santin A, Coma E, et al. Association between timing of intensive care unit admission and outcomes for emergency department patients with community-acquired pneumonia. Crit Care Med 2009;37(11):2867–74.

40. Haller G, Myles PS, Wolfe R, et al. Validity of unplanned admission to an intensive care unit as a measure of patient safety in surgical patients. Anesthesiology 2005; 103(6):1121–9.

41. Frost SA, Alexandrou E, Bogdanovski T, et al. Unplanned admission to intensive care after emergency hospitalisation: risk factors and development of a nomogram for individualising risk. Resuscitation 2009;80(2):224–30.

42. Kennedy M, Joyce N, Howell MD, et al. Identifying infected emergency department patients admitted to the hospital ward at risk of clinical deterioration and intensive care unit transfer. Acad Emerg Med 2010;17(10):1080–5.

43. Whittaker SA, Fuchs BD, Gaieski DF, et al. Epidemiology and outcomes in patients with severe sepsis admitted to the hospital wards. J Crit Care 2015; 30(1):78–84.

44. Jessen MK, Mackenhauer J, Hvass AMSW, et al. Predictors of intensive care unit transfer or death in emergency department patients with suspected infection. Eur J Emerg Med 2015;22(3):176–80.

45. Shapiro NI, Wolfe RE, Moore RB, et al. Mortality in Emergency Department Sepsis (MEDS) score: a prospectively derived and validated clinical prediction rule. Crit Care Med 2003;31(3):670–5.

46. Caterino JM, Jalbuena T, Bogucki B. Predictors of acute decompensation after admission in ED patients with sepsis. Am J Emerg Med 2010;28(5):631–6.

47. Glickman SW, Cairns CB, Otero RM, et al. Disease progression in hemodynamically stable patients presenting to the emergency department with sepsis. Acad Emerg Med 2010;17(4):383–90.

48. Tang Y, Choi J, Kim D, et al. Clinical predictors of adverse outcome in severe sepsis patients with lactate 2-4 mM admitted to the hospital. QJM 2015;108(4): 279–87.

49. Tsai JCH, Cheng CW, Weng SJ, et al. Comparison of risks factors for unplanned ICU transfer after ED admission in patients with infections and those without infections. ScientificWorldJournal 2014;2014(5):1–10.

50. Delgado MK, Liu V, Pines JM, et al. Risk factors for unplanned transfer to intensive care within 24 hours of admission from the emergency department in an integrated healthcare system. J Hosp Med 2012;8(1):13–9.

51. Kahn JM, Goss CH, Heagerty PJ, et al. Hospital volume and the outcomes of mechanical ventilation. N Engl J Med 2006;355(1):41–50.

52. Peelen L, de Keizer NF, Peek N, et al. The influence of volume and intensive care unit organization on hospital mortality in patients admitted with severe sepsis: a retrospective multicentre cohort study. Crit Care 2007;11(2):R40.

53. Guérin C, Reignier J, Richard JC, et al. Prone positioning in severe acute respiratory distress syndrome. N Engl J Med 2013;368(23):2159–68.

54. Papazian L, Forel JM, Gacouin A, et al, ACURASYS Study Investigators. Neuromuscular blockers in early acute respiratory distress syndrome—supplementary index. N Engl J Med 2010;393(12):1107–16.

55. Chalfin DB, Trzeciak S, Likourezos A, et al. Impact of delayed transfer of critically ill patients from the emergency department to the intensive care unit. Crit Care Med 2007;35(6):1477–83.

56. Faine BA, Noack JM, Wong T, et al. Interhospital transfer delays appropriate treatment for patients with severe sepsis and septic shock. Crit Care Med 2015; 43(12):2589–96.

Antimicrobial Stewardship in the Management of Sepsis

Michael S. Pulia, MD, MS[a],*, Robert Redwood, MD, MPH[b],
Brian Sharp, MD[c]

KEYWORDS

- Antimicrobial stewardship • Antibiotics • Sepsis • Clinical decision support
- Biomarkers • Rapid pathogen identification assays • Quality measures
- Emergency medicine

KEY POINTS

- Antimicrobial stewardship refers to efforts aimed at enhancing judicious prescribing of these unique therapeutic agents in health care settings.
- Inappropriate use of antimicrobials represents a global threat to public health and a direct threat to individual patient safety.
- Sepsis is a life-threatening, complex clinical syndrome without a gold standard diagnostic test and thus represents a unique clinical dilemma with regard to antimicrobial stewardship.
- Recent literature questioning the clinical impact of time to antimicrobials in sepsis before the onset of shock and improving the definition of sepsis may have a positive impact on antimicrobial stewardship.
- Electronic health record clinical decision support, biomarkers, and rapid pathogen identification assays have tremendous potential to enhance antimicrobial stewardship in sepsis care and should be a focus of future research efforts.

INTRODUCTION

The term antimicrobial stewardship is often mistakenly considered to only include efforts to reduce or restrict use of these agents. A more comprehensive view includes a focus on the "4 Ds" of optimal antimicrobial therapy coined by

Cempra Pharmaceuticals: Advisory Board Member, Consultant; Thermo Fisher Scientific: Advisory Board Member, Consultant (M.S. Pulia). No financial disclosures (R. Redwood, B. Sharp).
[a] Emergency Medicine Antimicrobial Stewardship Program, BerbeeWalsh Department of Emergency Medicine, University of Wisconsin School of Medicine and Public Health, 800 University Bay Drive, Suite 310, Madison, WI 53705, USA; [b] Antibiotic Stewardship Committee, Divine Savior Healthcare, 2817 New Pinery Road, Portage, WI 53901, USA; [c] The American Center, BerbeeWalsh Department of Emergency Medicine, University of Wisconsin School of Medicine and Public Health, 800 University Bay Drive, Suite 310, Madison, WI 53705, USA
* Corresponding author.
E-mail address: mspulia@medicine.wisc.edu

Emerg Med Clin N Am 35 (2017) 199–217
http://dx.doi.org/10.1016/j.emc.2016.09.007
emed.theclinics.com

Joseph and Rodvold[1] in 2008: drug, dose, de-escalation, and duration. The focus here is on getting the right antimicrobial in the right dose to the right patient for the right amount of time. The opposite of optimal antimicrobial therapy is often referred to as inappropriate or overuse. These terms can refer to a range of practices, such as prescribing when no antimicrobial was indicated, prescribing an overly broad-spectrum agent, or prescribing an excessive length of therapy. In some instances, such as bronchitis, the right antimicrobial is no antimicrobial. In cases of septic shock, the right antimicrobial is broad-spectrum coverage of all likely pathogens. Both of these scenarios represent widely accepted approaches to antimicrobial stewardship. Unfortunately, when it comes to suspected sepsis in the emergency department (ED) setting, the ideal approach to the antimicrobial management is less clear.

The timely administration of antimicrobial agents with activity against the causative pathogen has been a cornerstone of sepsis management long before it was included in the original Surviving Sepsis consensus guidelines.[2] Based on the literature linking time and appropriateness of antimicrobials to mortality in sepsis,[3–7] the ED implementation of this concept has been to rapidly cover all potential pathogens with broad-spectrum agents. De-escalation of therapy is left to occur days later after the patient has stabilized or when pathogen information is available.

The problem with this approach stems from a lack of a true gold standard for diagnosing the complex syndrome that is sepsis and the corresponding inaccuracy of widely used diagnostic criteria. The Sepsis 2.0 definition of 2 systemic inflammatory response syndrome (SIRS) criteria plus suspected infection suffers from poor discriminant validity due to a lack of specificity for both infection and the occurrence of adverse outcomes.[8–10] The combination of flawed diagnostic criteria with incredible time pressure to provide broad-spectrum antimicrobial therapy is troubling from the stewardship perspective, as it is not uncommon for patients with otherwise uncomplicated cases of common infections (eg, influenza, pneumonia, or pyelonephritis) to meet this widely used definition of sepsis.

Emerging literature that questions the optimal timing and clinical impact of antimicrobial agents in sepsis before the onset of shock may relax some of the pressure on emergency providers and allow more judicious and targeted administration in response to clinical judgment and patient trajectory rather than rigid definitions.[11–14] Also, recently updated definitions of sepsis and septic shock appear to offer an improved ability to identify septic patients at risk for adverse outcomes and thus most likely in need of early broad-spectrum antimicrobials.[9,15] As these definitions were developed with hospital mortality as the primary outcome variable,[15] their value as broad screening tools for sepsis in the ED and impact on antimicrobial stewardship will require further study. Unfortunately, these promising developments for antimicrobial stewardship in sepsis exist in sharp contrast to the recently implemented Centers for Medicare and Medicaid Services (CMS) ED Sepsis Quality Measure, which codifies poor performing and outdated definitions of sepsis and links them to mandated use of a specific list of broad-spectrum agents.

The discussion around more judicious use of antimicrobials in sepsis also must include data that suggest that up to 30% of patients diagnosed with sepsis in US EDs do not receive antibiotics before admission.[16] There is clearly much work to be done in both defining what constitutes optimal antimicrobial use in sepsis and the development of implementation strategies that facilitate their appropriate administration. The aim of this article was to provide an overview of antimicrobial resistance, evidence-based antimicrobial stewardship interventions for the ED, and potential future directions with regard to antimicrobial use in sepsis care. Due to a paucity of interventional research aimed at improving antimicrobial use in sepsis, aside from enhancing time to administration, much of this information is gleaned from interventional ED stewardship research involving other types of infection.

PUBLIC HEALTH IMPLICATIONS OF ANTIMICROBIAL OVERUSE

Antimicrobial resistance is a naturally occurring phenomenon in which antimicrobials exert selective pressure on pathogens that, in turn, develop defense mechanisms against that antimicrobial agent's mode of attack.[17] Overuse and misuse of antimicrobials has accelerated this natural process, resulting in multidrug-resistant organisms or "super bugs," as well as a general trend toward antimicrobial resistance outpacing humankind's ability to develop novel, effective antimicrobials.[18]

Although the root causes of antimicrobial resistance are multifold and include antimicrobial overuse in the agricultural and veterinary sectors; the use of antimicrobials in human medicine is a key cause of nosocomial-resistant organisms like *Clostridium difficile,* methicillin-resistant *Staphylococcus aureus* (MRSA), and vancomycin-resistant *Enterococcus.*[19] Worldwide there are 700,000 annual deaths attributable to nosocomial-resistant organisms.[20] If the trend continues at the current rate, antimicrobial resistance will have cost the global economy more than $100 *trillion* by 2050.[20] A 2014 review commissioned by the prime minister of the United Kingdom warns of "a return to the dark age of medicine" in which routine medical care like childbirth and outpatient surgery are risky undertakings and cancer chemotherapy or organ transplantation is no longer possible.[20]

In the United States, conservative estimates of morbidity and mortality attributable to antimicrobial resistance place the annual number of illnesses at 2,049,442 and the annual number of deaths at 23,000.[19] Regarding resource management, sequelae of antimicrobial resistance costs the United States between $21 and $34 billion annually and subjects US citizens to more than 8 million additional patient-days in the hospital.[17] The World Health Organization, US Centers for Disease Control and Prevention (CDC), European Medicines Agency, Institute of Medicine, World Economic Forum, Society for Healthcare Epidemiology of America, the Infectious Diseases Society of America, and most recently the White House have identified antimicrobial resistance as a pressing threat to global public health.[21–23] The CDC's *Get Smart for Healthcare Campaign* calls the improved use of antimicrobials "an important patient safety and public health issue as well as a national priority" and encourages a shift toward more judicious antimicrobial use.[24] In an effort to support public health agencies, hospitals, and clinicians in the fight against antimicrobial-resistant organisms, the CDC provides a variety of resources to promote stewardship activities, including assessment tools for antimicrobial use and a workshop on the core elements of hospital antimicrobial stewardship programs.[25]

PATIENT SAFETY IMPLICATIONS OF ANTIMICROBIAL OVERUSE

Although much of the emphasis around antimicrobial stewardship is related to the public health concerns of increasing resistance, it also should be regarded as a means of enhancing individual patient safety.[26,27] Examples of negative sequelae related to antimicrobials are pervasive in the medical literature and include adverse reactions, drug-drug interactions, and nosocomial-resistant pathogens (ie, *C difficile*). Although evidence-based infection control practices are firmly established within the lexicon of patient safety,[28] antimicrobial stewardship has only recently begun to garner similar institutional attention and support.[27]

Adverse drug events are injuries resulting from drug-related medical interventions and are estimated to account for more than 700,000 annual ED visits in the United States.[29] Shehab and colleagues[26] found that approximately 20% of ED visits for adverse drug events (more than 140,000 ED visits per year) were related to antimicrobial use. In an 11-year national data analysis, antimicrobials by category accounted for the highest number (27.5%) of all pediatric adverse drug events occurring in the outpatient setting.[30] Most of these visits were allergic reactions with clinical presentations ranging from mild rash to life-threatening anaphylaxis. The incidence of adverse drug events related to antimicrobials is likely underestimated, as many patients may not seek out medical attention for less severe episodes. For example, antimicrobial-associated diarrhea is estimated to occur in 30% of outpatient courses and is a contributing factor in nonadherence.[31,32] Additional serious adverse drug reactions associated with antimicrobials include retinal detachment,[33] tendon injury,[34] and encephalopathy.[35] Observational studies have also found an association between the macrolide class of antimicrobials and an increased risk of arrhythmias and sudden cardiac death.[36,37]

Drug-drug interactions with antimicrobials are common and, in many cases, related to changes in the activity of the cytochrome P450 isoenzymes, especially CYP3A.[38] Symptoms of drug interactions can range from disruptive (unwanted pregnancy resulting from an interaction with oral contraceptives)[39] to life-threatening (arrhythmias with amiodarone, QT prolongation with antipsychotics, and coagulopathies with warfarin).[40–43] Concurrent use of warfarin and antimicrobials deserves special mention, as these interactions are common and can result in intracranial hemorrhage or fatal gastrointestinal bleeding. Warfarin-antimicrobial interactions are particularly risky in the elderly population and can result in a sixfold increase in the odds of being hospitalized for bleeding complications.[42] Of the antimicrobials that interact with warfarin, common medications like trimethoprim/sulfamethoxazole, metronidazole, fluconazole, ciprofloxacin, levofloxacin, azithromycin, and clarithromycin are the most significant.[44]

Nosocomial-resistant pathogens are increasingly prevalent in hospitals throughout the United States. *C difficile* is widely recognized as one of the more virulent of these pathogens, infecting more than 500,000 patients annually and causing 15,000 annual deaths.[41,45] In the elderly, 1 in 11 patients older than 65 dies within a month of being diagnosed.[19] *C difficile* is classified by the CDC as an "urgent threat" to patient safety and is 7 to 10 times more likely to be found in patients who have recently taken antimicrobials.[19]

ANTIMICROBIAL STEWARDSHIP IN THE EMERGENCY DEPARTMENT

The ED is increasingly recognized as the nexus of the US health care system, serving as a 24/7 diagnostic center and entry point for most hospital admissions.[46] As such, the ED is also increasingly viewed as playing a strategic role in public health initiatives, such as curbing antimicrobial resistance.[47] As plans for outpatient care, facility-based long-term care, and inpatient care often begin in the ED, careful decisions about antimicrobial use are crucial in the ED.[48] Emergency providers (EPs) have 2 key opportunities to practice antimicrobial stewardship. First, the seemingly simple choice of whether or not to prescribe antimicrobials requires significant clinical judgment. Given the lack of diagnostic tests that can rapidly distinguish bacterial from viral infections, as well as logistical barriers to using a watch-and-wait strategy in the ED, EPs must rely heavily on clinical gestalt and evidence-based guidelines in making this determination. Second, after deciding to prescribe an antimicrobial, the choices of drug, dose, and duration represent additional opportunities for stewardship and require careful consideration of factors such as infection type, local resistance patterns, patient allergies, and cost.

As a proactive response to the epidemic of antimicrobial resistance, many EDs have implemented evidence-based care pathways[49–51] or antimicrobial stewardship intervention bundles.[52–58] Furthermore, basic antimicrobial stewardship principles are appearing as either optional or required performance measures for state and/or federal quality metric reporting.[59] For example, the American College of Emergency Physicians recently highlighted the 2016 CMS Physician Quality Reporting System (PQRS), which includes 2 antimicrobial stewardship measures: #93, avoidance of inappropriate systemic antibiotic therapy for acute otitis externa, and #116, avoidance of antibiotic treatment in adults with acute bronchitis.[60] At the hospital level, the Joint Commission promotes 16 standards and 1 National Patient Safety Goal related to antimicrobial stewardship.[59]

As antimicrobial stewardship becomes increasingly tied to ED quality reporting and value-based payment, it is imperative that these quality metrics are based on high levels of evidence. The desire to reduce the trend of global antimicrobial resistance and enhance patient safety with quality metrics must be balanced by acknowledging diagnostic uncertainty and inadequate access to follow-up care; 2 factors EPs cite as primary drivers of antimicrobial overuse.[61,62]

ANTIMICROBIAL STEWARDSHIP INTERVENTIONS FOR SEPSIS IN THE EMERGENCY DEPARTMENT

The available literature involving antimicrobial stewardship interventions in the ED is scant when compared with what is reported for inpatient and ambulatory care settings.[63,64] It is also highly fragmented in terms of intervention type(s), target disease, and antimicrobial stewardship outcome of interest. Although guidelines exist regarding optimal selection of initial antimicrobials based on the most likely source of sepsis, local resistance patterns, and patient-level risk factors for multidrug-resistant infections,[65–71] we were able to find only a handful of interventional studies targeting this outcome.

Intervention Bundles

The 4 identified studies, which included appropriateness of empiric antimicrobials for sepsis as an outcome measure, each used intervention bundles and were published between 2006 and 2010.[54,55,72,73] As there is considerable overlap between these studies in terms of design (pre-post), elements included in the intervention bundle (eg, provider education, standardized order sets, and care pathways) and overarching objective (improved adherence to Surviving Sepsis Campaign guidelines), we have selected the largest US-based and international studies for detailed discussion. From a practical perspective, when interpreting the results of these studies, it is impossible to determine the impact of each intervention bundle element on the observed outcomes. Knowing which bundle elements are highest yield would be of great value to those tasked with implementation of antimicrobial stewardship programs but unfortunately this information is not readily available. On the contrary, one could also argue that education is a foundational part of any new health care intervention and that the similar approaches used in each study combined with a shared goal (improved standardization of sepsis care) make them easily adoptable.

Micek and colleagues[72] examined the impact of an educational program and standardized paper-based order set for 120 patients (60 pre, 60 post) with septic shock at a single US academic medical center. The order set included a detailed list of recommended antimicrobials divided by probable source of infection, and appropriate initial antimicrobial treatment in the ED was a primary outcome measure. Appropriate therapy was defined by positive culture results being treated based on in vitro susceptibility results at the time of identification. This metric improved from 72% to 87% ($P = .043$) after implementation of the intervention bundle.

Levy and colleagues[73] published results from an international, bundle-based approach to improve adherence with the initial Surviving Sepsis Campaign guidelines.[74] The intervention targeted patients with severe sepsis (2 SIRS plus organ dysfunction)[8] and included the creation and dissemination of educational materials and sepsis care bundles, recruitment of clinician site champions, and the creation of a secure database for tracking outcomes. This study involved 165 sites in Europe, North America, and South America, and included more than 15,000 subjects. Among the various pre/post outcomes measures tracked was administration of broad-spectrum antibiotics within 6 hours, which improved from 60.4% to 67.9% ($P = .0002$). As there is no information provided on how broad spectrum was defined and no assessment of the appropriateness of antimicrobial selection based on the source of sepsis or culture results, it is difficult to gauge the exact impact of this intervention on stewardship beyond time to administration.

In summary, bundle-based interventions to enhance compliance with guidelines (Surviving Sepsis Campaign) appear to have a positive impact on the appropriateness of empiric antimicrobial therapy. The studies from Micek and colleagues[72] and Francis and colleagues are particularly informative due to the use of prespecified definitions of appropriate use, which were based on objective criteria (culture results, published guidelines, and local susceptibility patterns). As electronic health records (EHR) and computerized physician order entry have become ubiquitous in the time since the last of these studies was published (2010), we anticipate future studies examining bundle interventions to enhance the appropriateness of empiric antimicrobials for sepsis will focus on clinical decision support (CDS) within the EHR.

Emergency Department–Specific Antibiograms

The Surviving Sepsis Campaign guidelines recommend that empiric antimicrobial therapy is based on likely pathogen and local/hospital resistance patterns.[66] It is important to note that hospital antibiograms generated from inpatient cultures may not reflect the ED population. One study found that the susceptibility pattern of Escherichia coli in ED patients requiring admission for urinary tract infections did not match information on the hospital antibiograms.[75] EPs should advocate that an ED-specific antibiogram be generated and maintained to guide empiric antimicrobial selection in septic patients.

Emergency Department Pharmacist Programs

Based on their unique knowledge of pharmacologic therapies, pharmacists can offer significant contributions toward antimicrobial stewardship programs. The American

Society of Health-System Pharmacists has issued a statement that defines the prominent role hospital pharmacists should play in antimicrobial stewardship efforts.[76] Specifically, they can promote appropriate selection, provide consultation and feedback, and identify potential drug-drug interactions.[77] Although the presence of ED-based pharmacists has been demonstrated to reduce medication errors and facilitate optimal therapy in discharged patients,[78] there is a paucity of interventional research examining their direct impact on antimicrobial stewardship. Two studies have demonstrated an improvement in appropriateness of antimicrobial therapy for ED patients with a pharmacist-led culture review process.[79,80] However, the direct applicability of these findings is questionable, as patients diagnosed with sepsis in the ED are universally admitted and cultures are typically reviewed by the inpatient care team.

Cultures in the Emergency Department

The Surviving Sepsis Guidelines recommend obtaining any appropriate cultures in patients with suspected sepsis before administration of antimicrobial therapy, as long as these cultures do not cause a significant delay in the administration of appropriate antibiotic therapy. This recommendation also includes obtaining 2 sets of blood cultures, as well as obtaining any other cultures of appropriate sites (urine, cerebrospinal fluid [CSF], wounds, respiratory secretions, or other body fluids).[66] These recommendations have become generally accepted as typical practice and were also incorporated as part of the recent CMS SEP-1 sepsis quality measure.

Identification of a causative organism is essential in allowing inpatient providers to de-escalate antibiotics, which in turn has the potential to reduce costs, decrease the length of hospital stays, and help to control development of antibiotic resistance. Several studies have demonstrated the positive impact of culture review programs on antibiotic prescribing.[79–83] The benefit derived from tailored antimicrobial therapy in the case of true-positive blood cultures must be balanced with the potential for overuse due to frequent false positives resulting from bacterial contamination.[84] This concern, combined with multiple reports indicating blood cultures obtained in the ED are rarely positive (and typically do not impact management) in immunocompetent patients with uncomplicated bacterial infections,[85–89] has led to calls for culture use guidelines that are based on objective markers of infection severity.

Once a decision has been made to obtain blood cultures, every effort should be made to obtain the samples before the initiation of antimicrobial therapy. Failure to do so can result in sterilization of the blood and subsequent negative culture results even when bacteremia was present. Although 2 separate 15-mL sets of blood cultures have been shown to detect the pathogen in 80% to 99% of bloodstream infections,[90,91] a much lower sensitivity has been demonstrated after antibiotics are initiated.[92] Similarly, CSF sterilization has been shown to occur anywhere from 2 to 4 hours after administration of antibiotics.[93,94]

Electronic Health Record Alerts and Clinical Decision Support (CDS)

Delays in the recognition and initiation of treatment of septic shock have been associated with increased mortality.[13] The most recent Surviving Sepsis Guidelines recommend the routine screening of "seriously ill patients for severe sepsis to increase the early identification of sepsis and allow implementation of early sepsis therapy."[66]

Operational barriers including ED crowding and increasing ED volumes, combined with the potential for occult presentations of sepsis, can make the prompt recognition and delivery of effective ED sepsis care difficult. When surveyed, 18.2% of physicians and 15.8% of nurses rated the lack of sepsis recognition in ED triage as the greatest cause of delay to sepsis treatment.[95]

Recent attention has turned toward the use of CDS for sepsis recognition and treatment in the ED. Although historically this was in the form of paper-based algorithms and protocols, it is increasingly electronically integrated, as EHRs are ubiquitous throughout health care. By constantly assessing available data in a "digital screening," this has the potential to facilitate early sepsis detection or patient deterioration, as well as encouraging and facilitating optimal sepsis care.

CDS tools for the detection and treatment of sepsis have been studied in the ED,[96–101] as well as general care/medical units.[73,102–104] Many of the ED electronic CDS systems describe the predictive value of such applications on process measures, such as time to antibiotics or intravenous fluids. One study evaluating an electronic CDS system in the ED did find increased ordering of chest radiographs and blood cultures after the electronic CDS was implemented, but no statistically significant increase in the number of patients receiving antibiotics.[96] Another study found an increased number of sepsis diagnoses with a higher percentage of obtaining blood cultures.[105]

There also has been research evaluating CDS with antimicrobial prescribing. This has been shown to successfully assist with antimicrobial prescribing in a variety of care settings,[106,107] such as the intensive care unit[108] and outpatient clinics.[109]

As electronically integrated CDS for sepsis care becomes increasingly used in EDs throughout the country, further study will be needed to determine its effect on utilization of antibiotics (decision to treat and spectrum). Additional work also may be merited to evaluate how to best integrate antimicrobial prescribing support within the CDS systems currently being implemented in the ED so as to achieve a balance between improved sepsis detection and antibiotic stewardship.

Biomarkers and Rapid Pathogen Diagnostic Assays

The greatest potential for a major breakthrough in antimicrobial stewardship for sepsis management exists within the rapidly advancing field of molecular diagnostics. From an antimicrobial stewardship perspective, the ideal assay is one that rapidly and accurately rules out bacterial infection as the cause of illness. For cases of suspected sepsis in the ED, an assay with performance characteristics that allowed discrimination between infectious and noninfectious causes of SIRS would be incredibly valuable. Additionally, the ability to rapidly identify viral or bacterial pathogens and susceptibility patterns would assist EPs with the decision to treat and optimal antimicrobial selection.[110]

C-reactive protein (CRP) and procalcitonin (PCT) are the 2 most extensively studied acute phase protein biomarkers in sepsis. CRP is produced in the liver and upregulated in response to inflammatory conditions via cytokines (primarily interleukin-6). It is widely available and frequently used in a clinical context to determine the likelihood of infection.[111] PCT, the prohormone of calcitonin, is ubiquitously produced in response to bacterial infection.[111]

Although there are sufficient data to support an adverse prognostic implication of elevated CRP and PCT in patients with sepsis,[112,113] the clinical utility of these biomarkers in the management of sepsis in the ED is an area of considerable controversy.[114,115]

Likely due to a superior kinetic profile and specificity for bacterial infections as compared with CRP,[116–122] PCT is the only biomarker that has been studied extensively as an antimicrobial stewardship intervention in the ED. A Cochrane review concluded that PCT has demonstrated efficacy in reducing antimicrobial use for respiratory tract infections in the ED without increasing adverse outcomes.[123] The 2012 Surviving Sepsis Guidelines include a recommendation for the use of low PCT levels to guide antimicrobial de-escalation in the intensive care unit when no evidence of infection is found. PCT has recently received Food and Drug Administration approval for use as a prognostic assay for ED patients with sepsis.[66,124] However, when discussing the utilization of PCT in the ED to guide antimicrobial management in sepsis, it is important to note that PCT performed only moderately well in identifying ED patients with bacteremia (area under the curve of 0.84, 95% confidence interval [CI] 0.75–0.90)[125] and distinguishing infectious from noninfectious SIRS (0.85, 95% CI 0.81–0.88).[126]

The bottom line is that despite some promising candidates, there is no single biomarker that has demonstrated adequate individual diagnostic performance characteristics to rule in or rule out sepsis.[127] This is likely because sepsis is a complex syndrome that evolves as it progresses rather than a measurable, single pathologic process.

The impact of pathogen identification on antimicrobial stewardship for suspected sepsis in the ED is currently bound by the limited number of relevant, rapidly available assays. Rapid influenza assays have been extensively studied in the pediatric ED population in terms of impact on antimicrobial prescribing. Unfortunately, we were unable to identify any study specifically examining impact on patients who met sepsis criteria. In addition to influenza assays, there are several studies examining the feasibility and impact of rapid MRSA identification assays on antimicrobial stewardship for purulent skin and soft tissue infections treated in the ED. These assays are capable of reliably identifying MRSA in purulent drainage in approximately 1 hour and feasibility studies indicate they can be incorporated into ED workflow without impacting important flow metrics.[128–130] Although not yet studied for this indication, these assays may have a role in helping to tailor initial antimicrobial therapy in cases of sepsis due to skin and soft tissue infections.

IMPACT OF CENTERS FOR MEDICARE AND MEDICAID SERVICES EMERGENCY DEPARTMENT SEPSIS QUALITY MEASURE ON ANTIMICROBIAL STEWARDSHIP

On October 1, 2015, CMS began to require reporting of the Severe Sepsis/Septic Shock Early Management Bundle (SEP-1).[131] Although this measure has the potential to reduce the mortality, morbidity, and hospital length of stay for patients with sepsis, there is also potential for an impact on antibiotic utilization and antibiotic stewardship in the ED.

SEP-1 requires the administration of broad-spectrum antibiotics from a prespecified list within the first 3 hours of care to patients with severe sepsis/septic shock. The SEP-1 definition of severe sepsis/septic shock includes a "suspected source of clinical infection, 2 or more manifestations of systemic infection (SIRS criteria), and the presence of sepsis-induced organ dysfunction," including a lactate greater than 2.[66] This more inclusive definition of severe sepsis has the potential to lead to reflexive overuse of broad-spectrum antibiotics without room for application of clinical discretion. For a detailed discussion on SEP-1, see Jeremy S. Faust and Scott D. Weingart's article, "The Past, Present, and Future of the Centers for Medicare and Medicaid Services Quality Measure SEP-1, the Early Management Bundle for Severe Sepsis/Septic Shock," in this issue.

Many groups have expressed their concern over potential for overutilization of antibiotics due to SEP-1. In a letter sent to CMS, the American Hospital Association, America's Essential Hospitals, Association of American Medical Colleges, and Federation of American Hospitals expressed concern that the measure will "promote the overuse of the antibiotics that are our last line of defense against drug-resistant bacteria" and that requiring reporting on this measure "runs counter to the tenets of effective antimicrobial stewardship."[132]

Given the high level of concern among professional societies about the impact of SEP-1 on antibiotic stewardship, it is useful to reexamine lessons from another antibiotic-prescribing, process-based quality measure that had unanticipated consequences. In 2002, the Joint Commission and CMS endorsed PN-5b as one of their initial "core measures." PN-5b required that the first dose of antibiotics for pneumonia be administered within 4 hours of presentation to the ED. This was based on 2 large retrospective studies that demonstrated an association between the timing of antibiotic administration and improved outcomes in patients with community-acquired pneumonia.[133,134] However, subsequent studies began to demonstrate the unintended negative impact of PN-5b on antibiotic stewardship, including the administration of antibiotics to many patients who ultimately did not have pneumonia or any other infectious process.[135,136] One such study revealed that that more than half of ED physicians who were surveyed endorsed prescribing antibiotics to patients who they did not believe had pneumonia so as to comply with the CMS guideline (almost half of these more than 3 times a month).[137] Medical directors of academic medical centers surveyed had instituted operational responses to this measure that included policies for administration of antibiotics before chest radiograph if pneumonia was suspected (37%).[138] A variety of pressures including financial and social pressures likely led to adoption of this "shoot first and ask questions later" mentality of giving antibiotics to any patient who "might have" pneumonia. The timeline was first loosened to a 6-hour window and then ultimately withdrawn completely.

Quality measures are an important vehicle to improve health care. Process of care measures, such as SEP-1 or PN-5b, are much easier to identify and measure than clinical outcomes. Unfortunately, these are often shown to generate unanticipated consequences. Similar to the PN-5b measure, we will need to closely monitor the effect that the SEP-1 measure has on antibiotic utilization, especially because it involves the use of broad-spectrum antibiotics.

SUMMARY

Sepsis management in the ED is an incredibly dynamic landscape with massive implications for antimicrobial stewardship. This is an important issue both from a public health (ie, increasing global bacterial resistance) and patient safety perspective (eg, adverse drug reactions, C difficile). The broad-spectrum agents used in suspected cases of sepsis make it absolutely essential that we continue to refine the definitions of sepsis such that we can more accurately identify who is in need of immediate antimicrobials and who might be safely observed for clinical progression. Definitions aside, investing in new rapid biomarkers and organism identification assays is worthwhile, as they provide EPs with objective data regarding the presence and severity of bacterial illness while also allowing optimal pathogen targeting. Intelligent CDS tools embedded in the EHR that can synthesize patient-level clinical data, the ED antibiogram, and best practice guidelines also possess great potential for improving stewardship. Ultimately, the most effective antimicrobial stewardship intervention for sepsis will likely be a bundle composed of traditional quality improvement strategies (eg, education, audit, and feedback) combined with rapid diagnostics and CDS (**Table 1**). Recently implemented quality measures targeting ED sepsis management have the potential to adversely impact antimicrobial stewardship in the ED and need to be closely monitored.

Table 1
Summary of antimicrobial stewardship interventions in the emergency department

Intervention	Rationale
Emergency department antibiogram	Resistance patterns observed in the emergency department may differ from that observed in inpatient units
Educational and audit/feedback programs	• Ensure baseline level of awareness among clinical staff regarding antimicrobial stewardship for condition of interest (eg, sepsis) • Tailoring individual feedback based on specific cases or practice patterns as compared with group may encourage behavior change
Standardized care pathways	• Assist providers in optimizing the use of antimicrobials using available best practice, evidence-based guidelines • Decreases variability of antimicrobial prescribing and selection decisions among various providers
Cultures before antimicrobial therapy	• Yield of clinical cultures (eg, blood, urine, cerebrospinal fluid) declines rapidly following antimicrobial therapy • Culture results are a primary tool for antimicrobial stewardship after emergency department care (eg, de-escalation of broad-spectrum agents started for suspected sepsis)
Clinical decision support embedded in the electronic health record	• Enhance early detection of sepsis • Support compliance with quality measures • Assist with optimal antimicrobial selection
Biomarkers and organism identification assays	• Procalcitonin to guide antimicrobial therapy in respiratory tract infections (nonseptic) • Rapid influenza assays to identify potential viral etiology for the presence of systemic inflammatory response syndrome criteria

REFERENCES

1. Joseph J, Rodvold KA. The role of carbapenems in the treatment of severe nosocomial respiratory tract infections. Expert Opin Pharmacother 2008;9(4): 561–75.

2. Bochud P-Y, Bonten M, Marchetti O, et al. Antimicrobial therapy for patients with severe sepsis and septic shock: an evidence-based review. Crit Care Med 2004;32(11 Suppl):S495–512.

3. Gaieski DF, Mikkelsen ME, Band RA, et al. Impact of time to antibiotics on survival in patients with severe sepsis or septic shock in whom early goal-directed therapy was initiated in the emergency department. Crit Care Med 2010;38(4): 1045–53.

4. Kumar A, Roberts D, Wood KE, et al. Duration of hypotension before initiation of effective antimicrobial therapy is the critical determinant of survival in human septic shock. Crit Care Med 2006;34(6):1589–96.

5. Garnacho-Montero J, Garcia-Garmendia JL, Barrero-Almodovar A, et al. Impact of adequate empirical antibiotic therapy on the outcome of patients admitted to the intensive care unit with sepsis. Crit Care Med 2003;31(12): 2742–51.

6. Kumar A, Ellis P, Arabi Y, et al. Initiation of inappropriate antimicrobial therapy results in a fivefold reduction of survival in human septic shock. Chest 2009; 136(5):1237–48.

7. Paul M, Shani V, Muchtar E, et al. Systematic review and meta-analysis of the efficacy of appropriate empiric antibiotic therapy for sepsis. Antimicrob Agents Chemother 2010;54(11):4851–63.

8. Levy MM, Fink MP, Marshall JC, et al. 2001 SCCM/ESICM/ACCP/ATS/SIS International sepsis definitions conference. Crit Care Med 2003;31(4):1250–6.

9. Singer M, Deutschman CS, Seymour CW, et al. The third international consensus definitions for sepsis and septic shock (sepsis-3). JAMA 2016; 315(8):801.

10. Kaukonen K-M, Bailey M, Pilcher D, et al. Systemic inflammatory response syndrome criteria in defining severe sepsis. N Engl J Med 2015;372(17): 1629–38.

11. Casserly B, Hannigan A. Meta-analysis based on limited data shows no evidence to support the guideline recommendation for early administration of antibiotics in severe sepsis and septic shock. Evid Based Med 2015;20(6):214–5.

12. de Groot B, Ansems A, Gerling DH, et al. The association between time to antibiotics and relevant clinical outcomes in emergency department patients with various stages of sepsis: a prospective multi-center study. Crit Care 2015;19:194.

13. Puskarich MA, Trzeciak S, Shapiro NI, et al. Association between timing of antibiotic administration and mortality from septic shock in patients treated with a quantitative resuscitation protocol. Crit Care Med 2011;39(9):2066–71.

14. Sterling SA, Miller WR, Pryor J, et al. The impact of timing of antibiotics on outcomes in severe sepsis and septic shock: a systematic review and meta-analysis. Crit Care Med 2015;43(9):1907–15.

15. Seymour CW, Liu VX, Iwashyna TJ, et al. Assessment of clinical criteria for sepsis: for the third international consensus definitions for sepsis and septic shock (sepsis-3). JAMA 2016;315(8):762–74.

16. Filbin MR, Arias SA, Camargo CA Jr, et al. Sepsis visits and antibiotic utilization in U.S. emergency departments. Crit Care Med 2014;42(3):528–35.

17. WHO. Antimicrobial resistance: global report on surveillance 2014. WHO. Available at: http://www.who.int/drugresistance/documents/surveillancereport/en/. Accessed July 13, 2014.

18. Tanwar J, Das S, Fatima Z, et al. Multidrug resistance: an emerging crisis. Interdiscip Perspect Infect Dis 2014;2014:1–7. Available at: https://www.hindawi.com/journals/ipid/2014/541340/. Accessed October 4, 2016.

19. Threat Report 2013. Antimicrobial resistance. CDC. Available at: http://www.cdc.gov/drugresistance/threat-report-2013/. Accessed October 30, 2013.

20. Antimicrobial resistance: tackling a crisis for the health and wealth of nations. Publications: AMR Review. Available at: http://amr-review.org/sites/default/files/AMR%20Review%20Paper%20-%20Tackling%20a%20crisis%20for%20the%20health%20and%20wealth%20of%20nations_1.pdf. Accessed April 7, 2016.

21. Spellberg B, Srinivasan A, Chambers HF. New societal approaches to empowering antibiotic stewardship. JAMA 2016;315(12):1229–30.

22. Society for Healthcare Epidemiology of America, Infectious Diseases Society of America, Pediatric Infectious Diseases Society. Policy statement on antimicrobial stewardship by the Society for Healthcare Epidemiology of America (SHEA), the Infectious Diseases Society of America (IDSA), and the Pediatric Infectious Diseases Society (PIDS). Infect Control Hosp Epidemiol 2012;33(4): 322–7.

23. National Action Plan for Combating Antibiotic-Resistant Bacteria. Available at: https://www.whitehouse.gov/sites/default/files/docs/national_action_plan_for_ combating_antibotic-resistant_bacteria.pdf. Accessed June 17, 2015.

24. Pollack LA, Srinivasan A. Core elements of hospital antibiotic stewardship programs from the Centers for Disease Control and Prevention. Clin Infect Dis 2014; 59(Suppl 3):S97–100.

25. Core Elements - Implementation Resources - Get Smart for Healthcare - CDC. Available at: http://www.cdc.gov/getsmart/healthcare/implementation/core-elements.html#Developments. Accessed May 20, 2014.

26. Shehab N, Patel PR, Srinivasan A, et al. Emergency department visits for antibiotic-associated adverse events. Clin Infect Dis 2008;47(6):735.

27. Tamma PD, Holmes A, Ashley ED. Antimicrobial stewardship: another focus for patient safety? Curr Opin Infect Dis 2014;27(4):348–55.

28. Burke JP. Infection control—a problem for patient safety. N Engl J Med 2003; 348(7):651–6.

29. Budnitz DS, Pollock DA, Weidenbach KN, et al. National surveillance of emergency department visits for outpatient adverse drug events. JAMA 2006; 296(15):1858–66.

30. Bourgeois FT, Mandl KD, Valim C, et al. Pediatric adverse drug events in the outpatient setting: an 11-year national analysis. Pediatrics 2009;124(4): e744–50.

31. Barbut F, Meynard JL. Managing antibiotic associated diarrhoea. BMJ 2002; 324(7350):1345–6.

32. McFarland LV. Epidemiology, risk factors and treatments for antibiotic-associated diarrhea. Dig Dis 1998;16(5):292–307.

33. Raguideau F, Lemaitre M, Dray-Spira R, et al. Association between oral fluoroquinolone use and retinal detachment. JAMA Ophthalmol 2016;134(4):415–21.

34. Khaliq Y, Zhanel GG. Fluoroquinolone-associated tendinopathy: a critical review of the literature. Clin Infect Dis 2003;36(11):1404–10.

35. Bhattacharyya S, Darby RR, Raibagkar P, et al. Antibiotic-associated encephalopathy. Neurology 2016;86(10):963–71.

36. Cheng Y-J, Nie X-Y, Chen X-M, et al. The role of macrolide antibiotics in increasing cardiovascular risk. J Am Coll Cardiol 2015;66(20):2173–84.

37. Ray WA, Murray KT, Hall K, et al. Azithromycin and the risk of cardiovascular death. N Engl J Med 2012;366(20):1881–90.

38. Pai MP, Momary KM, Rodvold KA. Antibiotic drug interactions. Med Clin North Am 2006;90(6):1223–55.

39. Weaver K, Glasier A. Interaction between broad-spectrum antibiotics and the combined oral contraceptive pill. A literature review. Contraception 1999; 59(2):71–8.

40. Yap YG, Camm AJ. Drug induced QT prolongation and torsades de pointes. Heart 2003;89(11):1363–72.

41. Yap YG, Camm J. Risk of torsades de pointes with non-cardiac drugs. Doctors need to be aware that many drugs can cause qt prolongation. BMJ 2000; 320(7243):1158–9.

42. Baillargeon J, Holmes HM, Lin Y-L, et al. Concurrent use of warfarin and antibiotics and the risk of bleeding in older adults. Am J Med 2012;125(2):183–9.

43. Granowitz EV, Brown RB. Antibiotic adverse reactions and drug interactions. Crit Care Clin 2008;24(2):421–42.

44. Ghaswalla PK, Harpe SE, Tassone D, et al. Warfarin-antibiotic interactions in older adults of an outpatient anticoagulation clinic. Am J Geriatr Pharmacother 2012;10(6):352–60.

45. Lessa FC, Mu Y, Bamberg WM, et al. Burden of *Clostridium difficile* infection in the United States. N Engl J Med 2015;372(9):825–34.

46. Gonzalez Morganti K, Bauhoff S, Blanchard JC, et al. The evolving role of emergency departments in the United States. 2013. Available at: http://www.rand. org/pubs/research_reports/RR280.html. Accessed April 16, 2014.

47. Emergency Department as Community Microcosm, Data Hub: Q&A with Jeremy Brown. RWJF. 2013. Available at: http://www.rwjf.org/en/culture-of-health/2013/ 08/emergency_department.html. Accessed April 7, 2016.

48. May L, Cosgrove S, L'Archeveque M, et al. A call to action for antimicrobial stewardship in the emergency department: approaches and strategies. Ann Emerg Med 2013;62(1):69–77.e2.

49. Benenson R, Magalski A, Cavanaugh S, et al. Effects of a pneumonia clinical pathway on time to antibiotic treatment, length of stay, and mortality. Acad Emerg Med 1999;6(12):1243–8.

50. Marrie TJ, Lau CY, Wheeler SL, et al. A controlled trial of a critical pathway for treatment of community-acquired pneumonia. JAMA 2000;283(6):749–55.

51. Spiro DM, Tay K, Arnold DH, et al. Wait-and-see prescription for the treatment of acute otitis media: a randomized controlled trial. JAMA 2006;296(10):1235–41.

52. Ambroggio L, Thomson J, Murtagh Kurowski E, et al. Quality improvement methods increase appropriate antibiotic prescribing for childhood pneumonia. Pediatrics 2013;131(5):e1623–31.

53. Borde JP, Kern WV, Hug M, et al. Implementation of an intensified antibiotic stewardship programme targeting third-generation cephalosporin and fluoroquinolone use in an emergency medicine department. Emerg Med J 2015; 32(7):509–15.

54. De Miguel-Yanes JM, Muñoz-González J, Andueza-Lillo JA, et al. Implementation of a bundle of actions to improve adherence to the Surviving Sepsis Campaign guidelines at the ED. Am J Emerg Med 2009;27(6):668–74.

55. Francis M, Rich T, Williamson T, et al. Effect of an emergency department sepsis protocol on time to antibiotics in severe sepsis. CJEM 2010;12(4):303–10.

56. McIntosh KA, Maxwell DJ, Pulver LK, et al. A quality improvement initiative to improve adherence to national guidelines for empiric management of community-acquired pneumonia in emergency departments. Int J Qual Health Care 2011;23(2):142–50.

57. Ostrowsky B, Sharma S, DeFino M, et al. Antimicrobial stewardship and automated pharmacy technology improve antibiotic appropriateness for community-acquired pneumonia. Infect Control Hosp Epidemiol 2013;34(6): 566–72.

58. Percival KM, Valenti KM, Schmittling SE, et al. Impact of an antimicrobial stewardship intervention on urinary tract infection treatment in the ED. Am J Emerg Med 2015;33(9):1129–33.

59. Joint Commission joins White House effort to reduce antibiotic overuse. Jt Comm Perspect 2015;35(7):4, 11.

60. ACEP PQRS Quality details: 2016 regulatory highlights. Available at: https:// www.acep.org/Legislation-and-Advocacy/Federal-Issues/Quality-Issues/2016- Regulatory-Highlights/. Accessed April 7, 2016.

61. Get smart about antibiotics Vermont-antibiotic stewardship in emergency departments. Available at: http://healthvermont.gov/prevent/antibiotics/getsmart. aspx. Accessed July 16, 2014.

62. May L, Gudger G, Armstrong P, et al. Multisite exploration of clinical decision making for antibiotic use by emergency medicine providers using quantitative and qualitative methods. Infect Control Hosp Epidemiol 2014;35(9):1114–25.

63. Davey P, Brown E, Charani E, et al. Interventions to improve antibiotic prescribing practices for hospital inpatients. Cochrane Database Syst Rev 2013;(4):CD003543.

64. Arnold SR, Straus SE. Interventions to improve antibiotic prescribing practices in ambulatory care. Cochrane Database Syst Rev 2005;(4):CD003539.

65. Mandell LA, Wunderink RG, Anzueto A, et al. Infectious Diseases Society of America/American Thoracic Society consensus guidelines on the management of community-acquired pneumonia in adults. Clin Infect Dis 2007;44(Suppl 2): S27–72.

66. Dellinger RP, Levy MM, Rhodes A, et al. Surviving sepsis campaign: international guidelines for management of severe sepsis and septic shock: 2012. Crit Care Med 2013;41(2):580–637.

67. American Thoracic Society, Infectious Diseases Society of America. Guidelines for the management of adults with hospital-acquired, ventilator-associated, and healthcare-associated pneumonia. Am J Respir Crit Care Med 2005;171(4): 388–416.

68. Nicolle LE. Urinary tract infection. Crit Care Clin 2013;29(3):699–715.

69. Kumar A, Zarychanski R, Light B, et al. Early combination antibiotic therapy yields improved survival compared with monotherapy in septic shock: a propensity-matched analysis. Crit Care Med 2010;38(9):1773–85.

70. Pappas PG, Kauffman CA, Andes D, et al. Clinical practice guidelines for the management of candidiasis: 2009 update by the Infectious Diseases Society of America. Clin Infect Dis 2009;48(5):503–35.

71. Mermel LA, Allon M, Bouza E, et al. Clinical practice guidelines for the diagnosis and management of intravascular catheter-related infection: 2009 update by the Infectious Diseases Society of America. Clin Infect Dis 2009; 49(1):1–45.

72. Micek ST, Roubinian N, Heuring T, et al. Before-after study of a standardized hospital order set for the management of septic shock. Crit Care Med 2006; 34(11):2707–13.

73. Levy MM, Dellinger RP, Townsend SR, et al. The Surviving Sepsis Campaign: results of an international guideline-based performance improvement program targeting severe sepsis. Intensive Care Med 2010;36(2):222–31.

74. Dellinger RP, Carlet JM, Masur H, et al. Surviving sepsis campaign guidelines for management of severe sepsis and septic shock. Crit Care Med 2004; 32(3):858–73.

75. Fleming VH, White BP, Southwood R. Resistance of *Escherichia coli* urinary isolates in ED-treated patients from a community hospital. Am J Emerg Med 2014; 32(8):864–70.

76. Antimicrobial Stewardship Resources. Available at: http://www.ashp.org/ menu/PracticePolicy/ResourceCenters/Inpatient-Care-Practitioners/Antimicro bial-Stewardship. Accessed April 13, 2016.

77. Bishop BM. Antimicrobial stewardship in the emergency department challenges, opportunities, and a call to action for pharmacists. J Pharm Pract 2015;1–8.

Available at: http://jpp.sagepub.com/content/early/2015/05/29/0897190015585762.long. Accessed October 4, 2016.

78. Cesarz JL, Steffenhagen AL, Svenson J, et al. Emergency department discharge prescription interventions by emergency medicine pharmacists. Ann Emerg Med 2013;61(2):209–14.e1.

79. Baker SN, Acquisto NM, Ashley ED, et al. Pharmacist-managed antimicrobial stewardship program for patients discharged from the emergency department. J Pharm Pract 2012;25(2):190–4.

80. Randolph TC, Parker A, Meyer L, et al. Effect of a pharmacist-managed culture review process on antimicrobial therapy in an emergency department. Am J Health Syst Pharm 2011;68(10):916–9.

81. Acquisto NM, Baker SN. Antimicrobial stewardship in the emergency department. J Pharm Pract 2011;24(2):196–202.

82. Dumkow LE, Kenney RM, MacDonald NC, et al. Impact of a multidisciplinary culture follow-up program of antimicrobial therapy in the emergency department. Infect Dis Ther 2014;3(1):45–53.

83. Arbo MJ, Snydman DR. Influence of blood culture results on antibiotic choice in the treatment of bacteremia. Arch Intern Med 1994;154(23):2641–5.

84. Lin EC, Boehm KM. Positive predictive value of blood cultures utilized by community emergency physicians. ISRN Infect Dis 2013;1–5. Available at: http://dx.doi.org/10.5402/2013/135607. Accessed October 4, 2016.

85. Kelly AM. Clinical impact of blood cultures taken in the emergency department. J Accid Emerg Med 1998;15(4):254–6.

86. Mountain D, Bailey PM, O'Brien D, et al. Blood cultures ordered in the adult emergency department are rarely useful. Eur J Emerg Med 2006;13(2):76–9.

87. Munro PT, Howie N, Gerstenmaier JF. Do peripheral blood cultures taken in the emergency department influence clinical management? Emerg Med J 2007; 24(3):211–2.

88. Makam AN, Auerbach AD, Steinman MA. Blood culture use in the emergency department in patients hospitalized for community-acquired pneumonia. JAMA Intern Med 2014;174(5):803–6.

89. Benenson RS, Kepner AM, Pyle DN, et al. Selective use of blood cultures in emergency department pneumonia patients. J Emerg Med 2007;33(1):1–8.

90. Weinstein MP, Reller LB, Murphy JR, et al. The clinical significance of positive blood cultures: a comprehensive analysis of 500 episodes of bacteremia and fungemia in adults. I. Laboratory and epidemiologic observations. Rev Infect Dis 1983;5(1):35–53.

91. Lee A, Mirrett S, Reller LB, et al. Detection of bloodstream infections in adults: how many blood cultures are needed? J Clin Microbiol 2007;45(11):3546–8.

92. Tabriz MS, Riederer K, Baran J Jr, et al. Repeating blood cultures during hospital stay: practice pattern at a teaching hospital and a proposal for guidelines. Clin Microbiol Infect 2004;10(7):624–7.

93. Kanegaye JT, Soliemanzadeh P, Bradley JS. Lumbar puncture in pediatric bacterial meningitis: defining the time interval for recovery of cerebrospinal fluid pathogens after parenteral antibiotic pretreatment. Pediatrics 2001;108(5):1169–74.

94. Michael B, Menezes BF, Cunniffe J, et al. Effect of delayed lumbar punctures on the diagnosis of acute bacterial meningitis in adults. Emerg Med J 2010;27(6): 433–8.

95. Burney M, Underwood J, McEvoy S, et al. Early detection and treatment of severe sepsis in the emergency department: identifying barriers to implementation of a protocol-based approach. J Emerg Nurs 2012;38(6):512–7.

96. Nelson JL, Smith BL, Jared JD, et al. Prospective trial of real-time electronic surveillance to expedite early care of severe sepsis. Ann Emerg Med 2011;57(5):500–4.

97. Singer AJ, Taylor M, Domingo A, et al. Diagnostic characteristics of a clinical screening tool in combination with measuring bedside lactate level in emergency department patients with suspected sepsis. Acad Emerg Med 2014; 21(8):853–7.

98. Meurer WJ, Smith BL, Losman ED, et al. Real-time identification of serious infection in geriatric patients using clinical information system surveillance. J Am Geriatr Soc 2009;57(1):40–5.

99. Alsolamy S, Al Salamah M, Al Thagafi M, et al. Diagnostic accuracy of a screening electronic alert tool for severe sepsis and septic shock in the emergency department. BMC Med Inform Decis Mak 2014;14(1):105.

100. Nguyen SQ, Mwakalindile E, Booth JS, et al. Automated electronic medical record sepsis detection in the emergency department. Peer J 2014;2:e343.

101. Amland RC, Hahn-Cover KE. Clinical decision support for early recognition of sepsis. Am J Med Qual 2016;31(2):103–10.

102. Jones C, Currie-Cuyoy M, Jackson T. Code Sepsis: rapid identification and treatment of severe sepsis in floor patients [abstract]. J Hosp Med 2013; 8(Suppl 2). Available at: http://www.shmabstracts.com/abstract/code-sepsis-rapid-identification-and-treatment-of-severe-sepsis-in-floor-patients/. Accessed April 4, 2016.

103. Larosa JA, Ahmad N, Feinberg M, et al. The use of an early alert system to improve compliance with sepsis bundles and to assess impact on mortality. Crit Care Res Pract 2012;1–8. Available at: https://www.hindawi.com/journals/ccrp/2012/980369/. Accessed October 4, 2016.

104. Sawyer AM, Deal EN, Labelle AJ, et al. Implementation of a real-time computerized sepsis alert in nonintensive care unit patients. Crit Care Med 2011;39(3):469–73.

105. Whippy A, Skeath M, Crawford B, et al. Kaiser Permanente's performance improvement system, part 3: multisite improvements in care for patients with sepsis. Jt Comm J Qual Patient Saf 2011;37(11):483–93.

106. Shebl NA, Franklin BD, Barber N. Clinical decision support systems and antibiotic use. Pharm World Sci 2007;29(4):342–9.

107. Linder J, Schnipper JL, Volk LA, et al. Clinical decision support to improve antibiotic prescribing for acute respiratory infections: results of a pilot study. AMIA Annu Symp Proc 2007;468–72.

108. Sintchenko V, Iredell JR, Gilbert GL, et al. Handheld computer-based decision support reduces patient length of stay and antibiotic prescribing in critical care. J Am Med Inform Assoc 2005;12(4):398–402.

109. Samore MH, Bateman K, Alder SC, et al. Clinical decision support and appropriateness of antimicrobial prescribing: a randomized trial. JAMA 2005; 294(18):2305–14.

110. Stoneking LR, Patanwala AE, Winkler JP, et al. Would earlier microbe identification alter antibiotic therapy in bacteremic emergency department patients? J Emerg Med 2013;44(1):1–8.

111. Reinhart K, Bauer M, Riedemann NC, et al. New approaches to sepsis: molecular diagnostics and biomarkers. Clin Microbiol Rev 2012;25(4):609–34.

112. Jensen JU, Heslet L, Jensen TH, et al. Procalcitonin increase in early identification of critically ill patients at high risk of mortality. Crit Care Med 2006;34(10):2596–602.

113. Castelli GP, Pognani C, Meisner M, et al. Procalcitonin and C-reactive protein during systemic inflammatory response syndrome, sepsis and organ dysfunction. Crit Care 2004;8(4):R234–42.

114. Talan DA. Procalcitonin is not a useful biomarker of sepsis. Ann Emerg Med 2015;66(3):320–1.

115. Schuetz P, Mueller B. Procalcitonin: an effective screening tool and safe therapeutic decisionmaking aid for emergency department patients with suspected sepsis. Ann Emerg Med 2015;66(3):318–9.

116. Sakr Y, Burgett U, Nacul FE, et al. Lipopolysaccharide binding protein in a surgical intensive care unit: a marker of sepsis? Crit Care Med 2008;36(7):2014–22.

117. Monneret G, Labaune JM, Isaac C, et al. Procalcitonin and C-reactive protein levels in neonatal infections. Acta Paediatr 1997;86(2):209–12.

118. Meisner M, Tschaikowsky K, Palmaers T, et al. Comparison of procalcitonin (PCT) and C-reactive protein (CRP) plasma concentrations at different SOFA scores during the course of sepsis and MODS. Crit Care 1999;3(1):45–50.

119. Becker KL, Nylén ES, White JC, et al. Clinical review 167: Procalcitonin and the calcitonin gene family of peptides in inflammation, infection, and sepsis: a journey from calcitonin back to its precursors. J Clin Endocrinol Metab 2004; 89(4):1512–25.

120. Brunkhorst FM, Heinz U, Forycki ZF. Kinetics of procalcitonin in iatrogenic sepsis. Intensive Care Med 1998;24(8):888–9.

121. Eberhard OK, Haubitz M, Brunkhorst FM, et al. Usefulness of procalcitonin for differentiation between activity of systemic autoimmune disease (systemic lupus erythematosus/systemic antineutrophil cytoplasmic antibody-associated vasculitis) and invasive bacterial infection. Arthritis Rheum 1997;40(7):1250–6.

122. Meisner M, Tschaikowsky K, Hutzler A, et al. Postoperative plasma concentrations of procalcitonin after different types of surgery. Intensive Care Med 1998;24(7):680–4.

123. Schuetz P, Müller B, Christ-Crain M, et al. Procalcitonin to initiate or discontinue antibiotics in acute respiratory tract infections. Cochrane Database Syst Rev 2012;(9):CD007498.

124. Thermo Fisher Scientific announces expanded FDA clearance for its B·R·A·H·M·S PCT Sepsis Biomarker Business Wire. 2016. Available at: http://www.businesswire.com/news/home/20160301006265/en/Thermo-Fisher-Scientific-Announces-Expanded-FDA-Clearance. Accessed May 10, 2016.

125. Jones AE, Fiechtl JF, Brown MD, et al. Procalcitonin test in the diagnosis of bacteremia: a meta-analysis. Ann Emerg Med 2007;50(1):34–41.

126. Wacker C, Prkno A, Brunkhorst FM, et al. Procalcitonin as a diagnostic marker for sepsis: a systematic review and meta-analysis. Lancet Infect Dis 2013; 13(5):426–35.

127. Tsalik EL, Jaggers LB, Glickman SW, et al. Discriminative value of inflammatory biomarkers for suspected sepsis. The J Emerg Med 2012;43(1):97–106.

128. May LS, Rothman RE, Miller LG, et al. A randomized clinical trial comparing use of rapid molecular testing for *Staphylococcus aureus* for patients with cutaneous abscesses in the emergency department with standard of care. Infect Control Hosp Epidemiol 2015;36(12):1423–30.

129. Pulia M, Calderone M, Hansen B, et al. Feasibility of rapid polymerase chain reaction for detection of methicillin-resistant Staphylococcus aureus colonization among emergency department patients with abscesses. Open Access Emerg Med 2013;5:17–22.

130. Terp S, Krishnadasan A, Bowen W, et al. Introduction of rapid methicillin-resistant staphylococcus aureus polymerase chain reaction testing and antibiotic selection among hospitalized patients with purulent skin infections. Clin Infect Dis 2014;58(8):e129–32.

131. Baciak K. Sepsis care–what's new? The CMS Guidelines for Severe Sepsis and Septic Shock have arrived. emdocs. 2015. Available at: http://www.emdocs.net/sepsis-care-whats-new-the-cms-guidelines-for-severe-sepsis-and-septic-shock-have-arrived/. Accessed April 4, 2016.

132. AHA letter regarding SEP1. Available at: http://www.aha.org/advocacy-issues/letter/2015/150825-let-medgroups-cms.pdf. Accessed April 4, 2016.

133. Meehan TP, Weingarten SR, Holmboe ES, et al. A statewide initiative to improve the care of hospitalized pneumonia patients: the Connecticut Pneumonia Pathway Project. Am J Med 2001;111(3):203–10.

134. Houck PM, Bratzler DW, Nsa W, et al. Timing of antibiotic administration and outcomes for Medicare patients hospitalized with community-acquired pneumonia. Arch Intern Med 2004;164(6):637–44.

135. Welker JA, Huston M, McCue JD. Antibiotic timing and errors in diagnosing pneumonia. Arch Intern Med 2008;168(4):351–6.

136. Kanwar M, Brar N, Khatib R, et al. Misdiagnosis of community-acquired pneumonia and inappropriate utilization of antibiotics: side effects of the 4-h antibiotic administration rule. Chest 2007;131(6):1865–9.

137. Nicks BA, Manthey DE, Fitch MT. The Centers for Medicare and Medicaid Services (CMS) community-acquired pneumonia core measures lead to unnecessary antibiotic administration by emergency physicians. Acad Emerg Med 2009;16(2):184–7.

138. Pines JM, Hollander JE, Lee H, et al. Emergency department operational changes in response to pay-for-performance and antibiotic timing in pneumonia. Acad Emerg Med 2007;14(6):545–8.

The Past, Present, and Future of the Centers for Medicare and Medicaid Services Quality Measure SEP-1

The Early Management Bundle for Severe Sepsis/Septic Shock

Jeremy S. Faust, MD, MS[a],*, Scott D. Weingart, MD[b]

KEYWORDS

- Sepsis • Severe sepsis • Septic shock • CMS • Core measures • Quality
- Early goal-directed therapy • Shared decision-making

KEY POINTS

- The Centers for Medicare and Medicaid Services have enacted an executive branch rule (quality measure) known as SEP-1 that mandates the administration of a bundle that carefully prescribes precisely how patients with severe sepsis and septic shock must be treated in the early phases.
- CMS measures are meant to reflect best evidence and consensus practices. The provisions of SEP-1, however, are highly controversial among sepsis experts.
- CMS quality measures can fall under hospital-compare or value-based purchasing regimes. SEP-1 is currently hospital-compare, meaning that individual cases are not reimbursed differently depending on adherence. Rather a hospital's overall adherence is compared with others and rated publically.
- The definitions for severe sepsis and septic shock used in SEP-1 are not the same as those used in the four major prospective sepsis trials on which the measure was supposedly based.
- Some of the provisions of SEP-1 may be harmful to certain patients. The inclusion and exclusion criteria are not the same as the major prospective trials that were relied on.

Continued

The authors of this article have nothing to disclose.
[a] Department of Emergency Medicine, Brigham and Women's Hospital, Harvard Medical School, 10 Vining Street, Boston, MA 02115, USA; [b] Division of Emergency Critical Care, Department of Emergency Medicine, Stony Brook Hospital, 101 Nicolls Road, Stony Brook, NY 11704, USA
* Corresponding author.
E-mail address: jsfaust@gmail.com

Emerg Med Clin N Am 35 (2017) 219–231
http://dx.doi.org/10.1016/j.emc.2016.09.006
0733-8627/17/© 2016 Elsevier Inc. All rights reserved.

Continued

- The administrative burden of SEP-1 is unprecedented. To our knowledge, SEP-1 is the largest quality measure ever introduced by CMS by virtue of the number of required actions to achieve adherence.
- There are several contraindications to administering the SEP-1 bundle. We describe those and other approaches to avoid administering the provisions of SEP-1 to those who may be harmed by it.

INTRODUCTION

In October of 2015, the Centers for Medicare and Medicaid Services (CMS) enacted a new national quality measure on sepsis called the Early Management Bundle for Severe Sepsis/Septic Shock (SEP-1). SEP-1 was the end result of a colossal undertaking to standardize care for severe sepsis and septic shock regardless of the size of the emergency department (ED) where the patient is being treated. The final product deviates substantially from the original measure (stewarded by Henry Ford Hospital in Detroit, initially led by early goal directed therapy [EGDT] pioneer Dr Emmanuel Rivers) and does not necessarily follow the best current evidence available. Nevertheless, a thorough understanding of SEP-1 is crucial because all hospitals and emergency providers (EPs) will soon be accountable for meeting the requirements of this measure.

In brief, SEP-1 is the nation's first, and by law only, national quality measure on early management of sepsis care. It mandates that patients meeting criteria for SEP-1 must receive the bundle of care stipulated in the CMS Specifications Manual for National Hospital Inpatient Quality Measures. This measure applies to all US EDs.

This article provides a thorough review of the SEP-1 measure and all of the potential implications it may have on sepsis care provided in the United States. The measure has stirred up a great deal of controversy, which is not surprising given the complex nature of the sepsis disease process. The major concern is that hospitals may focus their attention on meeting compliance with the requirements of SEP-1 and consequently may stray from key patient-centered outcomes in sepsis. There is no question that the SEP-1 bundle is burdensome and much more complex than any previous core measure set forth by CMS. It remains to be seen if this will improve care of the patient with severe sepsis and septic shock in the ED.

A BRIEF HISTORY OF SEP-1

In 2003, the Surviving Sepsis Campaign (SSC) initiated work on guidelines on bundled sepsis care. The SSC group focused its efforts on ways to implement the tenets of the recently published EGDT trial, which focused on an aggressive, invasive, and protocol driven resuscitation of patients with severe sepsis and septic shock. The SSC was also cognizant of the recent Institute of Medicine report *To Err is Human*, which highlighted the impact of iatrogenic error in medicine. The best available evidence at the time suggested that EGDT and bundled care uniquely decreased mortality from severe sepsis and septic shock.

In 2008, Henry Ford Hospital and Dr Rivers succeeded in getting the National Quality Forum (NQF) to endorse their proposed sepsis bundle and embrace EGDT (NQF #0500).[1] Although the NQF is a feeder for CMS measures, a CMS measure did not materialize after initial NQF endorsement. In 2013, in accordance with new provisions of the Affordable Care Act, the Department of Health and Human Services identified sepsis as a priority for the following measure cycle. Simultaneously, NQF #0500 came up for its scheduled maintenance review. The new iteration of NQF #0500 now required the invasive components (eg, central venous catheter, arterial line) of EGDT and measurement of central venous pressure and central venous oxygen saturation. However, because the three largest sepsis trials ever were underway (ProCESS, ProMISe, and ARISE), it was decided that an ad hoc committee would reconvene when new data emerged.

When the landmark ProCESS trial demonstrated that EGDT performed no better than both a less-invasive protocol and usual care (ie, physician discretion determines care), the committee was forced to reconsider the portions of NQF that involved the most invasive portions of EGDT. Because CMS would likely now adopt the re-endorsed NQF #0500, many members of the NQF committee believed that it might be untenable to assess quality of sepsis care by provider compliance with EGDT. The NQF patient safety committee voted 11 to 7 to remove the invasive requirements of EGDT from the measure. Ultimately, the expensive and invasive aspects of the protocol (eg, central venous catheter, central venous pressure monitoring, and central venous oxygen saturation monitoring) were now optional. EPs were also given the option of documenting certain physical examination features or cardiac ultrasound in place of these modalities. This compromise was approved and thus NQF #0500 was finally re-endorsed in September of 2014 (20 days before the ARISE trial confirmed the ProCESS findings).

NQF #0500 was thus cleared for final approval by CMS. However, to turn NQF #0500 into a measure that could be implemented, CMS subcontracted Mathematica Policy Research group and Tellegen to turn the measure into the specification manual and the data dictionary needed for future chart reviewers to assess adherence. The result was a 51-page specification manual accompanied by a 393-page guide. Within these documents lie the keys to understanding and implementing SEP-1 (version 5.1, which we use for this article, is the latest version available, for use July–December, 2016).

WHERE ARE THE TEETH?

CMS quality measures are federal regulations, enacted under the Department of Health and Human Services. The teeth of quality measure enforcement may be tied to either hospital-compare or value-based purchasing regimes. In hospital-compare, a hospital's overall adherence to CMS measures is reported and compared with other hospitals. However, it is the Joint Commission that carries the genuine threat to hospitals not complying with CMS measures at stipulated thresholds. If a Joint Commission survey of a hospital exposes poor compliance to CMS measures, that hospital risks losing its accreditation. Therefore, adherence to CMS measures is compulsory under threat of loss of accreditation, under a hospital-compare regime.

After a CMS measure has been in use for some time, it may also be used for value-based purchasing. In value-based purchasing, Medicare and/or Medicaid reimbursement for sepsis cases is directly tied to rates of measure adherence, even on a case-by-case basis. Therefore, if a patient's case qualifies for that measure, the hospital's adherence would determine whether or not the hospital would be reimbursed for that care. Currently, SEP-1 is a hospital-compare measure. It may become a part of value-based purchasing in fiscal year 2017 to 2018.

The metric of interest to CMS for SEP-1 is adherence to the measure, not mortality or other patient-centered outcomes. That is because it is an a priori assumption that adherence to the quality measure improves mortality. This assumption is derived from the lengthy process before measure approval, which includes a rigorous testing regime during NQF measure development.

If the measure development process is flawed, there is no immediate recourse after a measure has been endorsed by the NQF or adopted by CMS and the Department of Health and Human Services. However, in a process somewhat analogous to a phase IV clinical trial, CMS measures, like all federal regulations, are also eventually subject to retrospective review. These reviews often lead to changes in, and in some cases the repealing of, CMS measures. SEP-1 has not yet come up for such review.

WHAT IS SEP-1 AND WHICH PATIENTS MUST RECEIVE ITS PROVISIONS?

The language that CMS uses for inclusion and exclusion criteria for measure applications is worth reviewing. Because such measures are designed to assess overall hospital performance by way of adherence, CMS thinks in terms of statistics. Thus, "numerators" are the patients to whom providers/hospitals have "correctly" applied a measure, whereas "denominators" are the patients that CMS deems should have had the measure applied to them. The definitions of these populations are termed numerator statements and denominator statements. For SEP-1, the denominator statement therefore identifies the pool of patients who should have received the CMS sepsis bundle, whereas the numerator represents those who actually received it and had it properly documented.

The debate over which patients should be in the denominator group and what actions must be taken for the patient to be counted in the numerator, is the crucial focus for debate on sepsis care, and in any CMS measure (**Boxes 1** and **2**).

The SEP-1 numerator statement is the number of patients from the denominator population who had all of the actions in **Box 2** completed and documented properly. Because there are provisions for both severe sepsis and septic shock, there are two separate "clocks" in this measure. This means that there are interventions for patients that must be completed within 3 hours of presentation of severe sepsis. However, if septic shock is noted later, a separate "shock clock" is started. For interventions that must be completed within 3 hours of presentation of septic shock, it is the shock clock that must be used. This means that if severe sepsis was detected at 1 PM, the 3-hour bundle for severe sepsis would be due at 4 PM. If septic shock was detected

---

Box 1
CMS SEP-1 inclusion and exclusion criteria

Inclusion criteria (denominator statement)

Discharge age >17 and any of the following diagnoses:
  International Classification of Diseases-10-CM principal or other diagnosis code of sepsis
  Severe sepsis (CMS version only, see **Box 3**)
  Septic shock (CMS version only, see **Box 3**)

Exclusion criteria

Comfort care within 3 hours of presentation for severe sepsis or 6 hours for septic shock

Administrative contraindication to care (eg, patient refusals)

Length of stay >120 days

Transfer in from another acute care facility (see **Box 2**)

Patients with severe sepsis who expire within 3 hours of presentation

Patients with septic shock who expire within 6 hours of presentation

Patients receiving intravenous antibiotics >24 hours before presentation of severe sepsis

---

Box 2
CMS SEP-1 required actions for included patients (numerator statements)

CMS Sep-1 Severe Sepsis Requirements

Must meet all of within 3 hours of presentation:
   Initial lactate level measurement
   Broad-spectrum or other antibiotics administered
   Blood cultures drawn BEFORE antibiotics

And within 6 hours of presentation of severe sepsis:
   Repeat lactate level measurement (if initial elevated)

CMS Sep-1 Septic Shock Requirements

All must receive within 3 hours if septic shock present:
   Resuscitation with 30 mL/kg crystalloid fluids

If hypotension persists after fluid administration must receive within 6 hours of presentation:
   Vasopressors

If hypotension persists after fluids or initial lactate $\geq$4 mmol/L must receive within 6 hours of presentation:
   Repeat volume status and tissue perfusion assessment via:
      A focused examination including vital signs, cardiopulmonary examination, capillary refill, peripheral pulse evaluation, and skin examination
      OR
   Any two of the following four:
      Central venous pressure measurement
      Central venous oxygen measurement
      Bedside cardiovascular ultrasound
      Passive leg raise or fluid challenge

---

at 2:30 PM, the 3-hour bundle for septic shock would be due at 5:30 PM, and the 6-hour bundle at 8:30 PM (for an excellent graphic representation, see Ref.[2]).

Certain patients may be excluded from the denominator. When a permitted reason has been documented as to why a patient with a chart coded to have severe sepsis or septic shock diagnoses did not receive the appropriated SEP-1 bundle interventions, the case is not scored (ie, does not count in the hospital's statistics). That said, a permitted reason that is not properly documented does in fact count in the aggregate metrics. Thus, the case counts against a hospital's statistics for adherence if the exclusion criteria are not properly documented. Patients who may be excluded are outlined in **Box 1**.

Receiving credit for adherence to SEP-1 depends on four things: (1) performance of all the required actions, (2) correct documentation of these actions, (3) proper documentation of patients with permissible exclusion from the denominator, and (4) chart abstractors being able to find and interpret all of this documentation. Because SEP-1 is a composite measure, all of the intervention outlines must completed for a case to pass the measure and count favorably on hospital compare metrics. It is then up to chart abstractors and their hospitals to report the aggregate rate of adherence to CMS. This must all be done manually, because there are no software applications available for this bundle.

THE TROUBLE WITH COMPOSITE MEASURES AND POTENTIAL LEGAL IMPLICATIONS

Composite measures require perfect adherence for hospitals to be scored as compliant in each case. SEP-1 requires documentation of adherence to an astounding

141 specific actions or variables. These variables are represented by 20 separate flowcharts with multiple decision points within each tree. If an EP fails to perform or correctly document adherence to a single variable, the entire case is considered to be noncompliant (ie, "Rejected.") Proponents of protocolized care see this as vital, because strictly obeying such checklists is precisely what they believe reduces error and improves outcomes. Looking at this from a different perspective, if there is failure to document or perform even the smallest required variable, the EP no longer has any incentive to continue to adhere to or document adherence to the remainder of the measure, because the EP has already "failed" to comply. Alternatively, if measure adherence were to be changed and defined as, for example, greater than 90% adherence to the defined variables, one deviation from the protocol would not be akin to the falling house of cards.

To give a sense of how complex and potentially confusing this process is, consider the decision tree on only the *very first* of the 141 variable items of SEP-1. The abstractor judging measure adherence must first evaluate whether the patient was received from another hospital or an ambulatory surgical center. If the patient was received by an outside hospital or ambulatory surgical center, SEP-1 does not apply and the case is scored as "not in measure population." Such a case is not processed and the EP and that hospital need not have adhered to SEP-1. However, if documentation of a transfer was not properly completed, the case not only counts but is immediately scored as nonadherent. But it is not that simple, because some types of transfers exclude patients from SEP-1, whereas others do not (**Box 3**).

Thus, if a patient was not a transfer (or if it was either unclear if the patient was a transfer), the abstractor must progress from variable #1 to variable #2 of SEP-1. This process occurs for each of the 141 variables. Because SEP-1 has never actually been tested from an administrative standpoint, it is unclear what average rates of adherence to this measure will turn out to be nationally. We suspect the rates will be low. Although we do not believe that the measure is intentionally abstruse, the

---

Box 3
Inclusion and exclusion criteria of transfers for CMS SEP-1

Transfers included (CMS SEP-1 measure applies)

Urgent care center

Psychiatric or rehabilitation units (only if part of your hospital)

Dialysis centers (with some exceptions)

Same-day surgery centers within your hospital

Any clinic

Any skilled nursing facility

Transfers excluded (CMS SEP-1 measure does not apply)

Patients coming from long-term acute care (not nursing homes)

Any acute rehabilitation

Any outside psychiatric hospital

Cardiac catheterization laboratory (from an outside hospital)

Same-day surgery (from an outside hospital)

Patients brought to the ED as part of a mass casualty

process of turning a complicated algorithm on sepsis management into discrete data points that are adjudicated by nonphysician abstractors makes this sort of complexity inevitable.

In fact, the administrative burden that we have already alluded to may now pose a threat to the legality of SEP-1. Under Executive Order 13,563 (section 6), signed by President Obama in 2011, such agencies as CMS are required to create and implement an ongoing Retrospective Analyses of Existing Rules, with a particular eye toward rules that are determined to be "excessively burdensome." When such rules are identified, CMS is legally obligated to "modify, streamline, expand, or repeal them in accordance with what has been learned." Simply complying with the chart abstraction aspects of SEP-1 alone may be a practical impossibility and thus render this measure unworkable. This is especially true given how broad the inclusion population for SEP-1 is (ie, the expanded definition of severe sepsis that the NQF used for this measure, discussed later). For context, we must note that not all CMS measures are quite so burdensome, including even some controversial ones. For example, the newly adapted CMS measure on thrombolytic therapy administration for acute stroke (CMS measure STK-4), contains only 18 variables for abstraction, in comparison with the 141 variables required in SEP-1. Moreover, the burden of having to perform the SEP-1 measure on patients whom an EP believes may be hurt by its provisions (eg, the requirement of giving broad-spectrum intravenous antibiotics to a patient whose suspected source of severe sepsis is *Clostridium difficile*) is not a typical posture in other CMS measures. The STK-4 measure maintenance is guided by the Joint Commission's Stroke Measure Maintenance Technical Advisory Panel and this measure allows EPs to invoke clinical judgment to exclude patients from the measure. All that is required is an EP to document a reason for not initiating intravenous thrombolytics. Currently, no such provision exists for SEP-1 where an EP may determine a patient should be excluded from the measure.

CRITICISMS OF SEP-1

Because CMS is the single largest payer for health care in the United States, assessing and encouraging quality care seems like a logical endeavor.[3] CMS quality measures are the prime mechanism for this. Thus, it would seem reasonable that a CMS measure should be the result of settled science. In the case of SEP-1, however, numerous aspects of the measure do not logically follow what the literature suggests is best practice for care in severe sepsis and septic shock.

Consider a comparison with another CMS measure, AMI-1. AM1-is instructive for the quality of underlying research and the lower administrative and safety burden it places on EPs and hospitals. AMI-1 measures the percentage of patients presenting with acute myocardial infarction who received aspirin within 24 hours of presenting to the hospital. The only data element that must be reached for a patient to be successfully counted in the CMS numerator is "Was aspirin received within 24 hours before or 24 hours after hospital arrival?" The allowable answers are yes or no. The SEP-1 numerator, by contrast, contains 59 such elements (from which the previously mentioned 141 variables are derived). AMI-1 contains several permitted exclusion criteria and assesses adherence to a treatment with a well-established number needed to treat for mortality that comes from a study that will likely never be repeated.[4]

Conversely, SEP-1 does not reflect the best evidence in management of early severe sepsis and septic shock. This fact led the SEP-1 measure stewards to publicly consider withdrawing the entire measure after the ProCESS trial came out. At that time, Dr Sean Townsend (writing for the stewards) suggested waiting for the results of ProMISe and ARISE. He and others believed that ProMISe and ARISE might contradict ProCESS and thus EGDT would be retained in SEP-1.[5,6] If those trials confirmed Pro-CESS, the NQF committee would then need to determine whether to reject the entire measure. Despite this, the committee decided against waiting, and a compromise was made. This was fortuitous for the stewards because, ultimately, the two remaining trials showed no mortality benefit for bundled sepsis care. By confirming the findings of the ProCESS trial, a contradiction now existed for the data brought to the NQF at the time of re-endorsement of NQF #0500.[7] In sum, SEP-1 is the antithesis of CMS core measure AMI-1. AMI-1 has a foundation in high-quality literature demonstrating significant patient benefit and the measure is exceptionally straightforward and it is reasonable to expect hospitals of any size to comply with this measure. SEP-1, conversely, is exceptionally complex and as it is currently written, does not follow the best available evidence and it may not result in the overall CMS goal of improved patient outcomes.

One of the major criticisms for SEP-1 involves the definition of severe sepsis they opted to endorse and enforce. There are, to our knowledge, at least five definitions of severe sepsis that one might have selected from the past 25 years. First, there is the Society of Critical Care Medicine (SCCM)/1992 guideline, which defined severe sepsis as "sepsis associated with organ dysfunction, hypoperfusion abnormality, or sepsis-induced hypotension. Hypoperfusion abnormalities include lactic acidosis, oliguria, and acute alteration of mental status."[8] At that time, no other specific laboratory abnormalities were required, although the use of multiple organ disease scoring was seen as a prognostic tool.[8,9] For all intents and purposes, Rivers and colleagues[10] proposed the second definition of severe sepsis in their landmark EGDT trial as follows: two of four systemic inflammatory response syndrome criteria, suspicion of infectious etiology, and an initial blood lactate concentration greater than or equal to 4 mmol/L. The third option for a severe sepsis definition is the SCCM definition from 2001 to 2003.[11–13] In this definition, several upper-limit-of-normal parameters for organ dysfunction were proposed, to our knowledge, for the first time. For example, a sepsis-attributed rise in creatinine of 0.5 mg/dL was considered a sign of organ dysfunction. By 2012, the fourth severe sepsis definition was offered by the SSC and they stated that severe sepsis was met if a patient had sepsis plus one of nine qualifiers of end-organ damage (eg, elevated creatinine, thrombocytopenia, hypoxia, hypotension).[13,14] The authors of the 2012 SSC guideline site the 2001 to 2003 definitions of severe sepsis as a source for their nine qualifiers of end-organ damage. However, it is not clear that there was a solid literature basis for these specific criteria or the cutoffs (eg, platelets <100,000 μL, creatinine >2.0 mg/dL). Nevertheless, these qualifiers were adopted by NQF #0500 and ultimately the SEP-1 measure (**Box 4**). Finally, there is the 2016 SCCM/European Society of Intensive Care Medicine consensus definitions, which have removed the term "severe sepsis" entirely.[15]

Unfortunately the NQF #0500 and now CMS SEP-1 definition of severe sepsis was never studied as part of River's EGDT trial or the ARISE, ProMISe, or ProCESS trials. These trials used a lactate greater than 4 mmol/L as the inclusion criteria for patients enrolled with severe sepsis. Conversely, the SEP-1 inclusion of a lactate greater than 2 mmol/L in the severe sepsis cohort is not consistent with the best prospective evidence available today.

A major concern regarding the severe sepsis definition of SEP-1 is the potential for excessive use of broad-spectrum antibiotics. As the measure stands, broad-spectrum antibiotics must be given within 3 hours of patient presentation if a patient has a lactate greater than 2 mmol/L (or any one of the other severe sepsis qualifiers). Although there is evidence to show benefit of early antibiotics in patients with septic shock, there is

---

Box 4
CMS SEP-1 definitions of severe sepsis (and upper limits of normal for organ failure) and septic shock

Severe Sepsis

Documentation of suspected or "possible" source of infection

AND

$\geq$2 systemic inflammatory response syndrome manifestations

AND

Organ dysfunction evidenced by any one of the following:
  Systolic blood pressure <90 OR mean arterial pressure <65, OR a systolic blood pressure decrease of more than 40 mm Hg
  Acute respiratory failure as evidenced by a new need for invasive or noninvasive mechanical ventilation
  Creatinine >2.0 OR urine output <0.5 mL/kg/hour for 2 hours
  Bilirubin >2 mg/dL
  Platelet count <100,000
  International normalized ratio >1.5 or activated partial thromboplastin time >60 seconds (nonanticoagulated patient)
  Lactate >2 mmol/L

Septic Shock

Documentation of severe sepsis present

AND

Hypotension persists in hour after the fluid bolus as evidenced by:
  Systolic blood pressure <90 OR mean arterial pressure <65, OR a systolic blood pressure decrease of more than 40 mm Hg.
  OR
  Tissue hypoperfusion present by initial lactate level $\geq$4 mmol/L

---

only one lower quality study to demonstrate benefit of early administration of antibiotics for severe sepsis.[14–18] This is the crux of the major complaint about SEP-1 from the Infectious Diseases Society of America (IDSA). They, along with other organizations, believe that the current SEP-1 inclusion criteria will lead to antibiotic shortages and increased drug-resistant organisms. Furthermore, the IDSA and other organizations have registered on-record dissents that there are no exclusion criteria for suspected *C difficile* as the source of severe sepsis or septic shock. Treating undifferentiated severe sepsis with broad-spectrum intravenous antibiotics is a known cause and exacerbating factor for *C difficile*. Although the latest version of SEP-1 addresses this concern, the new requirement demands laboratory-confirmed proof of *C difficile*, which is often impossible in the ED and SEP-1-imposed timeframe. The IDSA further noted an objection because the chart of approved broad-spectrum antibiotics was developed after NQF endorsement (ie, During CMS development of the specification manual) and thus there was never a comment period for the antibiotic specifications in the measure (the required CMS comment period came after NQF endorsement but before CMS released its manual containing the list of approved antibiotics). In sum, the IDSA believes that SEP-1 represents a large threat to antibiotic stewardship.

As we have alluded, septic shock has also been redefined in NQF #0500 and thus in CMS SEP-1. Our main concern is that an initial lactate of greater than 4 mmol/L has, since EGDT, defined severe sepsis, not septic shock. This matters because patients with septic shock are subjected to a more aggressive bundle in SEP-1. We are unaware of any randomized controlled trials that used these definitions. Thus, this bundle seems to widen the denominator without evidence of benefit.

Box 5 outlines some suggested changes (author recommendations) to improve SEP-1. These suggestions would help bring SEP-1 more in line with the 2016 SCCM/European Society of Intensive Care Medicine consensus definitions of sepsis and septic shock. Furthermore, these changes would bring SEP-1 closer in line with current best evidence by limiting the interventions to only evidence-based ones and by excluding patients excluded in the previous high-quality studies on which the measure relies.

APPLYING SEP-1 TO PATIENTS WHO MIGHT BE HARMED BY IT

Some patients are excluded from the measure and thus their sepsis cases are not to be scored. Such cases do not count against EPs and hospitals, if a permitted exclusion criterion is properly documented. However, the permissible exclusion criteria for SEP-1 are narrow (see **Box 1**). It seems logical to permit an EP to document that their clinical judgment suggests that a patient should not be included in the SEP-1 protocol. However, the current measure does not afford EPs this autonomy, a point of significant contention for many. For many EPs, this alone renders the current measure untenable given the complexity of sepsis.

One potential opportunity for improvement is to involve the patient in a shared decision-making model especially in situations where harm may done by the SEP-1 measure. Shared decision-making is one of modernity's most ethical responses to the paternalism that plagued medicine of the past. For example, a patient's refusal to receive any portion of the protocol qualifies as a permissible administrative contraindication to the protocol (although the most recent iteration of the measure has some exceptions to this). Does a patient with severe systolic dysfunction or end-stage renal disease realize that 30 mL/kg may not be appropriate when considering these comorbid conditions if they would otherwise qualify for the SEP-1 measure? Why not engage the patient in a shared-decision making model so the patient may be educated on the risk of fluid overload with the aggressive fluid resuscitation regime of SEP-1. Although physicians should not use the patient "opt-out" as a means to avoid the SEP-1 measure uniformly, there are circumstances where the potential for harm mandates that the physician consider the benefits and risks to protocolized care for the individual patient.

Box 5
Recommendations for bringing CMS SEP-1 consistent with best evidence

Limit inclusion criteria to severe sepsis and septic shock studied in EGDT, ProCESS, ProMISe, and ARISE

Exclude patients who were excluded in EGDT and subsequent trials

Eliminate the requirement to draw blood cultures

Limit the antibiotic requirement within 3 hours to the new definition of septic shock

Keep the 20–30 mL/kg of fluid for the CMS patients with septic shock

Allow clinicians to document why particular patients should be permitted to be excluded from fluid intervention (eg, presence of ventricular assist device, exceedingly low cardiac ejection fraction)

Keep the vasopressors for patients with persistent hypotension after fluid resuscitation

Eliminate the focused re-examination

Furthermore, we also notice that among the permitted exclusion criteria for severe sepsis and septic shock is the "directive for comfort care." A note that the EP has "discussed comfort care with family on arrival prior to onset of septic shock" is a permitted exclusion. Thus, the patient or family need not have decided on comfort care. Rather, a documentation of a discussion of comfort care suffices for exclusion. This is, of course, in addition to other allowable documentation, such as noting that the family or patient requests comfort measures only, an order exists for hospice evaluation or consultation, or wording that states "comfort measures only recommendation" in the provider documentation.

SUMMARY

Every EP and hospital throughout the country will be held accountable for SEP-1 and as such, a thorough knowledge of this measure is imperative. Each CMS core measure is designed to improve patient care and allow patients some reassurance that common disease processes, such as sepsis, will be treated within parameters of accepted standard care at any size hospital in this country. However, sepsis is perhaps the most difficult disease process encountered in emergency medicine and thus it is not surprising that a core measure on sepsis is extraordinarily complex and potentially counterproductive to providers' efforts to optimally care for the sickest patients with sepsis. That said, according to CMS, new versions of SEP-1 are released every 6 months and it is possible that future changes to the measure may be significant. In the meantime, each provider and hospital has to be careful that their efforts to satisfy SEP-1 do not adversely impact patient outcomes in sepsis.

Those interested in checking on revisions to SEP-1 and future directions of this measure can check: https://www.qualitynet.org/dcs/ContentServer?c=Page&page name=QnetPublic%2FPage%2FQnetTier2&cid=1141662756099.

WHERE TO GET FURTHER INFORMATION

Because transparency in government regulations is required, CMS must provide a public forum for answers to questions in addition to the required comment periods during measure development at the NQF. Several administrative and clinical questions are answered at https://cms-ip.custhelp.com/(found under the "Hospital Inpatient Measures and Data Element Abstraction" tab). Additionally, anyone can posit a question and expect an answer. Other helpful resources include the following:

- SEP-1 Fact Sheet (CMS publication): http://www.mhanet.com/mhaimages/ Sepsis_FactSheet.pdf (or Google "Fact Sheet SEP-1: Early Management Bundle).
- SEP-1 Frequently Asked Questions (CMS publication): http://www.mhanet.com/ mhaimages/Sepsis_FAQ.pdf (or Google "Frequently Asked Questions SEP-1: Early Management Bundle).
- CMS SEP-1 Specifications Manual: https://www.qualitynet.org/dcs/Content Server?c=Page&pagename=QnetPublic%2FPage%2FQnetTier2&cid=1141662 756099
- Department of Health and Human Services Regulations Toolkit: http://www.hhs. gov/regulations/regulations-toolkit/index.html#additional
- CMS Pre-Rule Making Process (as required under the Affordable Care Act): https:// www.cms.gov/Medicare/Quality-Initiatives-Patient-Assessment-Instruments/ QualityMeasures/Pre-Rule-Making.html
- Executive Order 13,563 (President Barack Obama): https://www.gpo.gov/fdsys/ pkg/FR-2011-01-21/pdf/2011-1385.pdf

- Press with Two Clocks Scheme: https://prezi.com/1qp7kbctjnqi/sep-1-cms-sepsis-core-measure/

REFERENCES

1. National Quality Forum. NQF #0500. Severe sepsis and septic shock: management bundle. Available at: https://webcache.googleusercontent.com/search?q=cache:3LdfFfGPZUsJ:https://www.qualityforum.org/WorkArea/linkit.aspx%3FLinkIdentifier%3Did%26ItemID%3D71548+&cd=1&hl=en&ct=clnk&gl=us. Accessed May 1, 2016.

2. Cantrell E.. SEP-1 CMS sepsis core measure by Eric Cantrell on Prezi. Available at: https://prezi.com/1qp7kbctjnqi/sep-1-cms-sepsis-core-measure/. Accessed May 1, 2016.

3. RoadmapOverview_OEA_1-16.pdf. Available at: . https://www.cms.gov/Medicare/Quality-Initiatives-Patient-Assessment-Instruments/QualityInitiativesGenInfo/downloads/RoadmapOverview_OEA_1-16.pdf. Accessed May 1, 2016.

4. ISIS-2 (Second International Study of Infarct Survival) Collaborative Group. Randomised trial of intravenous streptokinase, oral aspirin, both, or neither among 17,187 cases of suspected acute myocardial infarction: ISIS-2. ISIS-2 (Second International Study of Infarct Survival) Collaborative Group. Lancet 1988; 2(8607):349–60.

5. National Quality Forum Conference call transcript. Moderator: Andrew Lyzenga July 14, 2014 2:00 p.m. Available at: http://webcache.googleusercontent.com/search?q=cache:iU06oQkE27wJ:www.qualityforum.org/Projects/n-r/Patient_Safety_Endorsement_Maintenance/Meeting_Transcript_07142014.aspx+&cd=1&hl=en&ct=clnk&gl=us. Accessed May 1, 2016.

6. Townsend S.. Letter to Consensus Standards Approval Committee (CSAC), 2014. Available at: http://www.qualityforum.org/Projects/n-r/Patient_Safety_Endorsement_Maintenance/Sutter_Health_Comment_Letter.aspx. Accessed June 13, 2016.

7. Levy MM, Dellinger RP, Townsend SR, et al. The Surviving Sepsis Campaign: results of an international guideline-based performance improvement program targeting severe sepsis. Crit Care Med 2010;38(2):367–74.

8. Bone RC, Sibbald WJ, Sprung CL. The ACCP-SCCM Consensus conference on sepsis and organ failure. Chest 1992;101(6):1481–3.

9. Marshall JC, Cook DJ, Christou NV, et al. Multiple organ dysfunction score: a reliable descriptor of a complex clinical outcome. Crit Care Med 1995;23(10): 1638–52.

10. Rivers E, Nguyen B, Havstad S, et al. Early Goal-Directed Therapy in the Treatment of Severe Sepsis and Septic Shock. N Engl J Med 2001;345:1368–77.

11. Dellinger RP, Levy MM, Rhodes A, et al. Surviving Sepsis Campaign: international guidelines for management of severe sepsis and septic shock: 2012. Crit Care Med 2013;41(2):580–637.

12. Levy MM, Fink MP, Marshall JC, et al. 2001 SCCM/ESICM/ACCP/ATS/SIS International Sepsis Definitions Conference. Intensive Care Med 2003;29(4):530–8.

13. Adapted 2013 SSC-Guidelines-Table-2.png (PNG Image, 865 × 365 Pixels). Available at: http://i1.wp.com/emcrit.org/wp-content/uploads/2015/06/ssc-guidelines-table-2.png. Accessed May 1, 2016.

14. de Groot B, Ansems A, Gerling DH, et al. The association between time to antibiotics and relevant clinical outcomes in emergency department patients with various stages of sepsis: a prospective multi-center study. Crit Care 2015;19:194.

15. Kumar A, Roberts D, Wood KE, et al. Duration of hypotension before initiation of effective antimicrobial therapy is the critical determinant of survival in human septic shock. Crit Care Med 2006;34(6):1589–96.

16. Gaieski DF, Mikkelsen ME, Band RA, et al. Impact of time to antibiotics on survival in patients with severe sepsis or septic shock in whom early goal-directed therapy was initiated in the emergency department. Crit Care Med 2010;38(4): 1045–53.

17. Puskarich MA, Trzeciak S, Shapiro NI, et al, Emergency Medicine Shock Research Network (EMSHOCKNET). Association between timing of antibiotic administration and mortality from septic shock in patients treated with a quantitative resuscitation protocol. Crit Care Med 2011;39(9):2066–71.

18. Ferrer R, Martin-Loeches I, Phillips G, et al. Empiric antibiotic treatment reduces mortality in severe sepsis and septic shock from the first hour: results from a guideline-based performance improvement program. Crit Care Med 2014; 42(8):1749–55.

... ...

... ...

Index

Note: Page numbers of article titles are in **boldface** type.

A

Abdominal pain, in intraabdominal infections, 49
Acute-phase reactants, in sepsis, 116
Africa, sepsis care in, 165
Antibiotic regimens, empiric, in sepsis, 27, 28–30
Antibiotic therapy, blood and tissue cultures before, 31–32
    in sepsis, **25–40**
        selection of, 26–31
        timing of, 26–31
    pharmacokinetic/pharmacodynamic considerations in, 37–38
Antibiotics, administration of, in pediatric sepsis and septic shock, 133
    in general workup in sepsis, 46, 47
Antimicrobial agents, before onset of shock, 200
    for survival in sepsis, 161
    overdose of, patient safety implications of, 201–202
        public health implications of, 201
    timely administration of, 200
Antimicrobial stewardship, in emergency department, 202–207, 209
        impact of Centers for Medicare and Medicaid Services on, 207–208
    in management of sepsis, **199–217**
Arterial system, systemic, effect of vasopressors and inotropes on, 76

B

Biomarkers, and rapid pathogen diagnostic assays, 206–207
Blood and tissue cultures, before antibiotic therapy, 31–32
Blood culture, yield, according to infection, 32
Bloodstream, infections of, sepsis and, 53–54
Brazil, sepsis in, 164–165
Bundled care, for surviving sepsis in community, 160
    guidelines of Surviving Sepsis Campaign and, 17

C

Cardiac biomarkers, in sepsis, 116–117
Centers for Medicare and Medicaid Services, 5–6
    impact on antimicrobial stewardship, 207–208
    quality measure SEP-1, **219–231**
        application to patients who might be harmed, 228–229
        bringing it consistent with best evidence, 228
        composite measures and legal implications of, 223–225
        criticisms of, 225–228

Emerg Med Clin N Am 35 (2017) 233–239
http://dx.doi.org/10.1016/S0733-8627(16)30107-9
0733-8627/17

Moving?

Make sure your subscription moves with you!

To notify us of your new address, find your **Clinics Account Number** (located on your mailing label above your name), and contact customer service at:

Email: journalscustomerservice-usa@elsevier.com

800-654-2452 (subscribers in the U.S. & Canada)
314-447-8871 (subscribers outside of the U.S. & Canada)

Fax number: 314-447-8029

Elsevier Health Sciences Division
Subscription Customer Service
3251 Riverport Lane
Maryland Heights, MO 63043

*To ensure uninterrupted delivery of your subscription, please notify us at least 4 weeks in advance of move.

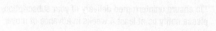

Printed and bound by CPI Group (UK) Ltd, Croydon, CR0 4YY

08/05/2025

01864696-0003